THROMBOPHILIA

Edited by **Andrea Luigi Tranquilli**

Thrombophilia
Edited by Andrea Luigi Tranquilli

Published by InTech
Janeza Trdine 9, 51000 Rijeka, Croatia

Publishing Process Manager Marina Jozipovic

Technical Editor Teodora Smiljanic

Cover Designer InTech Design Team

Additional hard copies can be obtained from orders@intechopen.com

Thrombophilia, Edited by Andrea Luigi Tranquilli
p. cm.
978-953-307-872-4

For EU product safety concerns:
IN TECH d.o.o., Prolaz Marije Krucifikse Kozulić 3, 51000 Rijeka, Croatia,
info@intechopen.com or visit our website at intechopen.com.

Meet the editor

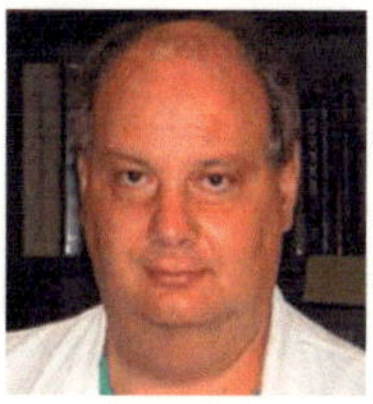

Professor Andrea Luigi Tranquilli graduated Medicine with honors at Catholic University of Rome, in 1979. He was Board certified as a Specialist in Gynecology and Obstetrics with honors at Catholic University of Rome in 1983. From 1983 to 1998 he was the Assistant at the Gynecology and Obstetrics Clinique of Ancona. In 1998 he was appointed Associate Professor of Gynecology and Obstetrics at the University of Polytechnics. Since 2005 he works as a Professor at the Gynecology and Obstetrics University Politecnica Marche. Currently he chairs the Department of Clinical Sciences at the same University. Prof. Tranquilli is a member of many scientific societies, among others, the American College of Obstetrics and Gynecology, Society for Maternal-Fetal Medicine, Italianan Association for Gynecology and Obstetrics, Association of Gynecological Universities of Italy. He is the Elected President (2012-14) of the International Society for the Study of Hypertension in Pregnancy, and Co-Editor in Chief of the Journal "Pregnancy Hypertension". He is also a reviewer of main Journals in the field and a member of several Editorial Boards. His main scientific interest has always been focused on maternal and fetal medicine. In recent years he has been developing a line of research on maternal and fetal aspects of thrombophilia.

Contents

Preface

Thrombophilia is a condition in which the blood tends to hypercoagulate and form clots. Such tendency is enhanced under special conditions like the prolonged immobility, surgical stress, and pregnancy.

Although it is conceivable that thrombophilia carriers are mostly prone to thrombotic events, those events are rare, and not necessarily a person who carries the risk will ever undergo one of them in the whole lifetime. Thombophilia is not a disease. It is only a condition that creates greater risks in special situations. There are inherited and acquired thrombophilias. The biologic research focused on the first has rapidly expanded in recent years, for the availability of genetic tests and molecular biology. Those tests allowed to design a new epidemiology of this phenomenon and to establish new connections between thrombotic events and the carrier status.

Pregnancy has become one of the most studied conditions with surprising results. Two situations are of crucial interest in pregnancy. Venous thromboembolism and its correlates is the first. Venous thromboembolism in pregnancy and puerperium is still one of the leading causes of maternal mortality. It increases with maternal age (and maternal age is increasing in industrial countries) and with caesarean section (this is constantly increasing as well). The second situation is the association between thrombophilia and medical and obstetric disorders in pregnancy (hypertension, preeclampsia, placental abruptio, intrauterine growth restriction, intrauterine fetal death, but also miscarriage and recurrent miscarriage), that is the placental involvement with fetal outcomes, besides the maternal thrombotic involvement. Those associations triggered an extraordinary scientific interest and the tendency to follow two clinical shortcuts: the idea of a large, universal, screening, and the pharmacologic prophylactic intervention. Not having yet large randomized clinical studies, today the indications are somehow empirical, and many of the most recent guidelines give controversial and often restrictive statements, mostly money saving-oriented and non-beneficially proved.

The aim of this book was to go deep in the problem and give to the reader a chance to form his/her own opinion in studying and treating patients at risk or carrier of a thrombophilic state. I hope we were able to accomplish this mission.

This book is dedicated to Prof. Pietro Leoni MD, Professor of Hematology in Ancona, and to my wife Monica.

Andrea Luigi Tranquilli
Department of Obstetrics and Gynecology,
Polytechnic University of Marche, Ancona,
Italy

Part 1

Thrombophilia

1

Inherited Thrombophilia: Past, Present, and Future Research

Jorine S. Koenderman and Pieter H. Reitsma
Leiden University Medical Center
The Netherlands

1. Introduction

Thrombophilia is defined as a disorder of hemostasis in which there is a tendency for the occurrence of thrombosis in veins or arteries due to abnormalities in blood composition, blood flow, or the vascular wall. The pathogenesis of venous versus arterial thrombosis is very distinct and these are often considered as separate diseases. The term thrombophilia is most often used in combination with venous thrombosis. VTE encompasses mainly deep vein thrombosis and pulmonary embolism.

Venous thromboembolism is a common disease with an annual age-dependent incidence of 1-3 individuals per 1000 per year (Naess et al, 2007). VTE is a serious disease with a thirty day case-fatality rate of 6.4% after a first VTE event and this rate is twice as high for pulmonary embolism (9.7%) than for deep vein thrombosis (4.6%) (Naess et al, 2007). VTE can also lead to complications like post-thrombotic syndrome that is characterized by pain and ulceration.

Although both sexes are equally affected by a first VTE, men have a more than 2-fold higher risk for a recurrent VTE as compared to women (Douketis et al, 2011).

VTE is a complex common disease in which multiple risk factors, both acquired and genetic, are involved in the development of the disease. Many acquired risk factors have been identified such as surgery, immobilization, trauma, oral contraceptive or hormone replacement therapy use, pregnancy, malignancy, and advanced age.

This chapter will focus on the genetic risk factors for VTE that have been identified to date and the research methods that were used to identify these factors in the past as well as new technological innovations used for the discovery of new genetic risk factors for VTE.

2. Past

2.1 Thrombophilia as monogenetic disease

In 1937, Nygaard and Brown introduced the designation "essential thrombophilia"in a report describing five cases of vascular disease characterized by recurrent episodes of acute occlusion in the large and small vessels of extremities, heart, kidney, and brain (Nygaard & Brown, 1937). In 1956 a survey of the literature that described a familial tendency for thrombosis was published that also used the term thrombophilia, now to indicate the hereditary nature of the disease (Jordan & Nandorff, 1956). Such a connection between inheritance and thrombosis was described as early as in 1911 (Schnitzler, 1926). Further studies into the genetic predisposition to thrombosis at the time were hampered by the lack of suitable tests and limited insight in the pathophysiology of VTE. Thrombophilia was considered a monogenetic disease starting with the identification of a family with hereditary antithrombin deficiency in 1965 (Egeberg, 1965).

In 1969, another heritable trait was found to be associated with thrombosis risk: non-O blood group. Blood group O is less often seen in thrombosis patients than one of the other blood groups (Jick et al, 1969). Protein C and protein S deficiencies were identified as genetic risk factors in thrombosis patients following the unraveling of the protein C anticoagulant system in the late 1970s and 1980s (Griffin et al, 1981; Schwarz et al, 1984). With improvement in DNA technology, mutations in the genes for antithrombin, protein C, and protein S that caused the deficiency states could be identified. In the 1990s activated protein C resistance and the Factor V Leiden mutation were discovered as well as the prothrombin mutation 20210G>A (Bertina et al, 1994; Poort et al, 1996). The prevalences of these known 'classic' genetic risk factors are represented in table 1.

	Prevalence		
Genetic risk factor	General population	VTE patients	Thrombophilia families
AT deficiency	0.0002-0.002%	1%	4%
PC deficiency	0.2-0.4%	3-5%	6%
PS deficiency	0.03-0.13%	1-5%	6%
Factor V Leiden	1-15%	10-50%	45%
Prothrombin 20210G>A	1-3%	6%	10%
Non-O blood group	57%	73%	

Table 1. Prevalences of major risk factors for VTE.

2.1.1 Antithrombin deficiency

Antithrombin (AT) deficiency was first described in a Scandinavian family in which several family members presented with thrombotic events and relatively low levels of AT in plasma. Heterozygous AT deficiency is a rare disorder with a prevalence of 1:500-1:5000 in the general population (Tait et al, 1994; Wells et al, 1994). AT deficiency is inherited as an autosomal dominant trait. Most cases are heterozygous and homozygous AT deficiency is hardly compatible with life and probably embryonic lethal. Heterozygous AT deficiency is observed in 4% of the thrombophilia families and in 1% of consecutive deep vein thrombosis patients (Lane et al, 1996).

DNA analyses resulted in the identification of loss of function mutations in the AT gene (*SERPINC1*) in people with AT deficiency. AT deficiency can be divided in two subtypes: type I (quantitative deficiency) and type II (qualitative deficiency). Type I deficiency is characterized by a reduction of activity and protein levels and accounts for 80% of the symptomatic patients with AT deficiency. Type I deficiencies are most commonly caused by short deletions and insertions and to a lesser extend by point mutations. Deletions are scattered throughout the AT gene, but three regions are often affected (codon 81, codon 106/107, codon 244/245). Recently, also large deletions (more than 30 bp) were identified in 8% of the AT deficient patients by using multiplex ligation-dependent probe amplification analysis (Luxembourg et al, 2011).

Type II deficiency is characterized by low activity and normal protein levels. Type II deficiencies result most often from single base pair substitutions that affect the reactive domain (type IIa) and heparin-binding domain (type IIb). Type IIc, a category including so-called pleiotropic defects, is often caused by mutations located in the strand Ic that impair the function of the reactive domain (Patnaik & Moll, 2008). The Human Gene Mutation Database describes at present 235 different mutations in the AT gene (Stenson et al, 2009).

Considering all known inherited thrombophilias, AT deficiency appears to lead to the highest risk for VTE. Risk for developing VTE depends on an individual's family history, presence of other mutations, and the subtype of AT deficiency. In particular subtype IIb confers a lower risk than the other subtypes (Finazzi et al, 1987). Risk estimates for developing VTE in the presence of AT deficiency are mainly based on family studies and these show a 10-20 fold increased risk (Lijfering et al, 2009; Mahmoodi et al, 2010; van Boven & Lane, 1997). The risk for developing a recurrent VTE is 10.5% per year without long-term anticoagulant treatment. With long-term anticoagulant treatment it still is 2.7% per year (Vossen et al, 2005).

2.1.2 Protein C deficiency

In 1981 the first patient with protein C (PC) deficiency and recurrent venous thromboembolism was described (Griffin et al, 1981). The prevalence of PC deficiency in the general population is 0.2-0.4% and 3-5% for VTE patients, although variation is observed among different study populations (Franco & Reitsma, 2001).

Homozygous or compound heterozygous PC deficiency is very rare and causes severe thromboembolic disease and purpura fulminans in newborns (Marlar & Mastovich, 1990). Heterozygous PC deficiency is more frequently observed and is associated with an increased risk to develop venous thromboembolism. The inheritance pattern of heterozygous PC deficiency is not as clear as that of AT deficiency. In general PC deficiency is inherited as an autosomal dominant disorder, but often with incomplete penetrance. For homozygous and compound heterozygous PC deficiency recessive inheritance patterns seems to fit better (Bafunno & Margaglione, 2010; Bereczky et al, 2010).

PC deficiency is primarily caused by loss of function mutation in the protein C gene (*PROC*). Mutations are very heterogeneous and the majority are single nucleotide substitutions in the coding regions of *PROC* (Bereczky et al, 2010).

PC deficiency is generally subdivided into two types: type I (quantitative deficiency) and type II (qualitative deficiency). Most PC deficiencies are type I and result mainly from single nucleotide substitutions in the coding regions of *PROC*. Type II deficiency is observed in 10-15% of the cases and often results from missense mutations in regions encoding for the Gla-domain, the propeptide, or the serine protease domain. In total, 275 distinct mutations in the *PROC* gene have been entered into the HGMD database (Stenson et al, 2009). However, still in 10-30% of families with PC deficiency no mutations have been found (Koeleman et al, 1997).

Heterozygous PC deficiency is associated with an increased risk for VTE. Risk estimates for the development of VTE depend on the population studied and vary between a 3 and 11 fold enhanced risk. The annual recurrent incidence rate is rather high with 5.1% in men and women combined. In men only, the recurrence risk is 10.8% per year (Vossen et al, 2005).

2.1.3 Protein S deficiency

Three years after the description of the first PC deficient patient, the first protein S (PS) deficient patient was reported. This patient also encountered recurrent VTE. (Schwarz et al,

1984). The prevalence of PS deficiency in the general Caucasian population is 0.03-0.13% and 1-5% in VTE patients, but these numbers vary between different populations (Franco & Reitsma, 2001). Especially in Asians, PS deficiency appears to be more prevalent than in Caucasians. In Asia, PS deficiency prevalences of 0.48-0.63% (general population), and 12.7% (VTE patients) have been claimed (Adachi, 2005).

Homozygous or compound heterozygous PS deficiency is rare and causes similar clinical symptoms as homozygous or compound heterozygous PC deficiency. Almost all PS deficiency cases are heterozygous. Heterozygous PS deficiency is usually inherited as an autosomal dominant trait and the mutation spectrum is rather heterogeneous.

Three subtypes of PS deficiency can be distinguished: type I (low activity, total, and free PS), type II (low activity), and type III (low activity and free PS). Type I PS deficiency is most frequently observed and often a consequence of missense mutations in the protein S gene (*PROS1*). Copy number variations were found in 33% of a group of missense negative patients with PS deficiency (Pintao et al, 2009). These copy number variations included deletion of the whole *PROS1* gene, partial gene deletions and partial duplications. In the Japanese population, one particular missense mutation, K196E, in the second EGF like domain of protein S is very abundant and was shown to be a risk factor for DVT (Kimura et al, 2006).

Type II PS deficiency is diagnosed in about 5% of the cases. This type of PS deficiency is mainly characterized by mutations in sequences of the *PROS1* gene that encode the Gla-domain and the EGF4-domain (Baroni et al, 2006). Type I and III deficiency often occur in the same family as phenotypic variants of the same genetic defect. An age-dependent increase of PS levels might play a role in these phenotypic expression variations (Simmonds et al, 1997). However, also families with only type III have been described. In the HGMD database 243 different mutations have been submitted at this moment.

Heterozygous PS deficiency is associated with a 5-11.5 fold increased risk of VTE in family-based studies, but this could not be confirmed in population-based studies (Rezende et al, 2004). The recurrence rate is, like for PC deficiency, also higher for men (10.5%) than for women (3.1%). This risk is not apparent in patients using anticoagulants for a long-term period (Vossen et al, 2005).

2.1.4 Blood group

During a drug surveillance program, patients treated with anticoagulants for venous thromboembolism showed to have more often blood group non-O than expected. Following this observation, a cooperative study was performed among women from the USA, UK, and Sweden that developed venous thrombosis while taking oral contraceptives, during pregnancy or the puerperium, or at other times. This study confirmed that there was a deficit of patients with blood group O, and the difference was larger when venous thromboembolism was associated with either oral contraceptive use or pregnancy (Jick et al, 1969).

Blood group O is associated with lower levels of von Willebrand Factor (VWF) and Factor VIII. Variation in plasma VWF levels were shown to be explained for 30% by ABO blood group (Orstavik et al, 1985). Blood group non-O is associated with a 2.6 fold increased risk for developing venous thrombosis. Blood group A is the main group responsible for the risk. The risk associated with VWF levels completely disappeared after adjustment for a particular blood group. However, the risk due to Factor VIII was not changed after adjustment for blood groups, which indicates that Factor VIII is an independent risk factor for venous thromboembolism (Tirado et al, 2005).

2.1.5 Activated protein C resistance and factor V Leiden

Activated protein C resistance (APCR) was identified in 1993 as an inherited abnormality that was highly prevalent in VTE patients within a family. In some family members, the activated partial thromboplastin time did not prolong by addition of activated PC to the plasma (Dahlback et al, 1993). This observation was referred to as activated protein C resistance and was later detected in 10-50% of VTE patients (Franco & Reitsma, 2001). With complementation tests, Bertina et al. discovered that APCR could be restored by adding coagulation factor V. A mutation in the factor V gene that is responsible for the APCR was identified in 1994 (Bertina et al, 1994). This mutation, often called factor V Leiden, causes a substitution of guanosine by adenosine at nucleotide position 1691, leading to an amino acid change from arginine to glutamine at position 506 of the protein. Factor V Leiden is a gain of function mutation because activated factor V is less sensitive to inactivation by APC, which facilitates the formation of more thrombin.

Factor V Leiden is quite prevalent in Caucasians (2-13%) (Bafunno & Margaglione, 2010), but varies among different geographical regions (Figure 1). The distribution of factor V Leiden is centered in Europe and extends into north India in the east. Factor V Leiden is introduced in America and Australia through emigration of Europeans. Factor V Leiden is prevalent in Europe and America, but also in Saudi Arabia and Israel. The mutation is rare in native populations from Eastern Asia, Africa, and America. In Basques and Inuit's from Greenland factor V Leiden is nearly absent. These populations represent autochthonous European groups that show limited mixing with other Europeans populations. Based on the worldwide distribution of the prevalences of factor V Leiden a single origin for this mutation has been hypothesized. Also haplotype analysis supports this hypothesis and factor V Leiden is therefore thought to be an founder mutation that occurred about 21,000 to 30,000 years ago (Zivelin et al, 1997). The factor V Leiden mutation might have arisen after the separation of Orientals and Caucasians as clear differences among races have been observed. (Bauduer & Lacombe, 2005; Herrmann et al, 1997; Rees, 1996)

In Europeans, factor V Leiden is the most common genetic defect involved in the etiology of VTE. Factor V Leiden is an autosomal dominant trait and heterozygotes have a 5 fold increased risk to develop VTE, while homozygotes have a 50 fold increased risk (Koster et al, 1993; Rosendaal et al, 1995).

Studies of the risk of developing recurrent venous thrombosis in the presence of factor V Leiden showed contradicting results. Most studies do not find an increased risk as compared to mutation negative subjects (Christiansen et al, 2005; De Stefano et al, 1999; Eichinger et al, 2002). Some studies found only an increased risk in men but not in women (Ridker et al, 1995; Vossen et al, 2005).

2.1.6 Prothrombin 20210G>A

The second most prevalent genetic abnormality causing thrombophilia was identified by a candidate gene approach in 1996 in patients from families with unexplained thrombophilia (Poort et al, 1996). This mutation is located in the 3'-untranslated region of the prothrombin gene, at position 20210. The nucleotide change from a guanosine to an adenosine causes no amino acid change, but probably positively affects polyadenylation and thereby increasing the mRNA and protein expression leading to increased plasma levels of prothrombin (Leitner et al, 2008). In heterozygous carriers the plasma levels of prothrombin are increased with 30% and in homozygous carriers with 70% (Bafunno & Margaglione, 2010).

Prothrombin 20210G>A is inherited as an autosomal dominant trait and is almost only observed in Caucasians from Europe. Outside Europe, only one case was observed in India (Rees et al, 1999). This mutation is found in 1-3% of the general population, in 6% of VTE patients, and in 10% of probands from thrombophilic families (Franco & Reitsma, 2001). This mutation was also suggested to originate from a single mutational event that occurred after the divergence of Africans from non-Africans and of Caucasoid from Mongoloid subpopulations, like the Factor V Leiden mutation (Zivelin et al, 1998).
Risk for venous thromboembolism is 2-5 fold increased in the presence of the prothrombin 20210G>A mutation. In combination with the Factor V Leiden mutation, risk showed a multiplicative effect and results in a 20 fold increased risk for VTE (Emmerich et al, 2001). Recurrence risk for VTE is not increased (Margaglione et al, 1999).

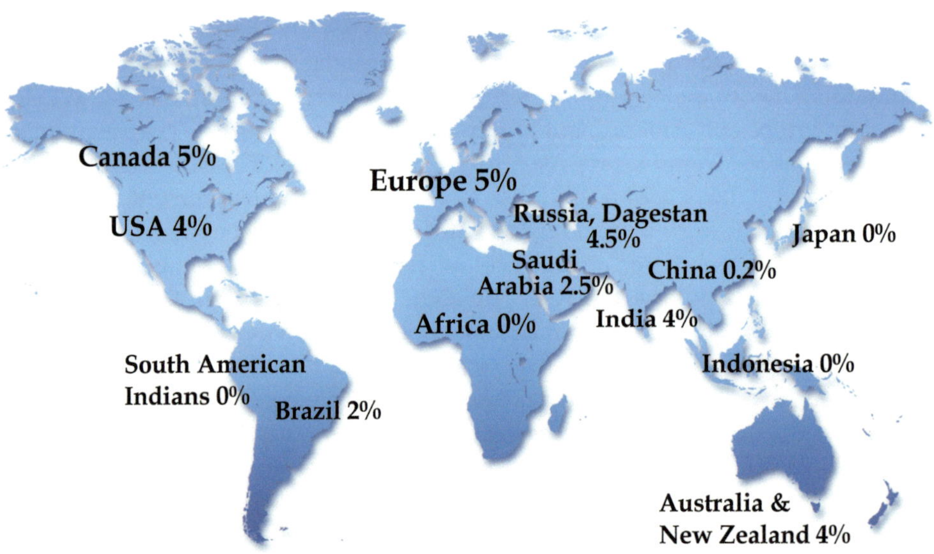

Fig. 1. World distribution of prevalences of factor V Leiden.

2.1.7 Fibrinogen γ variants

Fibrinogen consists of 3 polypeptides, Aα, Bβ, and γ, which are encoded by three separate genes. The gene for the fibrinogen γ polypeptide encodes two isoforms. The major mRNA form contains all 10 exons whereas the minor form (γ′) is the result of alternative splicing and includes intron 9 (de Moerloose et al, 2010). Approximately 10% of fibrinogen contains the minor isoform and this fibrinogen bears a high-affinity nonsubstrate-binding site for thrombin, which can cause an inhibition of thrombin activity (Mosesson, 2003).
Elevated levels of fibrinogen are associated with a 4 fold increased risk to develop a VTE (Kamphuisen et al, 1999), possibly by enhancing blood viscosity and platelet aggregation. An association study investigating linkage of haplotypes of the three fibrinogen genes showed that haplotype H2 of the *FGG* gene was associated with an increased risk for deep vein thrombosis (Uitte de Willige et al, 2005). This haplotype was also associated with

reduced fibrinogen γ′ levels and fibrinogen γ′ / total fibrinogen ratio, but not with fibrinogen levels. The risk conferred by this haplotype was proposed to result from SNP 10034C>T (rs2066865). About 6% of individuals carry the variant 10034C>T and this increases the risk for VTE two-fold in Caucasians (de Moerloose et al, 2010; Grunbacher et al, 2007; Uitte de Willige et al, 2009). In African Americans variant 10034C>T only increases the VTE risk marginally (Uitte de Willige et al, 2009). Variant 10034C>T is located in a GT-rich sequence region at the 3′-untranslated region of the *FGG* gene, which contains a putative cleavage stimulation factor binding site and is involved in the regulation of the polyadenylation signals (Uitte de Willige et al, 2007). Another variant, 9340T>C, was discovered to reduce VTE risk in Caucasians but not in African Americans. Variant 9340T>C reduces the risk approximately two-fold (Uitte de Willige et al, 2009).

3. Present

3.1 Thrombophilia as oligogenetic disease

With the discovery of deficiencies of protein S, protein C, and antithrombin, VTE was first suggested to be a monogenetic disease. However, in particular protein C deficiency showed variability in penetrance of the thrombotic phenotype within and between families, suggesting that additional genetic risk factors were present in these thrombosis prone families. This notion was confirmed with the finding of APC resistance. Individuals from families with protein S, protein C, or antithrombin deficiency but also APC resistance had a higher risk for VTE when they inherited combined defects rather than only one defect (Koeleman et al, 1994; van Boven et al, 1996). Thus, the penetrance of thrombosis increases in these protein C deficient families after introduction of the factor V Leiden allele in the pedigree (Brenner et al, 1996). Carriers of combinations of defects also presented with thrombosis earlier in life and more frequently. The same was observed in protein S deficient families, where combined defects of the protein S gene and either the Factor V Leiden mutation or the prothrombin 20210G>A were found in 40% (Koeleman et al, 1995; Zoller et al, 1995) and 30% (Castaman et al, 2000) of families, respectively. As a result, thrombophilia was then suggested to be an oligogenetic disease in which inherited predisposition results from 2 or more mutations in genes involved in blood clotting (Miletich et al, 1993).

The heritability of VTE was investigated in family and twin studies resulting in an estimated heritability of 50-60% (Heit et al, 2004; Larsen et al, 2003; Souto et al, 2000a). Heritability was also determined for individual coagulation factors involved in clot formation, like prothrombin (49-57%), factor V (44-62%), and von Willebrand Factor (34-75%) (de Lange et al, 2001; Souto et al, 2000b). In addition, 20-30% of consecutive VTE patients report one or more first-degree family members with VTE (Heijboer et al, 1990; van Sluis et al, 2006). These findings reaffirm that genetic risk factors do play an important role in the development of VTE.

An important question in the field remains whether there are a multitude of genetic risk factors that remain to be identified. In 13% of thrombophilia families already two or more genetic risk factors have been identified. In 60% and 27% of families 1 or no genetic factor was found, respectively (Bertina, 2001). This firmly suggests that we are still 'missing' genetic risk factors that predispose to venous thromboembolism.

3.2 Investigation of unexplained heritability

After establishing high levels of heritability in many complex diseases, including VTE, investigators concluded that many genetic risk factors remained to be discovered. New hypotheses were formulated to explain in which part of the genome sequence these missing genetic risk factors were to be found. One of these hypotheses was the 'common disease common variant (CDCV) hypothesis'. The CDCV hypothesis states that several common allelic variants - with appreciable frequency in the population and low penetrance - would account for the genetically determined variance in disease susceptibility of complex diseases like VTE. The central idea behind the CDCV hypothesis is that variants causing common diseases are reasonably frequent in the population, ranging from 1-10% (Collins et al, 1998; Lander, 1996). Other premises of this hypothesis are that the original mutation arose more than 100,000 years ago and that the model included absence of selection for or against these variants to make it possible for the variants to persist at a high frequency in the population. Evolutionary data suggests a proliferation of the human population from a rather small group of founders to 6 billion plus and this would be supplementary evidence for the CDCV theory. The mutation spectrum was likely to be narrow in the founders and a specific mutant could remain quite common during an expansion of the population (Iyengar & Elston, 2007).

Before the introduction of the CDCV hypothesis, new genetic determinants were investigated by linkage studies. Whole genome linkage studies have been performed in family studies with mini- and microsatellite markers, but later also with single nucleotide polymorphisms (SNPs). Linkage analysis assumes that many families share defects in the same locus, while there often is considerable locus heterogeneity in complex diseases, which will dilute linkage signals. Therefore, association studies of unrelated individuals using genotyping of a large set of single nucleotide polymorphisms (SNPs) are more appropriate to use for complex diseases. This approach is directly based on the CDCV hypothesis. With the finishing of the Human Genome Project (Collins et al, 2003) and the International HapMap Project (The International HapMap Consortium, 2005) and technological improvements, like microarrays, more genome wide association studies (GWAS) became feasible.

In the human genome around 20 million SNPs have been identified and validated (NCBI dbSNP Build 132). DNA sequences are inherited in blocks with high linkage disequilibrium. The pattern of SNPs in a block is called a haplotype. These blocks may contain a large number of SNPs, but determining only a few SNPs, so-called tagSNPs, are required to identify the haplotypes in a block. Especially the HapMap data has been employed as a source of information about haplotypes in different populations and tagSNPs. These tagSNPs were used in GWAS studies to examine genomes for association with a certain phenotype.

A GWAS study should be designed very carefully to prevent bias and other problems in the subsequent analyses. The study populations most used in GWASs are case-control studies. Cases and controls should have the same ethnicity and geographical background to avoid false positive results due to population-stratification. For case inclusion, strict criteria should be taken into account to prevent inclusion of phenocopies within the study population.

Type I errors, i.e. false-positive results, can be avoided by choosing an appropriate significance level. In GWAS studies, multiple tests are performed and the significance levels should be corrected for these multiple comparisons. One way is to apply the Bonferroni correction, which adjusts the significance level dependent on the number of independent comparisons that were performed (Johnson et al, 2010; Risch & Merikangas, 1996). The Bonferroni correction might be too strict when tested SNPs are in linkage disequilibrium and therefore should not be considered as independent comparisons. Type II errors, false negative results, can be avoided by using large sample sizes.

Positive results should be replicated in at least 2 other populations. The effect size and significance of a positive result is often overestimated in the first study. As a consequence, to replicate a claim, the sample size of the replication studies should be therefore larger than the original GWAS study.

The CDCV hypothesis was not accepted by the whole field. Opponents argued that in many complex diseases already a spectrum of disease associated rare variants had become known in direct contradiction of the CDCV hypothesis which states that only a few variants would account for the risk in complex diseases (Pritchard, 2001).

The alternative hypothesis put forward by opponents of the CDCV hypothesis was the 'common disease rare variant hypothesis (CDRV)' that argues that multiple rare variants, with relatively high penetrance, are the major contributors to genetic susceptibility to complex diseases. The rare variants would be more important because they were more likely to be functional or have phenotypic effects (Gorlov et al, 2008; Pritchard, 2001; Schork et al, 2009). Also the observation of familial clustering of complex diseases strengthened the CDRV hypothesis (Schork et al, 2009). This hypothesis gained increasing support when the genetic variation found with GWAS studies explained collectively only a small fraction of the heritability of any disease in the population.

GWAS studies are not powered for the detection of rare variants. The only strategy available to identify such rare variants is to sequence DNA directly, either in candidate genes or whole genome. To perform large studies with conventional Sanger sequencing is very costly, time consuming, and impossible in practise. With the introduction of next generation sequencing technologies, high-throughput sequencing of many genes became feasible and at a reasonably price.

Next generation sequencing can be used for de novo sequencing and re-sequencing purposes. For humans, re-sequencing is used because the reference sequence is already known from the Human Genome project (Collins et al, 2003) and will be further improved by the 1000 Genomes Project (The 1000 Genomes Project Consortium, 2010), which just finished the pilot study at the end of 2010.

Next generation sequencing was first used for targeted re-sequencing of candidate genes in just a few subjects. Nowadays, also whole exome sequencing can be performed for a reasonable price, although the samples sizes in most studies are still limited. The best, non-hypothesis driven, method would be whole genome sequencing, but this is still quite expensive especially when using large sample sizes.

Targeted re-sequencing of candidate genes was initially executed by first amplifying the target sequences by PCR and then sequence these PCR products with a next generation sequencer. The PCR steps are very time consuming and to accelerate the whole sample preparation process, a new method was developed: target enrichment. This method uses predesigned probes to enrich the DNA for the selected target genes and wash away remaining non-selected DNA sequences.

Next generation sequencers are improving constantly and are generating more and more reads with increasing read length. As a consequence, the total data output from one sequencing run is increasing and all these data need to be analyzed. The data analysis of the sequencing reactions remains a challenge. Especially the distinction of sequencing errors from real mutations is difficult and is best served by using a high coverage level, i.e. the same sequence is analysed multiple times. However, PCR errors that originated in the sample preparation phase cannot always be distinguished from real mutations and this problem is not solved by using higher coverage levels. Therefore, findings from next generation sequencing still have to be confirmed with Sanger sequencing.

In the next three sections, some genome wide linkage analysis studies, GWAS studies, and high-throughput sequencing studies in the field of thrombophilia will be discussed. High-throughput sequencing results for VTE are not available and therefore we will discuss some results from other complex diseases.

3.3 Results from genome wide linkage studies

Several genome wide linkage studies have been performed for venous thromboembolism. The first one was executed in the Genetic Analysis of Idiopathic Thrombophilia (GAIT) study (Souto et al, 2000a). The GAIT study consists of 21 extended Spanish pedigrees. Twelve of these families were selected through probands with idiopathic thrombophilia. The other 9 families were selected irrespective of any phenotype. Several genome scans were performed in the GAIT study. For the first scan 363 microsatellite markers were genotyped (Soria et al, 2002) while 485 microsatellite markers were used in the second scan (Lopez et al, 2008). Later, a scan employing 307,984 SNPs was performed (Buil et al, 2010; Malarstig et al, 2009). The investigators focussed on associations between genetic markers and intermediate phenotypes of VTE, like lipoprotein(a) levels (Lopez et al, 2008), factor XII levels (Soria et al, 2002), total plasma homocysteine (Malarstig et al, 2009), and C4BP plasma levels (Buil et al, 2010). In these studies quantitative trait loci were discovered, but these loci often included the structural gene for the investigated intermediate phenotype. The studies investigating total plasma homocysteine and C4BP plasma levels were combinations of linkage and association studies. In one of these, associations were found for SNPs near the *ZNF366* gene and the *PTPRD* gene, which might suggests novel pathways for homocysteine metabolism.

The second main genome wide linkage analysis was performed in the Kindred Vermont II study, which includes a single large pedigree with a high rate of VTE, partly due to type I protein C deficiency resulting from a single mutation in the protein C gene. Only a subset of the carriers of this mutation experienced a VTE and therefore a genome scan was performed including 375 microsatellite markers to investigate the presence of a second thrombophilic mutation in this pedigree (Hasstedt et al, 2004). Three potential gene loci were found and 109 genes within these loci were re-sequenced. Only one SNP in the *CADM1* gene was associated with VTE, but this association was limited to the subjects with PC deficiency (Hasstedt et al, 2009).

The GENES study included 22 families with unexplained thrombophilia (Wichers et al, 2009). Families were included through a proband with VTE and absence of known thrombophilic defects. This study found that the endogenous thrombin potential (ETP) was associated with VTE and therefore ETP was used as an intermediate phenotype for VTE. However, the heritability of ETP was mainly caused by only one large family (128 individuals). In this family, a genome wide linkage scan was performed for quantitative trait loci influencing ETP and other coagulation and fibrinolysis variables (Tanck et al, 2011). The highest LOD score (4.8) for PC levels was found on chromosome 20q11. Candidate gene analysis revealed that a locus of the *PROCR* gene is a genetic determinant for PC levels, as well as for soluble EPCR levels (Pintao et al, 2011).

3.4 Results from genome wide association studies

The first large scale association analysis for VTE had a multistage design (Bezemer et al, 2008). In the first stage 19,682 SNPs, selected based on their potential affect on gene function or expression, were genotyped in pooled DNA samples from the Leiden Thrombophilia Study (LETS), including 443 cases and 453 controls. This resulted in 1,206 SNPs that were significantly associated with VTE. These 1,206 SNPs were then replicated in pooled DNA samples from a subset of the Multiple Environmental and Genetic Assessment of Risk Factors for Venous Thrombosis (MEGA) study (1,398 cases and 1,757 controls). 104 SNPs were significantly associated with VTE in this population and these SNPs were subsequently genotyped in both populations again, but now in the individual samples. 18 SNPs remained associated and were replicated in another subset of the MEGA study. Eventually, four SNPs located in the *CYP4V2/KLKB1/F11* gene cluster and *GP6* and *SERPINC1* genes were consistently associated with VTE, as well as one SNP in the *FV* gene (Bezemer et al, 2010). Odds ratio's ranged from 1.10-1.49.

The second large-scale association analysis was a genome wide study, including 317,139 SNPs (Tregouet et al, 2009). These SNPs were genotyped in 453 cases and 1,327 controls and the significant results were replicated in two independent case-control studies. This study only found consistently associated SNPs with VTE in two known VTE susceptibility genes: *FV* and *ABO* blood group genes. The same authors also attempted to replicate the significant results found by Bezemer et al. in the two replication populations and confirmed the associations in the genes *CYP4V2* and *GP6*.

A genome wide association study investigating the intermediate phenotype plasma protein C levels was performed in a large population of individuals from European ancestry in the Atherosclerosis Risk in Communities (ARIC) study (Tang et al, 2010). In this study approximately 2.5 million SNPs were genotyped in 8048 subjects. Plasma protein C levels were associated with SNPs in the genes *GCKR, PROC, PROCR*, and *EDEM2*. All 4 loci were confirmed in a replication study including 1376 subjects. A fifth locus in gene BAZ1B was identified after pooling of the original study and replication study results.

3.5 High-through put sequencing results for complex diseases

High-throughput sequencing technology was first used to sequence a limited number of candidate genes. The first study that published next generation sequencing driven data investigated 10 candidate genes in type I diabetes (Nejentsev et al, 2009). These candidate genes were chosen based on positive association signals found in these genes with a GWAS. Exons and regulatory sequences of the 10 genes were sequenced in pools of DNA of 48 subject and 480 cases and 480 controls in total. Four rare variants were found in the gene *IFIH1*. Association analysis in over 30,000 participants showed that these variants were associated with a reduced risk with odds ratio's of 0.51-0.74.

Targeted re-sequencing was also performed for two intervals including the two candidate genes, *FAAH* and *MGLL*, for extreme obesity (Harismendy et al, 2010). These intervals were sequenced in 142 obese people and 147 controls. Rare variants were found in or near promoter sequences and other regulatory elements like transcriptional enhancers of these genes. The intervals including rare variants were associated with extreme obesity. Most of these variants had minor allele frequencies of <0.01.

For autism, whole exome sequencing was performed in 20 patients and their parents (O'Roak et al, 2011). Twenty-one de novo mutations were identified and 11 of these were protein altering. Most of the protein altering mutations were found in highly conserved amino acid residues. Potentially causative mutations were identified in 4 of the more severely affected subjects of the probands in the genes *FOXP1, GRIN2B, SCN1A*, and *LAMC3*.

4. Future directions

Future research of genetics for venous thrombosis and other complex diseases will be largely based on the technologies that are now becoming available. When the costs to perform high-throughput sequencing experiments decline further, larger populations can be sequenced, as well as larger regions of the genome. Nowadays, it is already possible to capture the whole exome of the human genome for sequencing, but this is still too expensive to be performed in larger study populations. The ultimate goal is to sequence the whole human genome. This would be the most unbiased method to investigate genetic risk factors, because there is no assumption made about the location of variants in the genome or any pathway that is involved in VTE. Sequencers can generate an increasing amount of data, but the limiting factor now is the data analysis and the interpretation of the results for the disease under investigation. Improvements are still required in this field to support research of rare variants in complex diseases.

Rare variants are probably not the only biological elements that account for the unexplained heritability for VTE. Future research should also focus on other mechanisms that influence gene regulation and gene expression. Non-coding RNA molecules can be involved in chromatin modification, transcriptional regulation, and translational efficiency. Genetic variability and expression of these non-coding RNA might also have an effect on the development of diseases. Epigenetic mechanisms, like DNA methylation, also participate in the regulation of gene expression in a heritable manner. These epigenetic changes are already associated with the aetiology of some diseases, like cancer, diabetes, and neurological disorders. Furthermore, it might be worthwhile to use pathway directed methods in the investigation of complex diseases. Variability in biological systems as a whole might be more important due to gene-gene interactions than the genetic variability in separate candidate genes in isolation and this might also be the reason why replication of results of association studies of candidate genes often fails.

If we get more insight from these data into the genetic architecture of venous thromboembolism and the pathways that are important in the development of this disease, personalized prediction and management might become reality.

5. Conclusion

Early studies of genetic risk factors for venous thromboembolism have revealed several genetic variations like the factor V Leiden and the prothrombin mutation, which increase the risk of developing venous thromboembolism. Based on studies in thrombophilia families that were showing variability in penetrance of the phenotype, thrombophilia was proposed to be an oligogenetic disease. However, the established genetic risk factors do not explain the total heritability for venous thromboembolism, suggesting that genetic risk factors remain to be discovered. Association studies have attempted to make such discoveries by searching for common susceptibility variants, but the contribution of these studies have been limited. Other studies have to be performed to find new genetic determinants for venous thromboembolism. The most recent hypothesis is that unique, rare variants can explain much of the genetic susceptibility for VTE. With the introduction of high-throughput sequencing technology, rare variants can now be directly identified by candidate gene or whole exome sequencing approaches. The data analysis remains the biggest challenge of these types of studies. The most appropriate and unbiased method to determine new genes and pathways involved in disease would be a whole genome sequencing approach, but financially it is not yet possible to do this in large study populations. Although the focus of research in complex diseases is now mostly on rare variants, we have to realize that the unexplained heritability for venous thromboembolism might also reside in other elements that do not change the DNA sequence, but influence gene expression and regulation through other biological mechanisms.

6. References

Adachi, T. (2005). Protein S and congenital protein S deficiency: the most frequent congenital thrombophilia in Japanese. *Curr.Drug Targets.*, Vol.6, No.5, pp. 585-592,

Bafunno, V. & Margaglione, M. (2010). Genetic basis of thrombosis. *Clin.Chem.Lab Med.*, Vol.48 Suppl 1, pp. S41-S51,

Baroni, M., Mazzola, G., Kaabache, T., Borgel, D., Gandrille, S., Vigano', D. S., Marchetti, G., di Iasio, M. G., Pinotti, M., D'Angelo, A., & Bernardi, F. (2006). Molecular bases of type II protein S deficiency: the I203-D204 deletion in the EGF4 domain alters GLA domain function. *J.Thromb.Haemost.*, Vol.4, No.1, pp. 186-191,

Bauduer, F. & Lacombe, D. (2005). Factor V Leiden, prothrombin 20210A, methylenetetrahydrofolate reductase 677T, and population genetics. *Mol.Genet.Metab*, Vol.86, No.1-2, pp. 91-99,

Bereczky, Z., Kovacs, K. B., & Muszbek, L. (2010). Protein C and protein S deficiencies: similarities and differences between two brothers playing in the same game. *Clin.Chem.Lab Med.*, Vol.48 Suppl 1, pp. S53-S66,

Bertina, R. M. (2001). Genetic approach to thrombophilia. *Thromb.Haemost.*, Vol.86, No.1, pp. 92-103,

Bertina, R. M., Koeleman, B. P., Koster, T., Rosendaal, F. R., Dirven, R. J., de, R. H., van der Velden, P. A., & Reitsma, P. H. (1994). Mutation in blood coagulation factor V associated with resistance to activated protein C. *Nature*, Vol.369, No.6475, pp. 64-67,

Bezemer, I. D., Bare, L. A., Arellano, A. R., Reitsma, P. H., & Rosendaal, F. R. (2010). Updated analysis of gene variants associated with deep vein thrombosis. *JAMA*, Vol.303, No.5, pp. 421-422,

Bezemer, I. D., Bare, L. A., Doggen, C. J., Arellano, A. R., Tong, C., Rowland, C. M., Catanese, J., Young, B. A., Reitsma, P. H., Devlin, J. J., & Rosendaal, F. R. (2008). Gene variants associated with deep vein thrombosis. *JAMA*, Vol.299, No.11, pp. 1306-1314,

Brenner, B., Zivelin, A., Lanir, N., Greengard, J. S., Griffin, J. H., & Seligsohn, U. (1996). Venous thromboembolism associated with double heterozygosity for R506Q mutation of factor V and for T298M mutation of protein C in a large family of a previously described homozygous protein C-deficient newborn with massive thrombosis. *Blood*, Vol.88, No.3, pp. 877-880,

Buil, A., Tregouet, D. A., Souto, J. C., Saut, N., Germain, M., Rotival, M., Tiret, L., Cambien, F., Lathrop, M., Zeller, T., Alessi, M. C., Rodriguez de, C. S., Munzel, T., Wild, P., Fontcuberta, J., Gagnon, F., Emmerich, J., Almasy, L., Blankenberg, S., Soria, J. M., & Morange, P. E. (2010). C4BPB/C4BPA is a new susceptibility locus for venous thrombosis with unknown protein S-independent mechanism: results from genome-wide association and gene expression analyses followed by case-control studies. *Blood,* Vol.115, No.23, pp. 4644-4650,

Castaman, G., Tosetto, A., Cappellari, A., Ruggeri, M., & Rodeghiero, F. (2000). The A20210 allele in the prothrombin gene enhances the risk of venous thrombosis in carriers of inherited protein S deficiency. *Blood Coagul.Fibrinolysis,* Vol.11, No.4, pp. 321-326,

Christiansen, S. C., Cannegieter, S. C., Koster, T., Vandenbroucke, J. P., & Rosendaal, F. R. (2005). Thrombophilia, clinical factors, and recurrent venous thrombotic events. *JAMA,* Vol.293, No.19, pp. 2352-2361,

Collins, F. S., Brooks, L. D., & Chakravarti, A. (1998). A DNA polymorphism discovery resource for research on human genetic variation. *Genome Res.,* Vol.8, No.12, pp. 1229-1231,

Collins, F. S., Morgan, M., & Patrinos, A. (2003). The Human Genome Project: lessons from large-scale biology. *Science,* Vol.300, No.5617, pp. 286-290,

Dahlback, B., Carlsson, M., & Svensson, P. J. (1993). Familial thrombophilia due to a previously unrecognized mechanism characterized by poor anticoagulant response to activated protein C: prediction of a cofactor to activated protein C. *Proc.Natl.Acad.Sci.U.S.A,* Vol.90, No.3, pp. 1004-1008,

de Lange, M., Snieder, H., Ariens, R. A., Spector, T. D., & Grant, P. J. (2001). The genetics of haemostasis: a twin study. *Lancet,* Vol.357, No.9250, pp. 101-105,

de Moerloose, P., Boehlen, F., & Neerman-Arbez, M. (2010). Fibrinogen and the risk of thrombosis. *Semin.Thromb.Hemost.,* Vol.36, No.1, pp. 7-17,

De Stefano, V., Martinelli, I., Mannucci, P. M., Paciaroni, K., Chiusolo, P., Casorelli, I., Rossi, E., & Leone, G. (1999). The risk of recurrent deep venous thrombosis among heterozygous carriers of both factor V Leiden and the G20210A prothrombin mutation. *N.Engl.J.Med.,* Vol.341, No.11, pp. 801-806,

Douketis, J., Tosetto, A., Marcucci, M., Baglin, T., Cosmi, B., Cushman, M., Kyrle, P., Poli, D., Tait, R. C., & Iorio, A. (2011). Risk of recurrence after venous thromboembolism in men and women: patient level meta-analysis. *BMJ,* Vol.342, pp. d813,

Egeberg, O. (1965). Inherited antithrombin deficiency causing thrombophilia. *Thromb.Diath.Haemorrh.,* Vol.13, pp. 516-530,

Eichinger, S., Weltermann, A., Mannhalter, C., Minar, E., Bialonczyk, C., Hirschl, M., Schonauer, V., Lechner, K., & Kyrle, P. A. (2002). The risk of recurrent venous thromboembolism in heterozygous carriers of factor V Leiden and a first spontaneous venous thromboembolism. *Arch.Intern.Med.,* Vol.162, No.20, pp. 2357-2360,

Emmerich, J., Rosendaal, F. R., Cattaneo, M., Margaglione, M., De, S., V, Cumming, T., Arruda, V., Hillarp, A., & Reny, J. L. (2001). Combined effect of factor V Leiden and prothrombin 20210A on the risk of venous thromboembolism--pooled analysis of 8 case-control studies including 2310 cases and 3204 controls. Study Group for Pooled-Analysis in Venous Thromboembolism. *Thromb.Haemost.,* Vol.86, No.3, pp. 809-816,

Finazzi, G., Caccia, R., & Barbui, T. (1987). Different prevalence of thromboembolism in the subtypes of congenital antithrombin III deficiency: review of 404 cases. *Thromb.Haemost.*, Vol.58, No.4, pp. 1094,

Franco, R. F. & Reitsma, P. H. (2001). Genetic risk factors of venous thrombosis. *Hum.Genet.*, Vol.109, No.4, pp. 369-384,

Gorlov, I. P., Gorlova, O. Y., Sunyaev, S. R., Spitz, M. R., & Amos, C. I. (2008). Shifting paradigm of association studies: value of rare single-nucleotide polymorphisms. *Am.J.Hum.Genet.*, Vol.82, No.1, pp. 100-112,

Griffin, J. H., Evatt, B., Zimmerman, T. S., Kleiss, A. J., & Wideman, C. (1981). Deficiency of protein C in congenital thrombotic disease. *J.Clin.Invest*, Vol.68, No.5, pp. 1370-1373,

Grunbacher, G., Weger, W., Marx-Neuhold, E., Pilger, E., Koppel, H., Wascher, T., Marz, W., & Renner, W. (2007). The fibrinogen gamma (FGG) 10034C>T polymorphism is associated with venous thrombosis. *Thromb.Res.*, Vol.121, No.1, pp. 33-36,

Harismendy, O., Bansal, V., Bhatia, G., Nakano, M., Scott, M., Wang, X., Dib, C., Turlotte, E., Sipe, J., Murray, S., Deleuze, J., Bafna, V., Topol, E., & Frazer, K. (2010). Population sequencing of two endocannabinoid metabolic genes identifies rare and common regulatory variants associated with extreme obesity and metabolite level. *Genome Biology*, Vol.11, No.11, pp. R118, ISSN 1465-6906

Hasstedt, S. J., Bezemer, I. D., Callas, P. W., Vossen, C. Y., Trotman, W., Hebbel, R. P., Demers, C., Rosendaal, F. R., & Bovill, E. G. (2009). Cell adhesion molecule 1: a novel risk factor for venous thrombosis. *Blood*, Vol.114, No.14, pp. 3084-3091,

Hasstedt, S. J., Scott, B. T., Callas, P. W., Vossen, C. Y., Rosendaal, F. R., Long, G. L., & Bovill, E. G. (2004). Genome scan of venous thrombosis in a pedigree with protein C deficiency. *J.Thromb.Haemost.*, Vol.2, No.6, pp. 868-873,

Heijboer, H., Brandjes, D. P., Buller, H. R., Sturk, A., & ten Cate, J. W. (1990). Deficiencies of coagulation-inhibiting and fibrinolytic proteins in outpatients with deep-vein thrombosis. *N.Engl.J.Med.*, Vol.323, No.22, pp. 1512-1516,

Heit, J. A., Phelps, M. A., Ward, S. A., Slusser, J. P., Petterson, T. M., & De, A. M. (2004). Familial segregation of venous thromboembolism. *J.Thromb.Haemost.*, Vol.2, No.5, pp. 731-736,

Herrmann, F. H., Koesling, M., Schroder, W., Altman, R., Jimenez, B. R., Lopaciuk, S., Perez-Requejo, J. L., & Singh, J. R. (1997). Prevalence of factor V Leiden mutation in various populations. *Genet.Epidemiol.*, Vol.14, No.4, pp. 403-411,

Iyengar, S. K. & Elston, R. C. (2007). The genetic basis of complex traits: rare variants or "common gene, common disease"? *Methods Mol.Biol.*, Vol.376, pp. 71-84,

Jick, H., Westerholm, B., Vessey, M., Lewis, G., Slone, D., Inman, W., Shapiro, S., & Worcester, J. (1969). Venous Thromboembolic Disease and ABO Blood Type: A Cooperative Study. *The Lancet*, Vol.293, No.7594, pp. 539-542, ISSN 0140-6736

Johnson, R. C., Nelson, G. W., Troyer, J. L., Lautenberger, J. A., Kessing, B. D., Winkler, C. A., & O'Brien, S. J. (2010). Accounting for multiple comparisons in a genome-wide association study (GWAS). *BMC.Genomics*, Vol.11, pp. 724,

Jordan, F. L. J. & Nandorff, A. (1956). The Familial Tendency in Thrombo-embolic Disease. *Acta Medica Scandinavica*, Vol.156, No.4, pp. 267-275, ISSN 0954-6820

Kamphuisen, P. W., Eikenboom, J. C., Vos, H. L., Pablo, R., Sturk, A., Bertina, R. M., & Rosendaal, F. R. (1999). Increased levels of factor VIII and fibrinogen in patients with venous thrombosis are not caused by acute phase reactions. *Thromb.Haemost.*, Vol.81, No.5, pp. 680-683,

Kimura, R., Honda, S., Kawasaki, T., Tsuji, H., Madoiwa, S., Sakata, Y., Kojima, T., Murata, M., Nishigami, K., Chiku, M., Hayashi, T., Kokubo, Y., Okayama, A., Tomoike, H., Ikeda, Y., & Miyata, T. (2006). Protein S-K196E mutation as a genetic risk factor for deep vein thrombosis in Japanese patients. *Blood,* Vol.107, No.4, pp. 1737-1738,

Koeleman, B. P., Reitsma, P. H., Allaart, C. F., & Bertina, R. M. (1994). Activated protein C resistance as an additional risk factor for thrombosis in protein C-deficient families. *Blood,* Vol.84, No.4, pp. 1031-1035,

Koeleman, B. P., Reitsma, P. H., & Bertina, R. M. (1997). Familial thrombophilia: a complex genetic disorder. *Semin.Hematol.*, Vol.34, No.3, pp. 256-264,

Koeleman, B. P., van, R. D., Hamulyak, K., Reitsma, P. H., & Bertina, R. M. (1995). Factor V Leiden: an additional risk factor for thrombosis in protein S deficient families? *Thromb.Haemost.*, Vol.74, No.2, pp. 580-583,

Koster, T., Rosendaal, F. R., de, R. H., Briet, E., Vandenbroucke, J. P., & Bertina, R. M. (1993). Venous thrombosis due to poor anticoagulant response to activated protein C: Leiden Thrombophilia Study. *Lancet,* Vol.342, No.8886-8887, pp. 1503-1506,

Lander, E. S. (1996). The new genomics: global views of biology. *Science,* Vol.274, No.5287, pp. 536-539,

Lane, D. A., Mannucci, P. M., Bauer, K. A., Bertina, R. M., Bochkov, N. P., Boulyjenkov, V., Chandy, M., Dahlback, B., Ginter, E. K., Miletich, J. P., Rosendaal, F. R., & Seligsohn, U. (1996). Inherited thrombophilia: Part 1. *Thromb.Haemost.*, Vol.76, No.5, pp. 651-662,

Larsen, T. B., Sorensen, H. T., Skytthe, A., Johnsen, S. P., Vaupel, J. W., & Christensen, K. (2003). Major genetic susceptibility for venous thromboembolism in men: a study of Danish twins. *Epidemiology,* Vol.14, No.3, pp. 328-332,

Leitner, J. M., Mannhalter, C., & Jilma, B. (2008). Genetic variations and their influence on risk and treatment of venous thrombosis. *Pharmacogenomics.*, Vol.9, No.4, pp. 423-437,

Lijfering, W. M., Brouwer, J. L., Veeger, N. J., Bank, I., Coppens, M., Middeldorp, S., Hamulyak, K., Prins, M. H., Buller, H. R., & van der Meer, J. (2009). Selective testing for thrombophilia in patients with first venous thrombosis: results from a retrospective family cohort study on absolute thrombotic risk for currently known thrombophilic defects in 2479 relatives. *Blood,* Vol.113, No.21, pp. 5314-5322,

Lopez, S., Buil, A., Ordonez, J., Souto, J. C., Almasy, L., Lathrop, M., Blangero, J., Blanco-Vaca, F., Fontcuberta, J., & Soria, J. M. (2008). Genome-wide linkage analysis for identifying quantitative trait loci involved in the regulation of lipoprotein a (Lpa) levels. *Eur.J.Hum.Genet.*, Vol.16, No.11, pp. 1372-1379,

Luxembourg, B., Delev, D., Geisen, C., Spannagl, M., Krause, M., Miesbach, W., Heller, C., Bergmann, F., Schmeink, U., Grossmann, R., Lindhoff-Last, E., Seifried, E., Oldenburg, J., & Pavlova, A. (2011). Molecular basis of antithrombin deficiency. *Thromb.Haemost.*, Vol.105, No.4, pp. 635-646,

Mahmoodi, B. K., Brouwer, J. L., Ten Kate, M. K., Lijfering, W. M., Veeger, N. J., Mulder, A. B., Kluin-Nelemans, H. C., & van der Meer, J. (2010). A prospective cohort study on the absolute risks of venous thromboembolism and predictive value of screening asymptomatic relatives of patients with hereditary deficiencies of protein S, protein C or antithrombin. *J.Thromb.Haemost.,* Vol.8, No.6, pp. 1193-1200,

Malarstig, A., Buil, A., Souto, J. C., Clarke, R., Blanco-Vaca, F., Fontcuberta, J., Peden, J., Andersen, M., Silveira, A., Barlera, S., Seedorf, U., Watkins, H., Almasy, L., Hamsten, A., & Soria, J. M. (2009). Identification of ZNF366 and PTPRD as novel determinants of plasma homocysteine in a family-based genome-wide association study. *Blood,* Vol.114, No.7, pp. 1417-1422,

Margaglione, M., D'Andrea, G., Colaizzo, D., Cappucci, G., del, P. A., Brancaccio, V., Ciampa, A., Grandone, E., & Di, M. G. (1999). Coexistence of factor V Leiden and Factor II A20210 mutations and recurrent venous thromboembolism. *Thromb.Haemost.,* Vol.82, No.6, pp. 1583-1587,

Marlar, R. A. & Mastovich, S. (1990). Hereditary protein C deficiency: a review of the genetics, clinical presentation, diagnosis and treatment. *Blood Coagul.Fibrinolysis,* Vol.1, No.3, pp. 319-330,

Miletich, J. P., Prescott, S. M., White, R., Majerus, P. W., & Bovill, E. G. (1993). Inherited predisposition to thrombosis. *Cell,* Vol.72, No.4, pp. 477-480,

Mosesson, M. W. (2003). Antithrombin I. Inhibition of thrombin generation in plasma by fibrin formation. *Thromb.Haemost.,* Vol.89, No.1, pp. 9-12,

Naess, I. A., Christiansen, S. C., Romundstad, P., Cannegieter, S. C., Rosendaal, F. R., & Hammerstrom, J. (2007). Incidence and mortality of venous thrombosis: a population-based study. *J.Thromb.Haemost.,* Vol.5, No.4, pp. 692-699,

Nejentsev, S., Walker, N., Riches, D., Egholm, M., & Todd, J. A. (2009). Rare variants of IFIH1, a gene implicated in antiviral responses, protect against type 1 diabetes. *Science,* Vol.324, No.5925, pp. 387-389,

Nygaard, K. K. & Brown, G. E. (1937). Essential thrombophilia: Report of five cases. *Archives of Internal Medicine,* Vol.59, No.1, pp. 82-106,

O'Roak, B. J., Deriziotis, P., Lee, C., Vives, L., Schwartz, J. J., Girirajan, S., Karakoc, E., Mackenzie, A. P., Ng, S. B., Baker, C., Rieder, M. J., Nickerson, D. A., Bernier, R., Fisher, S. E., Shendure, J., & Eichler, E. E. (2011). Exome sequencing in sporadic autism spectrum disorders identifies severe de novo mutations. *Nat.Genet.,* Vol.43, No.6, pp. 585-589,

Orstavik, K. H., Magnus, P., Reisner, H., Berg, K., Graham, J. B., & Nance, W. (1985). Factor VIII and factor IX in a twin population. Evidence for a major effect of ABO locus on factor VIII level. *Am.J.Hum.Genet.,* Vol.37, No.1, pp. 89-101,

Patnaik, M. M. & Moll, S. (2008). Inherited antithrombin deficiency: a review. *Haemophilia.,* Vol.14, No.6, pp. 1229-1239,

Pintao, M. C., Garcia, A. A., Borgel, D., Alhenc-Gelas, M., Spek, C. A., de Visser, M. C., Gandrille, S., & Reitsma, P. H. (2009). Gross deletions/duplications in PROS1 are relatively common in point mutation-negative hereditary protein S deficiency. *Hum.Genet.,* Vol.126, No.3, pp. 449-456,

Pintao, M. C., Roshani, S., de Visser, M. C., Tieken, C., Tanck, M. W., Wichers, I. M., Meijers, J. C., Rosendaal, F. R., Middeldorp, S., & Reitsma, P. H. (2011). High levels of protein C are determined by PROCR haplotype 3. *J.Thromb.Haemost.,* Vol.9, No.5, pp. 969-976,

Poort, S. R., Rosendaal, F. R., Reitsma, P. H., & Bertina, R. M. (1996). A common genetic variation in the 3'-untranslated region of the prothrombin gene is associated with elevated plasma prothrombin levels and an increase in venous thrombosis. *Blood,* Vol.88, No.10, pp. 3698-3703,

Pritchard, J. K. (2001). Are rare variants responsible for susceptibility to complex diseases? *Am.J.Hum.Genet.,* Vol.69, No.1, pp. 124-137,

Rees, D. C. (1996). The population genetics of factor V Leiden (Arg506Gln). *Br.J.Haematol.,* Vol.95, No.4, pp. 579-586,

Rees, D. C., Chapman, N. H., Webster, M. T., Guerreiro, J. F., Rochette, J., & Clegg, J. B. (1999). Born to clot: the European burden. *Br.J.Haematol.,* Vol.105, No.2, pp. 564-566,

Rezende, S. M., Simmonds, R. E., & Lane, D. A. (2004). Coagulation, inflammation, and apoptosis: different roles for protein S and the protein S-C4b binding protein complex. *Blood,* Vol.103, No.4, pp. 1192-1201,

Ridker, P. M., Miletich, J. P., Stampfer, M. J., Goldhaber, S. Z., Lindpaintner, K., & Hennekens, C. H. (1995). Factor V Leiden and risks of recurrent idiopathic venous thromboembolism. *Circulation,* Vol.92, No.10, pp. 2800-2802,

Risch, N. & Merikangas, K. (1996). The future of genetic studies of complex human diseases. *Science,* Vol.273, No.5281, pp. 1516-1517,

Rosendaal, F. R., Koster, T., Vandenbroucke, J. P., & Reitsma, P. H. (1995). High risk of thrombosis in patients homozygous for factor V Leiden (activated protein C resistance). *Blood,* Vol.85, No.6, pp. 1504-1508,

Schnitzler, J. (1926). Uber konstitutionelle und konditionelle mitbedingtheit post operativer vorkommnisse. *Wiener klinische Wochenschrift,* No.1, pp. 26,

Schork, N. J., Murray, S. S., Frazer, K. A., & Topol, E. J. (2009). Common vs. rare allele hypotheses for complex diseases. *Curr.Opin.Genet.Dev.,* Vol.19, No.3, pp. 212-219,

Schwarz, H. P., Fischer, M., Hopmeier, P., Batard, M. A., & Griffin, J. H. (1984). Plasma protein S deficiency in familial thrombotic disease. *Blood,* Vol.64, No.6, pp. 1297-1300,

Simmonds, R. E., Zoller, B., Ireland, H., Thompson, E., de Frutos, P. G., Dahlback, B., & Lane, D. A. (1997). Genetic and phenotypic analysis of a large (122-member) protein S-deficient kindred provides an explanation for the familial coexistence of type I and type III plasma phenotypes. *Blood,* Vol.89, No.12, pp. 4364-4370,

Soria, J. M., Almasy, L., Souto, J. C., Bacq, D., Buil, A., Faure, A., Martinez-Marchan, E., Mateo, J., Borrell, M., Stone, W., Lathrop, M., Fontcuberta, J., & Blangero, J. (2002). A quantitative-trait locus in the human factor XII gene influences both plasma factor XII levels and susceptibility to thrombotic disease. *Am.J.Hum.Genet.,* Vol.70, No.3, pp. 567-574,

Souto, J. C., Almasy, L., Borrell, M., Blanco-Vaca, F., Mateo, J., Soria, J. M., Coll, I., Felices, R., Stone, W., Fontcuberta, J., & Blangero, J. (2000a). Genetic susceptibility to thrombosis and its relationship to physiological risk factors: the GAIT study. Genetic Analysis of Idiopathic Thrombophilia. *Am.J.Hum.Genet.,* Vol.67, No.6, pp. 1452-1459,

Souto, J. C., Almasy, L., Borrell, M., Gari, M., Martinez, E., Mateo, J., Stone, W. H., Blangero, J., & Fontcuberta, J. (2000b). Genetic determinants of hemostasis phenotypes in Spanish families. *Circulation,* Vol.101, No.13, pp. 1546-1551,

Stenson, P. D., Mort, M., Ball, E. V., Howells, K., Phillips, A. D., Thomas, N. S., & Cooper, D. N. (2009). The Human Gene Mutation Database: 2008 update. *Genome Med.,* Vol.1, No.1, pp. 13,

Tait, R. C., Walker, I. D., Perry, D. J., Islam, S. I., Daly, M. E., McCall, F., Conkie, J. A., & Carrell, R. W. (1994). Prevalence of antithrombin deficiency in the healthy population. *Br.J.Haematol.*, Vol.87, No.1, pp. 106-112,

Tanck, M. W., Wichers, I. M., Meijers, J. C., Buller, H. R., Reitsma, P. H., & Middeldorp, S. (2011). Quantitative trait locus for protein C in a family with thrombophilia. *Thromb.Haemost.*, Vol.105, No.1, pp. 199-201,

Tang, W., Basu, S., Kong, X., Pankow, J. S., Aleksic, N., Tan, A., Cushman, M., Boerwinkle, E., & Folsom, A. R. (2010). Genome-wide association study identifies novel loci for plasma levels of protein C: the ARIC study. *Blood*, Vol.116, No.23, pp. 5032-5036,

The 1000 Genomes Project Consortium (2010). A map of human genome variation from population-scale sequencing. *Nature*, Vol.467, No.7319, pp. 1061-1073, ISSN 0028-0836

The International HapMap Consortium (2005). A haplotype map of the human genome. *Nature*, Vol.437, No.7063, pp. 1299-1320, ISSN 0028-0836

Tirado, I., Mateo, J., Soria, J. M., Oliver, A., Martinez-Sanchez, E., Vallve, C., Borrell, M., Urrutia, T., & Fontcuberta, J. (2005). The ABO blood group genotype and factor VIII levels as independent risk factors for venous thromboembolism. *Thromb.Haemost.*, Vol.93, No.3, pp. 468-474,

Tregouet, D. A., Heath, S., Saut, N., Biron-Andreani, C., Schved, J. F., Pernod, G., Galan, P., Drouet, L., Zelenika, D., Juhan-Vague, I., Alessi, M. C., Tiret, L., Lathrop, M., Emmerich, J., & Morange, P. E. (2009). Common susceptibility alleles are unlikely to contribute as strongly as the FV and ABO loci to VTE risk: results from a GWAS approach. *Blood*, Vol.113, No.21, pp. 5298-5303,

Uitte de Willige, S., de Visser, M. C., Houwing-Duistermaat, J. J., Rosendaal, F. R., Vos, H. L., & Bertina, R. M. (2005). Genetic variation in the fibrinogen gamma gene increases the risk for deep venous thrombosis by reducing plasma fibrinogen gamma' levels. *Blood*, Vol.106, No.13, pp. 4176-4183,

Uitte de Willige, S., Pyle, M. E., Vos, H. L., de Visser, M. C., Lally, C., Dowling, N. F., Hooper, W. C., Bertina, R. M., & Austin, H. (2009). Fibrinogen gamma gene 3'-end polymorphisms and risk of venous thromboembolism in the African-American and Caucasian population. *Thromb.Haemost.*, Vol.101, No.6, pp. 1078-1084,

Uitte de Willige, S., Rietveld, I. M., de Visser, M. C., Vos, H. L., & Bertina, R. M. (2007). Polymorphism 10034C>T is located in a region regulating polyadenylation of FGG transcripts and influences the fibrinogen gamma'/gammaA mRNA ratio. *J.Thromb.Haemost.*, Vol.5, No.6, pp. 1243-1249,

van Boven, H. H. & Lane, D. A. (1997). Antithrombin and its inherited deficiency states. *Semin.Hematol.*, Vol.34, No.3, pp. 188-204,

van Boven, H. H., Reitsma, P. H., Rosendaal, F. R., Bayston, T. A., Chowdhury, V., Bauer, K. A., Scharrer, I., Conard, J., & Lane, D. A. (1996). Factor V Leiden (FV R506Q) in families with inherited antithrombin deficiency. *Thromb.Haemost.*, Vol.75, No.3, pp. 417-421,

van Sluis, G. L., Sohne, M., El Kheir, D. Y., Tanck, M. W., Gerdes, V. E., & Buller, H. R. (2006). Family history and inherited thrombophilia. *J.Thromb.Haemost.*, Vol.4, No.10, pp. 2182-2187,

Vossen, C. Y., Walker, I. D., Svensson, P., Souto, J. C., Scharrer, I., Preston, F. E., Palareti, G., Pabinger, I., van der Meer, F. J., Makris, M., Fontcuberta, J., Conard, J., &

Rosendaal, F. R. (2005). Recurrence rate after a first venous thrombosis in patients with familial thrombophilia. *Arterioscler.Thromb.Vasc.Biol.,* Vol.25, No.9, pp. 1992-1997,

Wells, P. S., Blajchman, M. A., Henderson, P., Wells, M. J., Demers, C., Bourque, R., & McAvoy, A. (1994). Prevalence of antithrombin deficiency in healthy blood donors: a cross-sectional study. *Am.J.Hematol.,* Vol.45, No.4, pp. 321-324,

Wichers, I. M., Tanck, M. W., Meijers, J. C., Lisman, T., Reitsma, P. H., Rosendaal, F. R., Buller, H. R., & Middeldorp, S. (2009). Assessment of coagulation and fibrinolysis in families with unexplained thrombophilia. *Thromb.Haemost.,* Vol.101, No.3, pp. 465-470,

Zivelin, A., Griffin, J. H., Xu, X., Pabinger, I., Samama, M., Conard, J., Brenner, B., Eldor, A., & Seligsohn, U. (1997). A single genetic origin for a common Caucasian risk factor for venous thrombosis. *Blood,* Vol.89, No.2, pp. 397-402,

Zivelin, A., Rosenberg, N., Faier, S., Kornbrot, N., Peretz, H., Mannhalter, C., Horellou, M. H., & Seligsohn, U. (1998). A single genetic origin for the common prothrombotic G20210A polymorphism in the prothrombin gene. *Blood,* Vol.92, No.4, pp. 1119-1124,

Zoller, B., Berntsdotter, A., Garcia de, F. P., & Dahlback, B. (1995). Resistance to activated protein C as an additional genetic risk factor in hereditary deficiency of protein S. *Blood,* Vol.85, No.12, pp. 3518-3523.

2

Association of Haemostasis Activation Markers with Thrombophilia and Venous Thromboembolism

Tjaša Vižintin-Cuderman[1], Mojca Božič-Mijovski[1], Aleksandra Antović[2], Polona Peternel[1], Matija Kozak[1] and Mojca Stegnar[1]
[1]*Department of Vascular Diseases, University Medical Centre, Ljubljana,*
[2]*Karolinska Institute, Department of Clinical Sciences, Danderyd Hospital, Stockholm,*
[1]*Slovenia*
[2]*Sweden*

1. Introduction

Thrombophilia (TF) is defined as an inherited or acquired tendency to develop thrombosis. TF creates a state of hypercoagulability, i.e. haemostasis activation without actual clot formation which can be detected *in vitro* by specific laboratory techniques. Thrombosis as a clinical phenomenon, however, only occurs when the balance between pro-coagulant and anti-coagulant elements of haemostasis is disrupted to such an extent that it leads to clot formation in the circulating blood.

TF is most commonly associated with an increased risk of thrombosis in the venous system, i.e. venous thromboembolism (VTE). VTE is a common disease with an annual incidence of about 1 case per 1000 person-years and is a cause of substantial morbidity and mortality worldwide (White, 2003). Furthermore, it is a chronic disease that often recurs. A third of patients with first VTE, experience a recurrence within the next 5 to 8 years. Recurrence is best prevented since it is fatal in 5 % of patients and late sequelae, such as post-thrombotic syndrome, are also very common (Schulman et al, 2006). The standard treatment for acute VTE (unfractionated or low-molecular-weight heparin, followed by vitamin K antagonists for at least several months) reduces the risk of recurrence by 80 to 90 % (Kearon et al, 2008). Although ideally all patients should receive long-term treatment with vitamin K antagonists to reduce the risk of recurrence, one has to bear in mind the 2 -3 % annual incidence of major bleeding on anticoagulant treatment (Ansell et al, 2008). The duration of anticoagulant treatment should therefore be tailored individually to optimize the preventive action of treatment with the minimum risk of bleeding. The likelihood of recurrence varies among individuals and is strongly influenced by the presence of clinical risk factors. Patients whose first VTE was triggered by a circumstantial risk factor (provoked VTE) have a lower risk of recurrence than patients whose event was unprovoked (idiopathic VTE), or who carry persistent risk factors (Kearon et al, 2008). It is, however, arguable whether the level of risk estimated from clinical risk factors alone justifies long-term anticoagulation.

For a long time it was thought that screening for TF, a persistent risk factor for VTE, would facilitate clinical decision-making in determining the duration of anticoagulant treatment.

Over the past decades knowledge of TF has increased substantially, as did the number of individuals screened for TF. It was shown that when all known TF defects are considered, TF is found in about half of patients with the first VTE (Christiansen et al, 2005). However, routine TF screening is usually limited to those TF defects that carry a strong to moderate risk of VTE: antithrombin, protein C and protein S deficiencies, factor V Leiden, prothrombin G20210A mutation (inherited defects) and antiphospholipid antibodies (acquired defects). Testing for other TF defects, such as hyperhomocysteinaemia, high fibrinogen, increased factors VIII, IX, XI, dysfibrinogenaemia, reduced tissue factor pathway inhibitor and factor XIII polymorphisms is usually only performed in clinical studies (Stegnar, 2010).

TF status does not directly translate into an increased risk of either first or recurrent VTE (Christiansen et al, 2005). First of all, there is considerable variation in the magnitude of risk associated with different TF defects. Furthermore, the magnitude of risk a specific TF defect carries is not the same for first or for recurrent VTE. The most common TF defects, such as factor V Leiden and prothrombin G2021A mutation, carry a modest risk of both first and recurrent VTE (Ho et al, 2006). The rarely occurring deficiencies of antithrombin, protein C and protein S, historically believed to be very strong risk factors for first VTE, convey only a slightly higher risk for recurrence than factor V Leiden and prothrombin G2021A mutation (Christiansen et al, 2005; De Stefano et al, 2006).

The results of TF screening actually alter the clinical management only in selected groups of VTE patients (Stegnar, 2010). Moreover, since VTE is a multi-causal disease, there are usually other factors apart from TF that contribute to the development of VTE (Rosendaal 1999). It seems therefore that to assess VTE risk in individuals with TF an additional tool is needed. The aim of this article is to review the available evidence as to whether screening for hypercoagulability could represent such a tool.

2. Activation of haemostasis

The initial events in haemostasis involve activation of the endothelium and blood cells in response to vessel wall injury, which results in release of a variety of soluble factors involved in the control of haemostasis and cell adhesion. In this review, cell adhesion will be limited merely to cell adhesion molecules P-selectin, E-selectin, vascular cell adhesion molecule 1 (VCAM-1) and intercellular cell adhesion molecule 1 (ICAM-1) that mediate in the binding of endothelium and blood cells.

Blood coagulation is initiated by the release of tissue factor from activated endothelial and blood cells. Activated endothelial cells and platelets express P-selectin, which binds monocytes and macrophages. Bound monocytes and macrophages expose tissue factor to the circulation. Tissue factor forms a complex with circulating activated factor VII. This complex activates factor X to activated factor X (Xa) and factor Xa converts minor quantities of prothrombin into thrombin. In this process, prothrombin fragments 1+2 (F1+2) are released. These events are regulated by tissue factor pathway inhibitor, which neutralizes factor Xa and by antithrombin, which inactivates thrombin by forming thrombin-antithrombin (TAT) complexes. When the threshold level of thrombin is generated, thrombin activates platelets, as well as factors XIII, V, VIII and XI to augment its own generation. This is achieved by further conversion of factor X to factor Xa, using activated factors VIII and IX as cofactors. Factor Xa together with activated factor V (prothrombinase complex) converts the majority of prothrombin into thrombin. These events are regulated by activated protein C and its cofactor protein S, which neutralize activated factors V and VIII and so limit thrombin generation (Monroe & Hoffman, 2006).

Thrombin cleaves fibrinogen and fibrinopeptides A and B are released from alpha and beta polypeptide chains of fibrinogen. The resulting fibrin monomers polymerise to form soluble non-cross-linked fibrin, which is then cross-linked by activated factor XIII. The formation of fibrin triggers activation of the fibrinolytic system. Tissue-type plasminogen activator (t-PA), which is released by endothelial cells, activates plasminogen to plasmin. Plasmin degrades fibrin to fibrin degradation products of various molecular sizes. D-dimer, the smallest of the fibrin degradation products, retains the γ cross-links of the original fibrin. These events are regulated by several inhibitors of fibrinolysis: plasminogen activator inhibitors type 1 and 2 (PAI-1 and PAI-2), antiplasmin and thrombin activatable fibrinolysis inhibitor (Rijken & Lijnen, 2009).

3. Laboratory methods to detect activation of haemostasis

Activation of haemostasis (hypercoagulability) is ideally detected prior to the appearance of thrombotic phenomena. Laboratory recognition of hypercoagulability is, however, a very demanding task due to the complexity of the haemostatic system. It can be detected by global tests (global haemostasis screening assays) that provide an overview of the entire haemostatic system, including enzymes, cofactors and inhibitors. Another approach to detecting hypercoagulability is to measure specific substances (peptides, enzymes, enzyme-inhibitor complexes) that are liberated with activation of the coagulation and fibrinolysis systems *in vivo* (specific markers of haemostasis activation). The most recent method to assess hypercoagulability is to detect molecules that are released from activated endothelial and blood cells in response to injury of the vessel wall (markers of endothelial and platelet activation).

3.1 Global haemostasis screening assays

Activated partial thromboplastin time (aPTT) has been in use for more than half a century (Langdell et al, 1953). It is simple and the most widely used global haemostasis screening assay, sensitive to all coagulation factors except factor VII. The end-point of this assay is the formation of a fibrin clot, detected manually or automatically by measuring the optical density of plasma after addition of phospholipids and a surface activator such as celite. Clotting occurs when 3 - 5 % of the total amount of thrombin is produced (Brummel et al, 2002) and therefore subsequent haemostatic responses or possible abnormalities of the haemostatic process cannot be observed (Mann et al, 2003). Nonetheless, a strong association was found between shortened aPTT and increased risk of first (Tripodi et al, 2004) and recurrent VTE (Hron et al, 2006; Legnani et al, 2006). The increase in VTE risk was independent of TF status. Shortening of aPTT might be due to increased concentrations of factors VIII, IX and XI Legnani et al, 2006).

Thromboelastography (TEG) monitors haemostasis as a dynamic process, evaluating both clotting, fibrinolysis and platelet function. TEG variables are derived from a trace produced from measurement of the viscoelastic changes associated with clot formation and degradation (Sorensen et al, 2003).

Whilst the whole blood sample in a TEG cuvette remains liquid, the motion of the cuvette does not affect a pin which is suspended freely from a torsion wire. However, when the clot starts to form, the fibrin strands "couple" the motion of the cup to the motion of the pin, which is amplified and recorded. Several variables of the recording can be evaluated such as the reaction time, angle formed by the slope of the TEG trace, maximum amplitude and clot lysis index (Mallet & Cox, 1992).

TEG as a tool to measure hypercoagulability in the setting of VTE was only assessed in small studies. TEG showed a marked hypercoagulable profile in patients with acute VTE (Spiezia et al, 2008). Also in patients with a history of venous or arterial thrombosis, shorter clotting times and accelerated maximum velocity of clot propagation were measured (Hvitfeldt Poulsen et al, 2006). However, another study in patients with a history of cerebral vein thrombosis did not confirm these results (Koopman et al, 2009). TF, present in approximately half of the patients in these studies, did not influence TEG parameters. Similarly, in individuals with a personal or family history of VTE, hypercoagulable TEG was measured in 40 % of patients, but it did not correlate with TF status (O'Donnell et al, 2004). TEG therefore cannot be used as a screening test for TF, but it might be a useful adjunctive test, particularly in patients without known TF defects. Further studies are needed to determine whether TEG can be used to predict the recurrence of thrombotic events.

However, TEG is poorly standardized, has a high coefficient of variation and is influenced by many pre-analytical variables, which makes it less suitable for routine clinical use to assess hypercoagulability (Chen & Teruya, 2009). Besides, it is a whole blood assay and therefore frozen-thawed samples cannot be used.

Thrombin generation assay (TGA) reflects the potential of plasma to generate thrombin following *in vitro* activation of coagulation with tissue factor or other trigger (Hemker et al, 2002). The thrombin concentration is continuously monitored by adding a suitable thrombin substrate and formation of split products is detected by optical densitometry or fluorometry. The resulting thrombin generation curve and its three most important parameters of lag time, peak value and area under the curve or endogenous thrombin potential, reflect and integrate all pro- and anticoagulant reactions that regulate the formation and inhibition of thrombin (van Veen et al, 2008). However, TGA does not measure the final step of coagulation, i.e. fibrin formation. TGA is performed in plasma, is commercially available and relatively easy to use. It is, however, not standardized; it is influenced by many pre-analytical variables and there is a high inter-laboratory variability due to different reagents and their concentrations, making it difficult to establish reference ranges (Castoldi & Rosing 2011).

Thrombin generation is elevated in antithrombin deficiency (Wielders et al, 1997; Alhenc-Gelas et al, 2010), protein S deficiency (Castoldi et al, 2010), protein C deficiency (Hezard et al, 2007), in carriers of factor V Leiden (Hezard et al, 2006; Lincz et al, 2006) and prothrombin G202010 mutation (Kyrle et al, 1998; Lavigne-Lissalde et al, 2010). It is also associated with the presence of antiphospholipid antibodies (Liestol et al, 2007; Devreese et al, 2009) and increased levels of factors VIII (ten Cate-Hoek et al, 2008), IX and XI (Siegemund et al, 2004).

Elevated thrombin generation was also investigated as a risk factor for the first VTE event and its recurrence. It was shown that elevated thrombin generation was associated with a 1.7 – fold increased risk of first idiopathic VTE (van Hylckama Vlieg et al, 2007). The association between elevated thrombin generation and the risk of first VTE was confirmed in several other studies (Dargaud et al, 2006; Lutsey et al, 2009; Wichers et al, 2009). Furthermore, elevated thrombin generation identifies patients at risk of VTE recurrence. In one cohort it was shown that patients with low levels of thrombin generation after discontinuation of anticoagulant treatment had an almost 60 % lower risk of recurrence compared to patients with elevated thrombin generation (Hron et al, 2006). Subsequent studies have confirmed that patients at high risk of VTE recurrence can be identified by TGA (Hron et al, 2006; Tripodi et al, 2008; Besser et al, 2008; Eichinger et al, 2008).

Overall haemostasis potential (OHP) is based on repeated spectrophotometric registration of fibrin formation in two parallel samples of citrated plasma, to which small amounts of thrombin and t-PA (the first plasma sample) or only thrombin (the second plasma sample) are added. The areas under the fibrin formation curves obtained represent OHP (the first plasma sample with thrombin and t-PA) and overall coagulation potential (OCP, the second plasma sample with only thrombin added). Overall fibrinolytic potential (OFP) is calculated as the difference between OHP and OCP (He et al, 2001). The OHP assay is not commercially available and it is not yet standardized. It is, however, inexpensive, easy and fast to perform (Antović, 2008).

OHP has been shown to detect hypercoagulability in smaller studies. Increased OHP was found in 75 % of women with a history of pregnancy-provoked VTE. In women with concomitant TF (acquired activated protein C resistance or factor V Leiden) imbalance in haemostatic potential was more severe, since OHP was increased in all women (Antović et al, 2003). In another study, OHP also identified the hypercoagulable state in patients with lupus anticoagulants and a history of thrombotic events, regardless of concomitant anticoagulant therapy (Curnow et al, 2007). Using a modification of the original OHP assay (the coagulation inhibitor potential CIP assay), severe TF (deficiencies of antithrombin, protein C and protein S, homozygosity for factor V Leiden and combinations) could be detected with a sensitivity of 100 % and specificity of 70 - 80% (Andresen et al, 2002, 2004).

OHP was also studied during anticoagulant treatment for VTE. In a study of 70 patients with acute venous thrombosis given standard anticoagulant treatment (low-molecular-weight heparin followed by warfarin), OHP was significantly increased before treatment and greatly decreased during combined treatment with heparin and warfarin (overlapping period), while during warfarin only treatment OHP was about half that before treatment. After cessation of therapy, OHP values increased but remained lower than in the pre-treatment period. OHP levels did not differ between patients with or without TF (Vižintin-Cuderman et al, to be published).

3.2 Specific markers of haemostasis activation

F1+2 and TAT are markers of *in vivo* activity of factor X and thrombin. They are liberated during activation and generation of thrombin and are stable enough to be detected by laboratory methods, mainly enzyme-linked immunosorbent assays. However, they are extremely sensitive to *in vitro* artefacts. The quality of the sample and the reliability of the result depend on the technique of blood sampling and the experience of the person performing the procedure (Stegnar et al, 2007). Besides blood sampling, the different reagents used as well as the preparation and storage of the samples can influence the results (Greenberg et al 1994; Miller et al, 1995). Consequently, they are rarely used today. However, around twenty years ago they were tested in various small studies that gave contradictory results.

Increased F1+2 was found in individuals with antithrombin, protein C and S deficiencies (Demers et al, 1992; Mannucci et al, 1992), as well as in those with activated protein C (APC) resistance (Simioni et al, 1996; Bauer et al, 2000), prothrombin G20210A mutation (Bauer et al, 2000) antiphospholipid syndrome (Ames et al, 1996), hyperhomocysteinemia (Kyrle et al, 1997a) and increased levels of factor VIII (O'Donnell et al, 2001). Not all studies, however, confirmed the association of increased F1+2 levels with TF (Kyrle et al, 1998; Eichinger et al, 1999; Lowe et al, 1999).

TAT was increased in association with increased factor VIII levels (O'Donnell et al, 2001) and also with APC resistance in one study (Simioni et al, 1996), but not in two others (Eichinger et al, 1999; Lowe et al, 1999). Similarly, increased TAT was not associated with antithrombin (Demers et al, 1992), protein C and S deficiencies (Macherel et al, 1992) or with antiphospholipid syndrome (Ames et al, 1996).

In patients with acute VTE, F1+2 and TAT are elevated and normalize 2 to 4 days after introduction of heparin treatment (The DVTENOX study group, 1993; Stricker et al, 1999; Peternel et al, 2000). The levels of these markers remain low also during treatment with warfarin (Elias et al, 1993; Jerkemann et al, 2000; Vižintin-Cuderman et al, to be published). TF does not seem to influence F1+2 and TAT levels either during anticoagulant treatment or after its withdrawal (Cuderman et al, 2007; Vižintin-Cuderman et al, to be published).

There are few studies on the utility of these markers in assessing VTE recurrence risk. In two studies F1+2 was not associated with recurrence in patients with a history of VTE (Kyrle et al, 1997b, Vižintin-Cuderman et al, to be published). Two recent studies, however, showed that in patients with VTE increased F1+2 measured 1 month after withdrawal of anticoagulant treatment was associated with increased risk of recurrent thrombosis, irrespective of TF status (Poli, 2008, 2010).

D-dimer is a degradation product of cross-linked fibrin. It is marker of both activated coagulation and fibrinolysis. D-dimer is best known today as the biochemical gold standard for initial assessment of suspected VTE. It has a sensitivity of up to 95 % and a negative predictive value of nearly 100 % (Di Nisio et al, 2007) and is an integral part of diagnostic algorithms to exclude VTE (Righini et al, 2008).

In patients with acute VTE, D-dimer is elevated and decreases after 1 to 3 days of treatment, but remains above normal levels for at least the first week of treatment (The DVTENOX study group, 1993; Stricker et al, 1999; Peternel et al, 2002). This is probably due to prolonged fibrinolysis, which is independent of heparin therapy and thrombin generation, but it may also be partly due to the relatively long half-life of D-dimer (Mannucci, 1994). By the first month of treatment, D-dimer levels mostly return to normal and remain so throughout warfarin treatment (Elias et al, 1993; Meissner et al, 2000; Vižintin-Cuderman et al, to be published). One study showed that during anticoagulant treatment in patients with TF, D-dimer levels remain higher than in patients without TF, albeit not significantly (Vižintin-Cuderman et al, to be published). After discontinuation of anticoagulant treatment, D-dimer levels in patients with TF remain higher than in those without TF (Palareti et al, 2003, Vižintin-Cuderman et al, to be published).

D-dimer was also investigated as a risk factor of the first VTE event and its recurrence. In a population-based cohort study, D-dimer was associated with a 3-fold increased risk of the first VTE event (Cushman et al, 2003) and with a 2.2 - 3-fold increased risk of recurrent VTE (Andreescu et al, 2002; Palareti et al, 2003: Cosmi et al, 2005).

Moreover, D-dimer is a marker for predicting VTE recurrence after cessation of anticoagulant treatment (Verhovsek et al, 2008). Normal levels of D-dimer one month after cessation of anticoagulant treatment have been shown to have a high negative predictive value for VTE recurrence (Palareti et al, 2002; Eichinger et al, 2003). These results were tested in an interventional study in patients with unprovoked VTE. It was shown that elevated D-dimer one month after cessation of anticoagulant treatment significantly increases the risk of recurrent VTE, which can be reduced by resumption of anticoagulant therapy (Palareti et al, 2006). Interestingly, it was demonstrated that in patients with TF who have elevated D-dimer levels one month after cessation of anticoagulant treatment, the risk of recurrence is particularly high in comparison to patients with TF who have normal D-dimer. The difference was particularly important in carriers of common TF defects, such as factor V Leiden and prothrombin G20210A mutation (Palareti et al, 2003).

Surprisingly, there are few studies on the association of D-dimer with specific TF defects. Elevated D-dimer was found in carriers of factor V Leiden (Eichinger et al, 1999, Cuderman et al, 2007) and in the presence of antiphospholipid antibodies (Ames et al, 1996).

3.3 Markers of endothelial and platelet activation

P-selectin is a cell adhesion molecule that is expressed by platelets and endothelial cells upon their activation and is partly released in plasma in its soluble form. It can be measured in plasma by an enzyme-linked immunosorbent assay.

P-selectin levels are increased in acute VTE (Smith et al, 1999; Božič et al, 2002; Rectenwald et al, 2005; Ramacciotti et al, 2011). When P-selectin was tested as a possible marker for diagnosis of VTE, it was shown that a combination of the clinical prediction score and low P-selectin can be used to exclude VTE with a sensitivity and specificity similar to that of D-dimer. In addition, the combination of the clinical prediction score and high P-selectin has, unlike D-dimer, a very high positive predictive value in confirming acute VTE (Rectenwald et al, 2005; Ramacciotti et al, 2011).

After commencement of anticoagulant treatment for VTE, P-selectin levels decrease. A small study showed a decrease in P-selectin levels after 7 days of treatment with unfractionated heparin (Papalambros et al, 2004). In a study of 70 patients receiving low-molecular-weight heparin followed by warfarin, P-selectin levels decreased already after 3 days of treatment. Interestingly, one month after treatment discontinuation, P-selectin levels were not significantly higher than during treatment (Vižintin-Cuderman et al, to be published). Similarly, in another study there was no difference in P-selectin levels between patients receiving warfarin and those without anticoagulant therapy (Ay et al, 2007).

In patients with a history of VTE, elevated P-selectin is associated with increased risk of recurrence. Two case-control studies found that in patients at least 3 months after the onset of acute VTE, P-selectin levels were elevated compared to healthy controls (Blann et al, 2000; Ay et al, 2007). This result was confirmed in two prospective cohort studies that investigated P-selectin as a predictive marker for recurrence in patients with VTE (Kyrle et al, 2007; Vižintin-Cuderman et al, to be published). Similarly in another prospective cohort study, elevated P-selectin was a predictor of the occurrence of VTE in cancer patients (Ay et al, 2008).

There is not much evidence, however, on P-selectin levels in relation to specific TF defects. In a small study it was shown that P-selectin is elevated in patients with lupus anticoagulants and a history of VTE (Bugert et al, 2007). The presence of TF did not influence P-selectin levels during and after anticoagulant treatment in another study (Vižintin-Cuderman et al, to be published). Finally, TF status did not have any influence on P-selectin as a risk factor of VTE recurrence (Kyrle et al, 2007).

The association of **other markers of endothelial and platelet activation** (E-selectin, VCAM-1, ICAM-1, t-PA and PAI-1) with TF and VTE is poorly investigated. In a small study, E-selectin, VCAM-1 and ICAM-1 were not shown to be elevated in acute VTE (Bucek et al, 2003). However, elevated VCAM-1 levels were found in patients with acute VTE in two earlier studies (Smith et al, 1999, Božič et al, 2002). Elevated PAI-1 and t-PA levels were associated with increased risk of first or recurrent VTE in some studies (Schulman & Wiman, 1996; Meltzer et al, 2010), but not in others (Crowther et al, 2001; Folsom et al, 2003). The influence of TF on t-PA and PAI-1 levels was addressed in two small studies in patients with a history of VTE. No difference was found between patients with factor V Leiden (Stegnar et al, 1997) or hyperhomocysteinemia (Božič et al, 2000) and patients without these TF defects.

4. Conclusions

Assessment of haemostasis activation (hypercoagulability) is a very demanding task due to the complexity of the haemostatic system. However, it can be achieved either by global haemostasis screening assays that provide an overview of the entire haemostatic system, including enzymes, cofactors and inhibitors, or alternatively, by measuring specific haemostasis activation markers - peptides, enzymes or enzyme-inhibitor complexes that are liberated with the activation of coagulation, fibrinolysis, endothelial cells and platelets *in vivo*. Two global haemostasis screening assays (aPTT and TEG) have been used for many years, albeit their usefulness in detecting hypercoagulability and the risk of first and recurrent VTE seems to be limited due to insufficient clinical data, lack of standardization and the influence of pre-analytical factors. TGA and OHP are more promising. Both assays seem to be sensitive to TF defects and to be associated with the risk of VTE. Apart from D-dimer, other specific haemostasis activation markers, namely F1+2 and TAT, are extremely sensitive to *in vitro* artefacts and are rarely used today. However, around twenty years ago they were tested in various small studies that gave contradictory results. D-dimer is more robust and clinically useful for excluding VTE and also for detecting the risk of VTE after discontinuation of anticoagulant treatment. The risk of recurrence seems to be particularly high in patients with common TF defects, such as factor V Leiden and prothrombin G20210A mutation and high D-dimer. Finally, it has been shown that P-selectin, a marker of endothelial and platelet activation, can be used to exclude VTE with sensitivity and specificity similar to that of D-dimer. However, there is not much evidence on the association of P-selectin with specific TF defects.

5. References

Alhenc-Gelas M, Canonico M & Picard V.(2010). Influence of natural SERPINC1 mutations on *ex vivo* thrombin generation. *J Thromb Haemost*, Vol.8, No.4, (Apr 2010), pp.845–8

Ames PR, Tommasino C, Iannaccone L, Brillante M, Cimino R & Brancaccio V. (1996). Coagulation activation and fibrinolytic imbalance in subjects with idiopathic antiphospholipid antibodies - a crucial role for acquired protein S deficiency. *Thromb Haemost*, Vol.76, No.2, (Aug 1996), pp.190–4

Andreescu AC, Cushman M & Rosendaal FR. (2002). D-dimer as a risk factor for deep vein thrombosis: the Leiden Thrombophilia Study. *Thromb Haemost*, Vol. 87, No.1, (Jan 2002), pp.47–51

Andresen MS, Iversen N & Abildgaard U. (2002). Overall haemostasis potential assays performed in thrombophilic plasma: the effect of preactivating protein C and antithrombin. *Thromb Res*, Vol.108, No. 5-6, (Dec 2002), pp.323–8

Andresen MS, Abildgaard U, Liestøl S, Sandset PM, Mowinckel MC, Ødegaard OR, Larsen ML & Diep ML. (2004). The ability of three global plasma assays to recognize thrombophilia. *Thromb Res*, Vol.113, No.6, (2004), pp.411–7

Ansell J, Hirsh J, Hylek E, Jacobson A, Crowther M, Palareti G, & American College of Chest Physicians. (2008). Pharmacology and management of the vitamin K antagonists: American College of Chest Physicians Evidence-Based Clinical Practice Guidelines (8th Edition). *Chest*, Vol.133, No. 6 Suppl, (Jun 2008), pp. 160S–198S

Antović A, Blombäck M, Bremme K, Van Rooijen M & He S. (2003). Increased hemostasis potential persists in women with previous thromboembolism with or without APC resistance *J Thromb Haemost*, Vol.1, No.12, (Dec 2003), pp.2531–5

Antović A. (2008) Screening haemostasis – looking for global assays: the overall haemostasis potential (OHP) method – a possible tool for laboratory investigation of global haemostasis in both hypo- and hypercoagulable conditions. *Curr Vasc Pharm*, Vol.6, No.3, (Jul 2008), pp. 173–85

Ay C, Jungbauer LV, Sailer T, Tengler T, Koder S, Kaider A, Panzer S, Quehenberger P, Pabinger I & Mannhalter C. (2007). High concentrations of soluble P-selectin are associated with risk of venous thromboembolism and the P-selectin Thr715 variant. *Clin Chem*, Vol.53, No.7, (Jul 2007), pp.1235–43

Ay C, Simanek R, Vormittag R, Dunkler D, Alguel G, Koder S, Kornek G, Marosi C, Wagner O, Zielinski C & Pabinger I. (2008). High plasma levels of soluble P-selectin are predictive of venous thromboembolism in cancer patients: results from the Vienna Cancer and Thrombosis Study (CATS). *Blood*, Vol.112, No.7, (Oct 2008), pp.2703–8

Bauer KA, Humphries S, Smillie B, Li L, Cooper JA, Barzegar S, Rosenberg RG & Miller GJ. (2000). Prothrombin activation is increased among asymptomatic carriers of the prothrombin G20210A and factor V Arg506Gln mutations. *Thromb Haemost*, Vol.84, No.3, (Sep 2000), pp.396–400

Besser M, Baglin C, Luddington R, van Hylckama Vlieg A & Baglin T. (2008) High rate of unprovoked recurrent venous thrombosis is associated with high thrombin generating potential in a prospective cohort study. *J Thromb Haemost*, Vol.6, No.10, (Oct 2008), pp.1720–5

Blann AD, Noteboom WMP & Rosendaal FR. (2000). Increased soluble P-selectin levels following deep venous thrombosis: cause or effect? *Br J Haematol*, Vol.108, No.1, (Jan 2000), pp.191–3

Božič M, Stegnar M, Fermo I, Ritonja A, Peternel P, Stare J & D'Angelo A. (2000). Mild hyperhomocysteinemia and fibrinolytic factors in patients with history of venous thromboembolism. *Thromb Res*, Vol.100, No.4, (Nov 2000), pp.271–8

Božič M, Blinc A & Stegnar M. (2002). D-dimer, other markers of haemostasis activation and soluble adhesion molecules in patients with different clinical probabilities of deep vein thrombosis. *Thromb Res*, Vol.108, No.2-3, (Nov 2002), pp.107–14

Brummel KE, Paradis SG, Butenas S & Mann KG. (2002). Thrombin functions during tissue factor induced blood coagulation. *Blood*, Vol.100, No.1, (Jul 2002), pp.148–52

Bucek RA, Reiter M, Quehenberger P, Minar E & Baghestanian M. (2003). The role of soluble cell adhesion molecules in patients with suspected deep vein thrombosis. *Blood Coagul Fibrinolysis*, Vol. 14, No.7, (Oct 2003), pp.653–7

Bugert P, Pabinger I, Stamer K, Vormittag R, Skeate RC, Wahi MM & Panzer S. (2007). The risk for thromboembolic disease in lupus anticoagulant patients due to pathways involving P-selectin and CD154. *Thromb Haemost*, Vol.97, No.4, (Apr 2007), pp.573–80

Castoldi E, Maurissen LF, Tormene D, Spiezia L, Gavasso S, Radu C, Hackeng TM, Rosing J & Simioni P. (2010). Similar hypercoagulable states and thrombosis risk in type I and type III protein S-deficient individuals from families with mixed type I/III protein S deficiency. *Haematologica*, Vol.95, No.9, (Sep 2010), pp.1563–71

Castoldi E & Rosing J. (2011). Thrombin generation tests. *Thromb Res*, Vol.127, Suppl 3, (Feb 2011), pp.:S21–5

Chen A & Teruya J. (2009). Global hemostasis testing thromboelastography: old technology, new applications. *Clin Lab Med*, Vol.29, No.2, (Jun 2009), pp.391–407

Christiansen SC, Cannegieter SC, Koster T, Vandenbroucke JP & Rosendaal F.R. (2005). Thrombophilia, clinical factors, and recurrent venous thrombotic events. *JAMA*, Vol. 293, No.19, (May 2005), pp. 2352–61

Cosmi B, Legnani C, Cini M, Guazzaloca G & Palareti G. (2005). D-dimer levels in combination with residual venous obstruction and the risk of recurrence after anticoagulation withdrawal for a first idiopathic deep vein thrombosis. *Thromb Haemost*, Vol.94, No.5, (Nov 2005), pp.969–74

Crowther MA, Roberts J, Roberts R, Johnston M, Stevens P, Skingley P, Patrassi GM, Sartori MT, Hirsh J, Prandoni P, Weitz JI, Gent M & Ginsberg JS. (2001). Fibrinolytic variables in patients with recurrent venous thrombosis: a prospective cohort study. *Thromb Haemost*, Vol.85, No.3, (Mar 2001), pp. 390–4

Cuderman TV, Božič M, Peternel P & Stegnar M. (2008). Hemostasis activation in thrombophilic subjects with or without a history of venous thrombosis. *Clin Appl Thromb Hemost*, Vol.14, No.1, (Jan 2008), pp.55–62

Curnow JL, Morel-Kopp MC, Roddie C, Aboud M & Ward CM. (2007). Reduced fibrinolysis and increased fibrin generation can be detected in hypercoagulable patients using the overall hemostatic potential assay. *J Thromb Haemost*, Vol.5, No.3, (Mar 2007), pp.528–34

Cushman M, Folsom AR, Wang L, Aleksic N, Rosamond WD, Tracy RP & Heckbert SR. (2003). Fibrin fragment D-dimer and the risk of future venous thrombosis. *Blood*, Vol.101, No.4, (Feb 2003), pp.1243–8

Dargaud Y, Trzeciak MC, Bordet JC, Ninet J & Negrier C. (2006). Use of calibrated automated thrombinography +/− thrombomodulin to recognise the prothrombotic phenotype. *Thromb Haemost*, Vol.96, No.5, (Nov 2006), pp.562–7

Demers C, Ginsberg JS, Henderson P, Ofusu FA, Weitz JI & Blajchman MA. (1992) Measurement of markers of activated coagulation in antithrombin III deficient subjects. *Thromb Haemost*, Vol.67, No.5, (May 1992), pp.542–4

De Stefano V, Simioni P, Rossi E, Tormene D, Za T, Pagnan A & Leone G. (2006). The risk of recurrent venous thromboembolism in patients with inherited deficiency of natural anticoagulants antithrombin, protein C and protein S. *Haematologica*, Vol. 91, No.5, (May 2006), pp. 695–8

Devreese K, Peerlinck K, Arnout J & Hoylaerts MF. (2009). Laboratory detection of the antiphospholipid syndrome via calibrated automated thrombography. *Thromb Haemost*, Vol.101, No.1, (Jan 2009), pp.185-96

Di Nisio M, Squizzato A, Rutjes AW, Büller HR, Zwinderman AH & Bossuyt PM. (2007). Diagnostic accuracy of D-dimer test for exclusion of venous thromboembolism: a systematic review. *J Thromb Haemost*, Vol.5, No.2, (Feb 2007), pp.296-304

Eichinger S, Weltermann A, Philipp K, Hafner E, Kaider A, Kittl EM, Brenner B, Mannhalter C, Lechner K & Kyrle PA. (1999). Prospective evaluation of hemostatic system activation and thrombin potential in healthy pregnant women with and without factor V Leiden. *Thromb Haemost*, Vol.82, No.4, (Oct 1999), pp.1232-6

Eichinger S, Minar E, Bialonczyk C, Hirschl M, Quehenberger P, Schneider B, Weltermann A, Wagner O & Kyrle PA. (2003). D-dimer levels and risk of recurrent venous thromboembolism. *JAMA*, Vol.290, No.8, (Aug 2003), pp.1071-4

Eichinger S, Hron G, Kollars M & Kyrle PA. (2008). Prediction of recurrent venous thromboembolism by endogenous thrombin potential and D-dimer. *Clin Chem*, Vol.54, No.12, (Dec 2008), pp.2042-8

Elias A, Bonfils S, Daoud-Elias M, Gauthier B, Sié P, Boccalon H & Boneu B. (1993). Influence of long term oral anticoagulants upon prothrombin fragment 1+2, thrombin-antithrombinIII complex and D-dimer levels in patients affected by proximal deep vein thrombosis. *Thromb Haemost*, Vol.69, No.4, (Apr 1993), pp.302-5

Folsom AR, Cushman M, Heckbert SR, Rosamond WD & Aleksic N. (2003). Prospective study of fibrinolytic markers and venous thromboembolism. *J Clin Epidemiol*, Vol.56, No.6, (Jun 2003), pp.598-603

Greenberg CS, Hursting MJ, Macik BG, Ortel TL, Kane WH & Moore BM. (1994). Evaluation of preanalytical variables associated with measurement of prothrombin fragment 1.2. *Clin Chem*, Vol.40, No.10, (Oct 1994), pp.1962-9

He S, Antović A & Blombaeck M. (2001). A simple and rapid laboratory method for determination of haemostasis potential in plasma II. Modifications for use in routine laboratories and research work. *Thromb Res*, Vol.103, No.5, (Sep 2001), pp.355-61

Hemker HC, Giesen P, Al Dieri R, Regnault V, de Smed E, Wagenvoord R, Lecompte T & Béguin S. (2002). The calibrated automated thrombogram (CAT): a universal routine test for hyper- and hypocoagulability. *Patophysiol Haemost Thromb*, Vol.32, No.5-6, (Sep-Dec 2002), pp.249-53

Hézard N, Bouaziz-Borgi L, Remy MG, Florent B & Nguyen P. (2007). Protein C deficiency screening using a thrombin-generation assay. *Thromb Haemost*, Vol.97, No.1, (Jan 2007), pp.165-6

Hézard N, Bouaziz-Borgi L, Remy MG & Nguyen P. (2006). Utility of thrombin-generation assay in the screening of factor V G1691A (Leiden) and prothrombin G20210A mutations and protein S deficiency. *Clin Chem*, Vol.52, No.4, (Apr 2006), pp.665-70

Ho WK, Hankey GJ, Quinlan DJ & Eikelboom JW. (2006). Risk of recurrent venous thromboembolism in patients with common thrombophilia: a systematic review. *Arch Intern Med*, Vol 166, No 7, (Apr 2006), pp.729-36

Hron G, Eichinger S, Weltermann A, Quehenberger P, Halbmayer WM & Kyrle PA. (2006). Prediction of recurrent venous thromboembolism by the activated partial thromboplastin time. *J Thromb Haemost*, Vol.4, No.4, (Apr 2006), pp.752-6

Hvitfeldt Poulsen L, Christiansen K, Sørensen B & Ingerslev J. (2006). Whole blood thrombelastographic coagulation profiles using minimal tissue factor activation can display hypercoagulation in thrombosis-prone patients. *Scand J Clin Lab Invest*, Vol.66, No.4, (2006), pp.329-36

Jerkeman A, Astermark J, Hedner U, Lethagen S, Olsson CG & Berntorp E. (2000). Correlation between different intensities of anti-vitamin K treatment and coagulation parameters. *Thromb Res*, Vol.98, No.6, (Jun 2000), pp.467-71

Kearon C, Kahn SR, Agnelli G, Goldhaber S, Raskob GE, Comerota AJ & American College of Chest Physicians. (2008). Antithrombotic therapy for venous thromboembolic disease: American College of Chest Physicians Evidence-Based Clinical Practice Guidelines (8th Edition). *Chest*, Vol. 133, No. 6 Suppl, (Jun 2008), pp. 454S-545S

Koopman K, Uyttenboogaart M, Hendriks HG, Luijckx GJ, Cramwinckel IR, Vroomen PC, De Keyser J & van der Meer J. (2009). Thromboelastography in patients with cerebral venous thrombosis. *Thromb Res*, Vol.124, No.2, (Jun 2009), pp.185-8

Kyrle PA, Stuempflen A, Hirschl M, Bialonczyk C, Herkner K, Speiser W, Weltermann A, Kaider A, Pabinger I, Lechner K & Eichinger S. (1997a) Levels of prothrombin fragment F1+2 in patients with hyperhomocysteinemia and a history of venous thromboembolism. *Thromb Haemost*, Vol.78, No.5, (Nov 1997), pp.1327-31

Kyrle PA, Eichinger S, Pabinger I, Stuempflen A, Hirschl M, Bialonczyk C, Schneider B, Mannhalter C, Melichart M, Traxler G, Weltermann A, Speiser W & Lechner K. (1997b). Prothrombin fragment F1+2 is not predictive for recurrent venous thromboembolism. *Thromb Haemost*, Vol.77, No.5 (May 1997), pp.829-33

Kyrle PA, Mannhalter C, Beguin S, Stuempflen A, Hirschl M, Weltermann A, Stain M, Brenner B, Speiser W, Pabinger I, Lechner K & Eichinger S. (1998). Clinical studies and thrombin generation in patients homozygous or heterozygous for the G20210A mutation in the prothrombin gene. *Arterioscler Thromb Vasc Biol* , Vol.18, No.8, (Aug 1998), pp. 1287-91

Kyrle PA, Hron G, Eichinger S & Wagner O. (2007). Circulating P-selectin and the risk of recurrent venous thromboembolism. *Thromb Haemost*, Vol.97, No.6, (Jun 2007), pp.880-3

Langdell RD, Wagner RH & Brinkhous KM. (1953). Effect of antihemophilic factor on one-stage clotting tests; a presumptive test for haemophilia and a simple one-stage antihemophilic factor assay procedure. *J Lab Clin Med*, Vol.41, No.4, (Apr 1953), pp.637-47

Lavigne-Lissalde G, Sanchez C, Castelli C. Alonso S, Mazoyer ., Bal Dit Sollier C, Drouet L, Juhan-Vague ., Gris JC, Alessi MC & Morange PE. (2010). Prothrombin G20210A carriers the genetic mutation and a history of venous thrombosis contributes to thrombin generation independently of factor II plasma levels. *J Thromb Haemost*, Vol.8, No.5, (May 2010), pp.942-9

Legnani C, Mattarozzi S, Cini M, Cosmi B, Favaretto E & Palareti G. (2006). Abnormally short activated partial thromboplastin time values are associated with increased risk of recurrence of venous thromboembolism after oral anticoagulation withdrawal. *Br J Haematol*, Vol.134, No.2, (Jul 2006), pp.227-32

Liestøl S, Sandset PM, Mowinckel MC & Wisløff F. (2007). Activated protein C resistance determined with a thrombin generation-based test is associated with thrombotic events in patients with lupus anticoagulants. *J Thromb Haemost*, Vol.5, No.11, (Nov 2007), pp.2204–10.

Lincz LF, Lonergan A, Scorgie FE, Rowlings P, Gibson R, Lawrie A & Seldon M. (2006). Endogenous thrombin potential for predicting risk of venous thromboembolism in carriers of factor V Leiden. *Pathophysiol Haemost Thromb*, Vol.35, No.6, (2006), pp.435–9

Lowe GD, Rumley A, Woodward M, Reid E & Rumley J. (1991). Activated protein C resistance and the FV:R^{506}Q mutation in a random population sample. *Thromb Haemost*, Vol.81, No.6, (Jun 1991), pp.918–24

Lutsey PL, Folsom AR, Heckbert SR & Cushman M. (2009) Peak thrombin generation and subsequent venous thromboembolism: the Longitudinal Investigation of Thromboembolism Etiology (LITE) study. *J Thromb Haemost*, Vol.7, No.10, (Oct 2009), pp.1639–48

Macherel P, Sulzer I, Furlan M & Lammle B. (1992). Determination of thrombin-antithrombin-III-complex is not a suitable screening test for detecting deficiency of protein C or protein S. *Thromb Res*, Vol.66, No.6, (Jun 1992), pp.775–7

Mallett SV & Cox DJ. (1992). Thrombelastography. *Br J Anaesth*, Vol.69, No.3, (Sep 1992), pp.307–13

Mannucci PM, Tripodi A, Bottasso B, Baudo F, Finazzi G, De Stefano V, Palareti G,Manotti C, Mazzucconi MG & Castaman G. (1992). Markers of procoagulant imbalance in patients with inherited thrombophilic syndromes. *Thromb Haemost*, Vol.67, No.2, (Feb 1992), pp.200–2

Mannucci PM. (1994). Mechanisms, markers and management of coagulation activation. *Br Med Bull*, Vol.50, No.4, (Oct 1994), pp.851–70

Meissner MH, Zierler BK, Bergelin RO, Chandler WC, Manzo RA & Strandness DE Jr. (2000). Markers of plasma coagulation and fibrinolysis after acute deep venous thrombosis. *J Vasc Surg*, Vol.32, No.5, (Nov 2000), pp.870–80

Meltzer ME, Lisman T, de Groot PG, Meijers JC, le Cessie S, Doggen CJ & Rosendaal FR. (2010). Venous thrombosis risk associated with plasma hypofibrinolysis is explained by elevated plasma levels of TAFI and PAI-1. *Blood*, Vol.116, No.1, (Jul 2010), pp.113–21

Miller GJ, Bauer KA, Barzegar S, Foley AJ, Mitchell JP, Cooper JA & Rosenberg RD. (1995). The effects of quality and timing of venepuncture in markers of blood coagulation in healthy middle-aged men. *Thromb Haemost*, Vol.73, No.1, (Jan 1995), pp.82–6

Monroe DM & Hoffman M. (2006). What does it take to make the perfect clot? *Arterioscler Thromb Vasc Biol*, Vol.26, No.1, (Jan 2006), pp.41-8

O'Donnell J, Mumford AD, Manning RA & Laffan MA. (2001). Marked elevations of thrombin generation in patients with elevated FVIII:C and venous thromboembolism. *Br J Haematol*, Vol.115, No.3, (Dec 2001), pp.687–91

O'Donnell J, Riddell A, Owens D, Handa A, Pasi J, Hamilton G & Perry DJ. (2004). Role of the Thrombelastograph as an adjunctive test in thrombophilia screening. *Blood Coagul Fibrinolysis*, Vol.15, No.3, (Apr 2004), pp.207–11

Palareti G, Legnani C, Cosmi B, Guazzaloca G, Pancani C. & Coccheri S. (2002). Risk of venous thromboembolism recurrence: high negative predictive value of D-dimer performed after oral anticoagulation is stopped. *Thromb Haemost*, Vol.87, No.1, (Jan 2002), pp.7–12

Palareti G, Legnani C, Cosmi B, Valdré L, Lunghi B, Bernardi F & Coccheri S. (2003) Predictive value of D-dimer test for recurrent venous thromboembolism after anticoagulation withdrawal in subjects with a previous idiopathic event and in carriers of congenital thrombophilia. *Circulation*, Vol.108, No.3, (Jul 2003), pp.313–8

Palareti G, Cosmi B, Legnani C, Tosetto A, Brusi C, Iorio A, Pengo V, Ghirarduzzi A, Pattacini C, Testa S, Lensing AW, Tripodi A & PROLONG Investigators. (2006). D-dimer testing to determine the duration of anticoagulation therapy. *N Engl J Med*, Vol. 355, No.17, (Oct 2006), pp.1780–9.

Papalambros E, Sigala F, Travlou A, Bastounis E & Mirilas P. (2004). P-selectin and antibodies against heparin-platelet factor 4 in patients with venous or arterial diseases after a 7-day heparin treatment. *J Am Coll Surg*, Vol.199, No.1, (Jul 2004), pp.69–77

Peternel P, Terbižan M, Tratar G, Božič M, Horvat D, Salobir B & Stegnar M. (2002). Markers of hemostatic system activation during treatment of deep vein thrombosis with subcutaneous unfractionated or low-molecular weight heparin. *Thromb Res*, Vol.105, No.3, (Feb 2002), pp.241–6

Poli D, Antonucci E, Ciuti G, Abbate R & Prisco D. (2008). Combination of D-dimer, F1+2 and residual vein obstruction as predictors of VTE recurrence in patients with first VTE episode after OAT withdrawal. *J Thromb Haemost*, Vol.6, No.4, (Apr 2008), pp. 708–10

Poli D, Grifoni E, Antonucci E, Arcangeli C, Prisco D, Abbate R & Miniati M. (2010). Incidence of recurrent venous thromboembolism and of chronic thromboembolic pulmonary hypertension in patients after a first episode of pulmonary embolism. *J Thromb Thrombolysis*, Vol.30, No.3, (Oct 2010), pp.294–9

Ramacciotti E, Blackburn S, Hawley AE, Vandy F, Ballard-Lipka N, Stabler C, Baker N, Guire KE, Rectenwald JE, Henke PK, Myers DD Jr & Wakefield TW.(2011). Evaluation of Soluble P-Selectin as a Marker for the Diagnosis of Deep Venous Thrombosis. *Clin Appl Thromb Hemost*. 2011 May 17. [Epub ahead of print]

Rectenwald JE, Myers DD Jr, Hawley AE, Longo C, Henke PK, Guire KE, Schmaier AH & Wakefield TW. (2005). D-dimer, P-selectin, and microparticles:novel markers to predict deep venous thrombosis. A pilot study. *Thromb Haemost*, Vol.94, No.6, (Dec 2005), pp.1312–7

Righini M, Perrier A, De Moerloose P & Bounameaux H. (2008). D-Dimer for venous thromboembolism diagnosis: 20 years later. *J Thromb Haemost*, Vol.6, No.7, (Jul 2008), pp. 1059–71

Rijken DC, Lijnen HR. (2009). New insights into the molecular mechanisms of the fibrinolytic system. *J Thromb Haemost*, Vol.7, No.1, (Jan 2009), pp.4-13.

Rosendaal FR. (1999). Venous thrombosis: a multicausal disease. *Lancet*, Vol. 353, No. 9159, (Apr 1999), pp. 1167–73

Schulman S, Lindmarker P, Holmström M, Lärfars G, Carlsson A, Nicol P, Svensson E, Ljungberg B, Viering S, Nordlander S, Leijd B, Jahed K, Hjorth M, Linder O, & Beckman M. (2006). Post-thrombotic syndrome, recurrence, and death 10 years after the first episode of venous thromboembolism treated with warfarin for 6 weeks or 6 months. *J Thromb Haemost*, Vol. 4, No.4, (Apr 2006), pp. 734–42

Schulman S & Wiman B. (1996). The significance of hypofibrinolysis for the risk of recurrence of venous thromboembolism: Duration of Anticoagulation (DURAC) Trial Study Group. *Thromb Haemost*, Vol.75, No.4, (Apr 1996), pp.607-11.

Siegemund A, Petros S, Siegemund T, Scholz U, Seyfarth HJ & Engelmann L. (2004). The endogenous thrombin potential and high levels of coagulation factor VIII, factor IX and factor XI. *Blood Coagul Fibrinolysis*, Vol.15, No.3, (Apr 2004), pp.241-4

Simioni P, Scarano L, Gavasso S, Sardella C, Girolami B, Scudeller A & Girolami A. (1996). Prothrombin fragment 1+2 and thrombin-antithrombin complex levels in patients with inherited APC resistance due to factor V Leiden mutation. *Br J Haematol*, Vol.92, No.2, (Feb 1996), pp.435-41

Smith A, Quarmby JW, Collins M, Lockhart SM & Burnard KG. (1999). Changes in the levels of soluble adhesion molecules and coagulation factors in patients with deep vein thrombosis. *Thromb Haemost*, Vol.82, No.6, (Dec 1999), pp.1593-9

Sorensen B, Johansen P, Christiansen K, Woelke M & Ingerslev J. (2003). Whole blood coagulation thromboelastographic profiles employing minimal tissue factor activation. *J Thromb Haemost*, Vol.1, No.3, (Mar 2003), pp.551-8

Spiezia L, Marchioro P, Radu C, Rossetto V, Tognin G, Monica C, Salmaso L & Simioni P. (2008). Whole blood coagulation assessment using rotation thrombelastogram thromboelastometry in patients with acute deep vein thrombosis. *Blood Coagul Fibrinolysis*, Vol.19, No.5, (Jul 2008), pp.355-60

Stegnar M, Peternel P, Uhrin P, Cvelbar-Marinko T, Goršič-Tomažič K & Binder BR. (1997). Fibrinolysis in patients with the 1691G-A mutation in factot V gene and history of deep vein thrombosis. *Fibrinolysis Proteolysis*, Vol.11, No.4, (1997), pp.201-7

Stegnar M, Cuderman TV & Božič M. (2007). Evaluation of pre-analytical, demographic, behavioural and metabolic variables on fibrinolysis and haemostasis activation markers utilised to assess hypercoagulability. *Clin Chem Lab Med*, Vol.45, No.1, (2007), pp.40-6

Stegnar M. (2010). Thrombophilia screening-at the right time, for the right patient, with a good reason. *Clin Chem Lab Med*, Vol.48, Suppl 1, (Dec 2010), pp. S105-13

Stricker H, Marchetti O, Haeberli A & Mombeli G. (1999). Hemostatic activation under anticoagulant treatment: a comparison of unfractionated heparin vs. nadroparin in the treatment of proximal deep vein thrombosis. *Thromb Haemost*, Vol.82, No.4, (Oct 1999), pp.1227-31

ten Cate-Hoek AJ, Dielis AW, Spronk HM, van Oerle R, Hamulyák K, Prins MH & ten Cate H. (2008). Thrombin generation in patients after acute deep-vein thrombosis. *Thromb Haemost*, Vol.100, No.2, (Aug 2008), pp.240-5

The DVTENOX Study Group. (1993). Markers of hemostatic system activation in acute deep venous thrombosis-evolution during the first days of heparin treatment. *Thromb Haemost*, Vol.70, No.6, (Dec 1993), pp.909-14

Tripodi A, Chantarangkul V, Martinelli I, Bucciarelli P & Mannucci PM. (2004). A shortened activated partial thromboplastin time is associated with the risk of venous thromboembolism. *Blood*, Vol.104, No.12, (Dec 2004), pp.3631-4

Tripodi A, Legnani C, Chantarangkul V, Cosmi B, Palareti G & Mannucci PM. (2008). High thrombin generation measured in the presence of thrombomodulin is associated with an increased risk of recurrent venous thromboembolism. *J Thromb Haemost*, Vol.6, No.8, (Aug 2008), pp.1327-33 van Hylckama Vlieg A, Christiansen SC, Luddington R, Cannegieter SC, Rosendaal FR & Baglin TP. (2007). Elevated endogenous thrombin potential is associated with an increased risk of a first deep venous thrombosis but not with the risk of recurrence. *Br J Haematol*, Vol.138, No.6, (Sep 2007), pp.769-74

van Veen JJ, Gatt A & Makris M. (2008). Thrombin generation testing in routine clinical practice: are we there yet? *Br J Haematol*, Vol.142, No.6, (Sep 2008), pp.889-903

Verhovsek M, Douketis JD, Yi Q, Shrivastava S, Tait RC, Baglin T, Poli D & Lim W. (2008). Systematic review: D-dimer to predict recurrent disease after stopping anticoagulant therapy for unprovoked venous thromboembolism. *Ann Intern Med*, Vol.149, No.7, (Oct 2008), pp.481- 90.

Vižintin-Cuderman T, Božič-Mijovski M, Antović A, Peternel P, Kozak M & Stegnar M. Does the presence of thrombophilia modify hemostasis activation marker levels and overall hemostasis potential in patients treated for venous thrombosis? (to be published)

Wichers IM, Tanck MW, Meijers JC, Lisman T, Reitsma PH, Rosendaal FR, Büller HR & Middeldorp S. (2009). Assessment of coagulation and fibrinolysis in families with unexplained thrombophilia. *Thromb Haemost*, Vol.101, No.3, (Mar 2009), pp.465-70

Wielders S, Mukherjee M, Michiels J, Rijkers DT, Cambus JP, Knebel RW, Kakkar V, Hemker HC & Béguin S. (1997). The routine determination of the endogenous thrombin potential, first results in different forms of hyper- and hypocoagulability. *Thromb Haemost*, Vol.77, No.4, (Apr 1997), pp.629-36

White RH. (2003). The epidemiology of venous thromboembolism. *Circulation*, Vol.107, No.23, Suppl 1, (Jun 2003), pp. I4-8

3

Geographic and Ethnic Differences in the Prevalence of Thrombophilia

Lizbeth Salazar-Sanchez
Medicine School, Molecular Medicine Lab., CIHATA-UCR, San Juan de Dios Hospital, University of Costa Rica
Costa Rica

1. Introduction

Cardiovascular diseases and venous thromboembolism are multifactorial diseases. Risk factors result from genetics, environment and behavior. The concept of the multicausal disease has received much attention in recent years. One of the reasons is that some of the genetic risk factors concerning single point mutations are quite common in the general population. There are known molecular factors which increase the relative risk for disease, and others with protective effects. The genetic background is given by the combination of all these molecular markers.

Several genetic variants are currently identified as risk factors for venous and arterial thrombosis (myocardial infarction and deep venous thrombosis)(Table 1). Activated protein C (APC) resistance due to the factor V Leiden mutation (FVL) and the 20210 G>A mutation in the factor II (FII, Prothrombin) gene are well established causes of thrombophilia. Concerning the risk of myocardial infarction the results are different (Ozmen F et al., 2009).

The 677C>T mutation in the methylentetrahydrofolate reductase gene (MTHFR 677C>T), which causes a mild hyperhomocysteinemia, is considered to be a risk factor for coronary heart disease (Kluijtmans et al., 1997; Morita et al., 1997), venous thromboembolism and stroke (Frosst et al., 1995; Arruda et al., 1997; Margaglione et al., 1998, Khandanpour et al., 2009, Tug E et al., 2011), but the results are controversial.

New polymorphic markers of the FV gene were described in the last years (Lunghi et al., 1996; Bernardi et al.,1997; Castoldi et al., 1997; Castoldi, 2000). A specific factor V gene haplotype (HR2) was defined by five restriction polymorphisms in exon 13 and a sequence variation located in exon 16. The exon 13 markers include the Rsa I polymorphic site, the rare allele of which (R2) has been previously found to be associated with partial FV deficiency in the Italian population (Lunghi et al., 1996). The nucleotide change 4070 G>A underlying the R2 allele gives rise to an amino acid change His to Arg at position 1299. Bernardi et al. (1997) demonstrated that the FV gene marked by the HR2 haplotype, which was invariably found to underlie the R2 marker, is both able to contribute to a mild APC resistance phenotype and to interact synergistically with the FVL mutation Arg506Gln to produce a severe APC resistance phenotype. Carriers of the R2 allele are more frequent among patients of carotid endarterectomy (Marchetti et al., 1999) and the carriership of the R2 allele is associated with an increased risk for coronary artery disease (Hoekema et al., 1999; Hoekema et al., 2001) and venous thromboembolism (Bernardi et al., 1997; Faioni et al., 1999; Alhenc-Gelas et al., 1999).

For some new variants of clotting factors FVII, FXII and FXIII associations with venous and arterial thrombosis were reported. Within the FVII gene eight polymorphisms are known (Herrmann et al., 1998; Herrmann et al., 2000) and three of them influence the level of FVII activity: the insertion polymorphism of the promotor (Marchetti et al., 1993), a tandem repeat unit polymorphism within intron 7 (Marchetti et al., 1991; de Knijff et al., 1994; Mariani et al., 1994; Pinotti et al., 2000) and the Arg353Gln polymorphism of exon 8 (Green et al., 1991). Iacoviello et al. (1998) demonstrated in patients with myocardial infarction and family history of cardiovascular diseases, that the Gln353 allele of the Arg353Gln polymorphism and the 7(a) allele of the tandem repeat unit polymorphism of the hypervariable region 4 within intron 7 might have a protective effect on the risk of myocardial infarction. These alleles independently showed an effect in reducing the risk and both were associated with lower levels of FVII (Green et al., 1991; Mariani et al., 1994; Iacoviello et al., 1998; Domenico et al., 2000).

For severe factor XII deficiency, an increased predisposition to venous thromboembolic diseases and myocardial infarction has been reported. Some cohort studies have shown a high prevalence of slightly reduced FXII levels in patients of deep venous thrombosis or coronary heart diseases (Mannhalter et al., 1987; Halbmayer et al., 1994; Franco et al., 1999; Zito et al., 2000), but more association studies in this field are necessary. The C>T mutation at nucleotide 46 in the 5´untranslated region of FXII (FXII 46C>T) is associated with a diminished plasma FXII level (Kanaji et al., 1998; Kohler et al., 1999; Zito et al., 2000) and the role of this polymorphism as a thrombophilic risk factor is under discussion.

The G>T transition in exon 2 of the FXIII A subunit gene was reported to provide a protective effect against myocardial infarction (Kohler et al., 1998; Franco et al., 2000) and venous thrombosis (Catto et al., 1999; Franco et al., 1999; Rosendaal et al., 1999; Alhenc-Gelas et al., 2000; Franco et al., 2001), but also an increased predisposition to primary intracerebral hemorrhage (Catto et al., 1998; Reiner et al., 2001).

Many epidemiological studies have been performed to associate the presence (insertion, I) or absence (deletion, D) of a 287bp Alu repeat element in intron 16 of the ACE (Angiotensin Converting Enzyme) gene with the level of the circulating enzyme or cardiovascular pathophysiology. Some reports have found that the D allele confers increased susceptibility to cardiovascular diseases and myocardial infarction, others found no such association or even a beneficial effect (Rieder et al., 1999; Agerholm-Larsen et al., 2000). The same is true for cerebrovascular diseases, stroke or stenosis of carotids and venous thrombosis (Philipp et al., 1998; Della Valle et al., 2001). Markus et al. (1995) reported that the DD genotype is a risk factor for lacunar stroke but not for carotid atheroma. However, the precise role of the I/D polymorphism is not clear, so more association studies are necessary.

A series of studies have been carried out to elucidate the mechanisms of the athero-thrombotic pathology in the middle-age and older adults. However, few studies have examined the joint effect of interaction of environmental factors and molecular markers in the risk of thrombosis particularly among the young. However, these claims have been challenged. Based upon in this observation it was considered important to study the role of the risk factors and molecular markers for thrombosis in Hispanics living in Costa Rica, Central America. In the population of Costa Rica (CR) and its different ethnic groups the prevalence of molecular risk and protective factors are few reports until now. In order to estimate the role of these factors in this population it is necessary to know their prevalence and it will be interesting to compare with one Caucasian population as NE Germany, see Figure 1.

Subjects

Blood samples analyzed in this study were obtained from 732 CR-Indians belonging to six different tribes. Samples were collected from 133 Chorotega of the Matambu Indian locality; 157 Guaymi of the south area (San Vito, Coto Brus, Abrojo localities) and of the Pacific area (Osa); 150 Cabecar of the Atlantic Talamanca area (Chirripo, Amubri localities) and of the Pacific (Ujarras Indian locality); 110 Bribri of the Talamanca area (Bribi and Suretka localities); 153 Huetar of Quitirrisi and Zapaton Indian localities, as well as 29 Guatuso of the Guatuso Indian locality (figure 1).

In order to compare the results with European Caucasians blood samples were analyzed from 170 blood donors from northeastern Germany (NE-Germany).

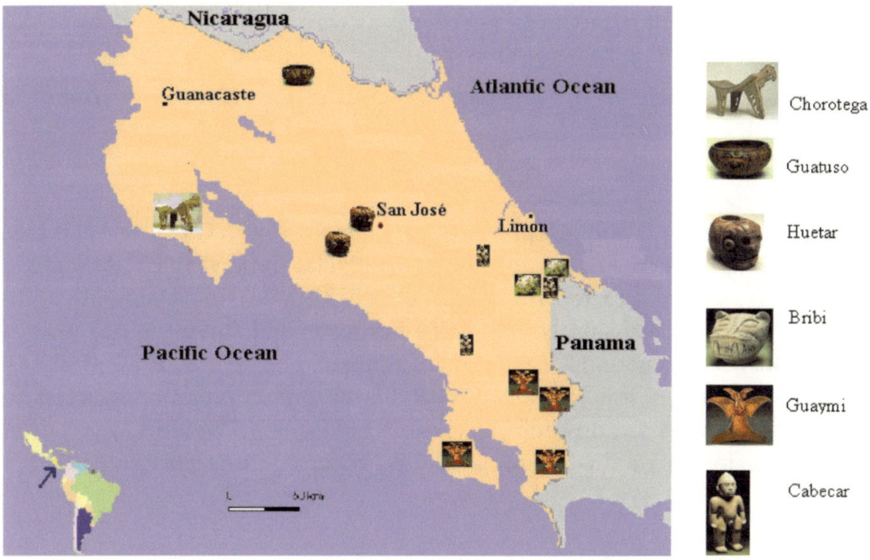

Fig. 1. The approximate geographic locations of the six tribes of CR Amerindians

2. A brief history of Costa Rican population

The current population of Costa Rica presents an ancestral gene combination of Amerindians (30%), Africans (10-15%) and Caucasians (50-60%) (Barrantes, 1998). In the pre-Columbian period, the human population in this area was composed of Amerindian tribes descending from the Na-dene and North-American Eskimos (Torroni et al., 1994). Four of the tribes studied (Guatuso, Guaymi, Cabecar, Bribri) belong to Chibcha-speaking tribes of lower Central America (Thompson et al., 1992; Barrantes, 1998). The Chibcha, which have been separated biologically and linguistically from other groups of this region, show differences in some aspects when compared to other North and South American groups of Indians (Barrantes et al., 1990; Thompson et al., 1992) and also have rare genetic variants and private polymorphisms.

The Chorotega, another tribe included in the present study (Figure 1), belong to the Mesoamerican culture with strong influences from the Aztec and Maya culture (Ibarra, 2001). At present, this tribe is located in the western Pacific area of the country.

The Huetar tribe inhabited the North-Central area of Costa Rica during the time of the Spanish Conquest. At the present time, they are located in the southwest of the country (Figure 1). During colonization, the admixture between Spanish colonizers, mostly from the south of Spain, and indigenous women began (Thiel, 1977; Ibarra, 2001).

In the 16th and 17th centuries Africans were firstly brought to Costa Rica by the transatlantic slave trade from western and Central Africa. The first settlement of Africans in Costa Rica was in the Pacific area (Meléndez and Duncan, 1989). From the beginning, this ethnic group participated in the admixture process with the Amerindians. The second important African migration to Costa Rica was into the Caribbean Area during the 18th and 20th centuries. This group of Africans migrated from the Antilles, principally from Jamaica, and settled in "Cahuita" in the Limon province at the Atlantic coast (Palmer, 2000).

Genotype prevalence and allele frequencies of the eleven molecular markers in Costa Rica Indians from six different tribes and Cr-Africans as well as blood donors from Costa Rica and NE Germany

The results of the prevalence of these molecular markers in this ethnic context are summarized in Table 1, 2, 3 and 4.

2.1 FII 20210G>A

The 20210A allele of the factor II polymorphism was extremely rare in CR-Indians (Table 2). Only one allele was detected in the Bribri and one in the Huetar Indians. In CR-Africans, the 20210A allele frequency was also extremely low (1 out of 578 alleles). In a cooperative study including more than 5500 healthy subjects from nine European and American countries, the overall prevalence of heterozygous FII carriers was estimated to be 2% (Rosendaal et al., 1998). In the same study a very low prevalence of the prothrombin mutation was reported for Africans and subjects of Asian descent (Rosendaal et al., 1998). Therefore, we conclude that the FII mutation found in CR-Indians and CR-Africans is of Caucasian origin, as suggested for FVL.

2.2 FV gene : FVL, FVHR2, FV IVS16

The factor V Leiden mutation is a known risk factor for venous thrombosis in Caucasians and has been discussed as a risk factor for arterial thrombosis. This mutation was rare in CR-Indians, with only five heterozygous FVL carriers detected among the Huetar. In the CR-Indian tribes without FVL, the frequency of the R2 allele of the HR2 haplotype was extremely high. It has been shown that this allele is associated with partial FV deficiency and acts synergistically with FVL (Bernardi et al., 1997; Lunghi et al., 1998). In various populations the R2 allele frequency ranged from 0.04 to 0.08; [Netherlands 0.040 (De Visser et al., 2000); England 0.055 (Luddington et al., 2000); Italy, India, Somalia 0.080 (Bernardi et al., 1997; Faioni et al., 1999;); Germany 0.070 (Hermann et al., 2001 and this study)]. The extremely high frequency of the R2 allele and the R1R2 and R2R2 genotypes in Bribri Indians is the highest reported so far. In the same CR Indian tribes with a high prevalence of the R2 allele, the D2 allele of FV IVS16 polymorphism was very rare.

The FVL mutation was likewise rare in the other CR groups analyzed (subpopulations of CR-Africans and in the CR blood donors). The R2 frequency of the HR2 haplotype was lower in the CR-Africans than in CR-Indians and CR-blood donors. However, in CR-Africans the rare R3 allele (His1254Arg) was also detected. This allele was first described in subjects from Somalia and in Greek Cypriotes and mimics the R2 polymorphism (His1299Arg) in subjects of African origin (Lunghi et al., 1998). The FVL mutation was not found in combination with the R2 or R3 allele in CR-Africans or CR-blood donors .

In the German group of 170 blood donors, 11 heterozygous FVL genotypes were detected. Eight of them had the R1R1 genotype and only three FVL heterozygotes had the R1R2 genotype. All the eleven FVL heterozygous subjects were also heterozygous for the D2

Polymorphism	Mutation	Localization	Genotype	Symbol	Phenotype Effect	References
Factor II Gene 20210 G>A	20210 G >A	Chromosome 11 3'-untranslated region	GG (wild type) GA (heterozygous) AA (homozygous)	GG GA AA	normal FII moderate increased FII increased FII	Poort et al. (1996)
Factor V Gene FV Leiden	R506Q 1691G>A	Chromosome 1 Exon 10	GG (wild type) GA (heterozygous) AA (homozygous)	GG GA AA	normal mild APC resistance APC resistance	Bertina et al. (1994)
FV HR2	H1299R 4070A>G	Exon 13	AA (wild type) AG (heterozygous) GG (homozygous)	R1R1 R1R2 R2R2	normal mild APC resistance mild APC resistance	Lunghi et al. (1996) Bernardi et al. (1997) Faioni et al. (1999)
	H1254R 3935A>G		AG (heterozygous)	R1R3	*	
FV IVS 16	IVS16+12 G>A	Intron 16	GG (wild type) GA (heterozygous) AA (homozygous)	D1D1 D1D2 D2D2	* * *	Castoldi et al. (1997)
Factor VII Gene FVII IVS 7	repeat 37 bp HVR4	Chromosome13 Intron 7	66 67 77 rare allele 4 5 8 9	bb ba aa rare allele 4 5 8 9	normal FVII: C reduced FVII: C strong reduced FVII:C increased FVII:C * * *	Marcheti et al. (1991) Bernardi et al. (1993)
FVII Arg353 Gln	Arg 353 Gln 10975 G>A	Exon 8	GG (wild type) GA (heterozygous) AA (homozygous)	M1M1 M1M2 M2M2	normal FVII: C reduced FVII: C strong reduced FVII:C	Green et al. (1991)
FVII IVS 1a FVII 73 G>A	73 G>A	Intron 1a	GG (wild type) GA (heterozygous) AA (homozygous)	GG GA AA	* * *	Herrmann et al. (1998); Wulff et al. (2000)
Factor XII Gene FXII 46 C> T	46 C >T	Chromosome 5 5'-untranslated region	CC (wild type) CT (heterozygous) TT (homozygous)	CC CT TT	normal FXII: C reduced FXII: C strong reduce FXII:C	Kanaji et al. (1998)
Factor XIII Gene FXIII Val34Leu	Val 34 Leu G>T	Chromosome 6 Exon 2 (XIII A-Subunit)	GG (wild type) GT (heterozygous) TT (homozygous)	ValVal ValLeu LeuLeu	Transglutaminase normal activity mild activity increased activity	Catto et al. (1999) Rosendaal et al. (1999)
MTHFR Gene MTHFR 677C>T	Ala >Val 677C>T	Chromosome 1	CC (wild type) CT (heterozygous) TT (homozygous)	CC CT TT	Homocysteine level normal normal mild increased	Kang et al. (1991) Frosst et al. (1995) Kluijtmans et al. (1999)

* Unknown effect.

Table 1. Characteristics of the different polymorphisms analyzed

POLYMORPHISMS	CHOROTEGA		GUATUSO		GUAYMI		CABECAR		BRIBRI		HUETAR		CR INDIANS Σ		GUANACASTE		LIMON		CR AFRICANS Σ		CR BLOOD DONORS		NE-GERMANY Caucasians	
	n	%	n	%	n	%	n	%	n	%	n	%	n	%	n	%	n	%	n	%	n	%	n	%
FII G>A 20210	133		29		157		149		110		152		730		179		110		289		392		170	
20210 GG	133	100.00	29	100.00	157	100.00	149	100.00	109	99.09	151	99.34	728	99.72	179	100.00	109	99.09	288	99 65	381	97.19	168	98.80
20210 GA	-		-		-		-		1	0.91	1	0.66	2	0.28	-		1	0.91	1	0.35	11	2.81	2	1.20
20210 AA	-		-		-		-		-		-		-		-		-		-		-		-	
f(G)	266	1.00*	58	1.00*	314	1.00*	298	1.00*	219	0.995*	303	0.997*	1458	0.998*	358	1.00*	219	0.995*	577	0.998*	773	0.986*	338	0.994*
f(A)									1	0.005*	1	0.003*	2	0.002*			1	0.005*	1	0.002*	11	0.014*	2	0.006*
FVL	132		29		156		149		110		153		729		179		113		292		392		1172	
1691 GG	132	100.00	29	100.00	156	100.00	149	100.00	110	100.00	148	96.73	724	99.31	178	99.44	111	98.23	289	98.97	383	97.70	1089	92.91
1691 GA	-		-		-		-		-		5	3.27	5	0.69	1	0.56	2	1.77	3	1.03	9	2.30	82	7.00
1691 AA	-		-		-		-		-		-		-		-		-		-		-		1	0.09
f(G)	264	1.00*	58	1.00*	312	1.00*	298	1.00*	220	1.00*	301	0.984*	1453	0.996*	357	0.997*	224	0.991*	581	0.995*	775	0.988*	2260	0.964*
f(A)											5	0.016*	5	0.004*	1	0.003*	2	0.009*	3	0.005*	9	0.012*	84	0.036*
FV-HR2 (His1299Arg)	133		23		156		149		110		153		724		178		114		292		377		358	
R1R1	70	52.63	12	52.17	126	80.77	82	55.03	45	40.91	111	72.55	446	61.60	138	77.53	103	90.35	241	82.54	303	80.37	308	86.03
R1R2	52	39.10	10	43.48	28	17.95	61	40.94	53	48.18	40	26.14	244	33.70	35	19.66	7	6.14	42	14.38	72	19.10	50	13.97
R2R2	11	8.27	1	4.35	2	1.28	6	4.03	12	10.91	2	1.31	34	4.70	1	0.56	-		1	0.34	2	0.53	-	
R1R3	-		-		-		-		-		-		-		4	2.25	4	3.51	8	2.74	-		-	
f(R1)	192	0.720*	34	0.739*	280	0.897*	225	0.755*	143	0.650*	262	0.856*	1136	0.785*	315	0.885*	217	0.952*	532	0.910*	678	0.899*	666	0.930*
f(R2)	74	0.278*	12	0.261*	32	0.103*	73	0.245*	77	0.350*	44	0.144*	312	0.215*	37	0.104*	7	0.031*	44	0.076*	76	0.101*	50	0.070*
f(R3)															4	0.011*	4	0.017*	8	0.014*				
FV-IVS16	133		25		157		149		109		153		726		179		114		293		94		170	
D1D1	130	97.74	24	96.00	156	99.36	148	99.33	108	99.08	142	94.77	708	97.52	165	92.18	93	81.57	258	88.05	88	93.61	146	85.90
D1D2	3	2.26	1	4.00	1	0.64	1	0.67	1	0.92	11	5.23	18	2.48	14	7.82	21	18.43	35	11.95	6	6.39	24	14.10
f(D1)	263	0.989*	49	0.980*	313	0.997*	297	0.997*	217	0.995*	295	0.964*	1434	0.988*	344	0.961*	207	0.908*	551	0.940*	182	0.968*	316	0.929*
f(D2)	3	0.011*	1	0.020*	1	0.003*	1	0.003*	1	0.005*	11	0.036*	18	0.012*	14	0.039*	21	0.092*	35	0.060*	6	0.032*	24	0.071*

*Allele frequency

Table 2 Prevalence of polymorphisms in the FII and FV genes in the different ethnic groups studied

POLYMORPHISMS	CHOROTEGA		GUATUSO		GUAYMI		CABECAR		BRIBRI		HUETAR		CR INDIANS Σ		GUANACASTE		LIMON		CR AFRICANS Σ		CR BLOOD DONORS		NE-GERMANY Caucasians	
	n	%	n	%	n	%	n	%	n	%	n	%	n	%	n	%	n	%	n	%	n	%	n	%
FVII IVS7	125		28		135		134		101		98		621		145		109		254		229		115	
(37bp repeat)																								
46 4b	2	1.60	-	-	-	-	-	-	-	-	-	-	2	1. 60	3	2. 07	-	-	3	1. 18	1	0. 44	-	-
47 4a	1	0.80	-	-	-	-	-	-	-	-	-	-	1	0. 80	-	-	1	0. 92	1	0. 39	-	-	-	-
55 55	-	-	-	-	-	-	-	-	-	-	-	-	-	-	-	-	-	-	-	-	1	0. 44	-	-
56 5b	-	-	-	-	-	-	-	-	1	0. 99	-	-	1	0. 16	-	-	-	-	-	-	-	-	-	-
57 5a	-	-	-	-	-	-	-	-	-	-	-	-	-	-	-	-	-	-	-	-	1	0. 44	-	-
66 bb	29	23.20	23	82.14	72	53. 33	69	51. 49	40	39. 61	46	46. 94	279	44. 93	58	40. 00	35	32 11	93	36. 61	106	46. 28	37	32. 17
67 ab	61	48.80	5	17.86	48	35. 55	54	40. 30	42	41. 58	44	44. 90	254	40. 90	59	40. 69	49	44. 95	108	42. 53	101	44. 10	54	46. 96
77 aa	30	24.00	-	-	15	11. 12	11	8. 21	18	17. 82	8	8. 16	82	13. 21	22	15. 17	19	17. 43	41	16. 15	18	7. 86	18	15. 65
86 8b	2	1.60	-	-	-	-	-	-	-	-	-	-	2	0. 32	2	1. 38	4	3. 67	6	2. 36	1	0. 44	4	3. 48
87 8a	-	-	-	-	-	-	-	-	-	-	-	-	-	-	1	0. 69	-	-	1	0. 39	-	-	1	0. 87
96 9b	-	-	-	-	-	-	-	-	-	-	-	-	-	-	-	-	1	0. 92	1	0. 39	-	-	1	0. 87
f(4)	3	0.012*	-	-	-	-	-	-	-	-	-	-	3	0. 002*	3	0. 010*	1	0. 005*	4	0. 008*	1	0. 002*	-	-
f(5)	-	-	-	-	-	-	-	-	1	0. 005*	-	-	1	0. 001*	-	-	-	-	-	-	3	0. 007*	-	-
f(6)	123	0.492*	51	0.911*	192	0. 711*	192	0. 716*	123	0. 609*	136	0. 694*	817	0. 658*	180	0. 621*	124	0. 569*	304	0. 598*	314	0. 686*	133	0. 578*
f(7)	122	0.488*	5	0.089*	78	0. 289*	76	0. 284*	78	0. 386*	60	0. 306*	419	0. 337*	104	0. 359*	88	0. 403*	192	0. 378*	139	0. 303*	91	0. 396*
f(8)	2	0.008*	-	-	-	-	-	-	-	-	-	-	2	0. 002*	3	0. 010*	4	0. 018*	7	0. 014*	1	0. 002*	5	0. 022*
f(9)	-	-	-	-	-	-	-	-	-	-	-	-	-	-	-	-	1	0. 005*	1	0. 002*	-	-	1	0. 004*
FVII 73G>A	123		27		152		136		94		60		592		114		104		218		51		72	
73GG	90	73.17	27	1.00	147	96.71	129	94.85	84	89.36	49	81.67	526	88.85	86	75.44	49	47.12	135	61.93	34	66.67	53	73.60
73GA	32	26.02	-	-	5	3.29	7	5.15	8	8.51	11	18.33	63	10.64	24	21.05	45	43.27	69	31.65	16	31.37	19	26.40
73AA	1	0.81	-	-	-	-	-	-	2	2.12	-	-	3	0.51	4	3.51	10	9.61	14	6.42	1	1.96	-	
f(G)	212	0.862*	54	1.00*	299	0.984*	265	0.974*	176	0.936*	109	0.908*	1115	0.942*	196	0.860*	143	0.688*	339	0.778*	84	0.824*	125	0.868*
f(A)	34	0.138*	-	-	5	0.016*	7	0.026*	12	0.064*	11	0.092*	69	0.058*	32	0.140*	65	0.312*	97	0.222*	18	0.176*	19	0.132*
FVII Arg353Gln	117		27		151		132		108		92		627		150		108		258		235		96	
ArgArg M1M1	88	75.21	27	100.00	148	98.01	119	90.15	96	88.89	74	80.43	552	88.04	122	81.33	78	72.22	200	77.52	175	74.47	71	73.95
ArgGln M1M2	29	24.79	-	-	3	1.99	13	9.85	12	11.11	18	19.57	75	11.96	23	15.33	27	25.00	50	19.38	57	24.25	22	22.92
GlnGln M2M2	-	-	-		-	-	-	-	-	-	-	-	-	-	5	3.34	3	2.78	8	3.10	3	1.28	3	3.13
f(Arg353) M1	205	0.876*	54	1.00*	299	0.990*	251	0.951*	204	0.944*	166	0.902*	1179	0.940*	267	0.890*	183	0.847*	450	0.872*	407	0.866*	164	0.854*
f(Gln353) M2	29	0.124*	-	-	3	0.010*	13	0.049*	12	0.056*	18	0.098*	75	0.060*	33	0.110*	33	0.153*	66	0.128*	63	0.134*	28	0.146*

*Allele frequency

Table 3. Prevalence of polymorphisms in the FVII gene in the different ethnic groups studied

POLYMORPHISMS	CHOROTEGA		GUATUSO		GUAYMI		CABECAR		BRIBRI		HUETAR		CR INDIANS Σ		GUANACASTE		LIMON		CR AFRICANS Σ		CR BLOOD DONORS		NE-GERMANY Caucasians	
	n	%	n	%	n	%	n	%	n	%	n	%	n	%	n	%	n	%	n	%	n	%	n	%
FXII 46C>T	127		26		153		106		95		84		591		93		49		142		55		97	
46 CC	62	48.82	12	46.15	56	36.60	24	22.64	49	51.58	30	35.71	233	39.42	33	35.48	11	22.45	44	30.99	24	43.63	67	69.07
46 CT	44	34.65	13	50.00	70	45.75	62	58.49	40	42.11	39	46.43	268	45.35	36	38.71	22	44.90	58	40.85	29	52.74	24	24.74
46 TT	21	16.53	1	3.85	27	17.65	20	18.87	6	6.31	15	17.86	90	15.23	24	25.81	16	32.65	40	28.16	2	3.63	6	6.19
f(C)	168	0.660*	37	0.710*	182	0.590*	110	0.520*	138	0.730*	99	0.590*	734	0.620*	102	0.548*	44	0.448*	146	0.514*	77	0.700*	158	0.814*
f(T)	86	0.340*	15	0.290*	124	0.410*	102	0.480*	52	0.270*	69	0.410*	448	0.380*	84	0.452*	54	0.551*	138	0.486*	33	0.300*	36	0.186*
FXIII Val34Leu	133		25		157		141		80		153		689		177		114		291		381		194	
Val34Val34	109	81.95	9	36.00	120	76.43	77	54.61	40	50.00	89	58.17	444	64.44	95	53.67	70	61.40	165	56.70	210	55.12	99	51.03
Val34Leu34	23	17.29	11	44.00	29	18.47	51	36.17	34	42.50	51	33.33	199	28.88	72	40.68	38	33.34	110	37.80	140	36.74	83	42.78
Leu34Leu34	1	0.76	5	20.00	8	5.10	13	9.22	6	7.50	13	8.50	46	6.68	10	5.65	6	5.26	16	5.50	31	8.14	12	6.19
f(Val34)	241	0.910*	29	0.580*	269	0.860*	205	0.730*	114	0.710*	229	0.750*	1087	0.790*	262	0.740*	178	0.780*	440	0.756*	560	0.734*	281	0.724*
f(Leu34)	25	0.040*	21	0.420*	45	0.140*	77	0.270*	46	0.290*	77	0.250*	291	0.210*	92	0.260*	50	0.220*	142	0.244*	202	0.266*	107	0.256*
ACE	133		25		157		150		110		153		728		179		113		292		351		194	
II	59	44.36	17	68.00	92	58.60	103	68.67	47	42.73	32	20.91	350	48.08	38	21.23	14	12.39	52	17.80	101	28.77	44	22.68
ID	68	51.13	7	28.00	56	35.67	43	28.67	56	50.91	83	54.25	313	42.99	108	60.34	57	50.44	165	56.51	163	46.44	91	46.91
DD	6	4.51	1	4.00	9	5.73	4	2.66	7	6.36	38	24.84	65	8.93	33	18.43	42	37.17	75	25.69	87	24.79	59	30.41
f(I)	186	0.670*	41	0.820*	240	0.764*	249	0.830*	150	0.682*	147	0.480*	1013	0.696*	184	0.514*	85	0.376*	269	0.461*	365	0.520*	179	0.461*
f(D)	80	0.330*	9	0.180*	74	0.236*	51	0.170*	70	0.318*	159	0.520*	443	0.304*	174	0.486*	141	0.624*	315	0.539*	337	0.480*	209	0.539*
MTHFR 677 C>T	133		29		157		147		110		153		729		179		111		290		392		170	
677 CC	18	13.53	1	3.45	9	5.73	5	3.40	10	9.09	21	13.73	64	8.78	48	26.82	74	66.67	122	42.00	107	27.30	84	49.94
677 CT	74	55.64	14	42.28	38	24.20	58	39.45	54	49.09	79	51.63	317	43.48	95	53.07	29	26.13	124	42.80	180	45.92	73	42.29
677 TT	41	30.83	14	48.25	110	70.07	84	57.15	46	41.82	53	34.69	348	44.74	36	20.11	8	7.20	44	15.20	105	26.78	13	7.70
f(C)	110	0.414*	16	0.276*	56	0.178*	68	0.231*	74	0.336*	121	0.395*	445	0.305*	191	0.534*	177	0.797*	368	0.634*	390	0.497*	241	0.709*
f(T)	156	0.587*	42	0.724*	258	0.822*	226	0.769*	146	0.664*	185	0.605*	1013	0.695*	167	0.466*	45	0.203*	212	0.366*	394	0.503*	99	0.291*

*Allele frequency

Table 4. Prevalence of polymorphism in the FXII, FXIII, ACE and MTHFR genes in the different ethnic groups studied

allele. On the other hand, only 45.80% of the D1D2 heterozygous subjects also had the heterozygous FVL genotype (Herrmann et al., unpublished).
The similar high frequency of the FV D2 allele in CR-Africans and in German Caucasians supports the hypothesis that this is a very old ancestral mutant allele (Bernardi et al., 1997; Castoldi et al., 1997), dating back to a time prior to the human migration out of Africa. The absence of FVL in native populations of Africa, eastern Asia, Australasia and in CR Indians is well known (Rees et al., 1995; Herrmann et al., 1997; Herrmann et al., 1999 and this study). The different distribution of the FVL and of the FVHR2 haplotypes supports the hypothesis that the HR2 haplotype is also older than FVL and represents an ancient set of mutations (Bernardi et al., 1997; Faioni, 2000). Both the R2 and the D2 mutations seem to have originated in a single mutation event in different ancestral wildtype alleles of the FV gene. The high frequency of the R2 allele in CR-Indians without FVL as well as the extremely low frequency of the D2 allele in the same Indian tribes (< 0.50%) seems to indicate that the R2 His1254Arg polymorphism is older than the FV IVS 16 polymorphism.
The „out of Africa" model of the origin of *Homo sapiens sapiens* provides a plausible explanation for the observed differences in the distribution of the three polymorphisms of FV gene among the different ethnic groups studied. This model suggests that non-African human populations were descended from an anatomically modern *H. sapiens* ancestor that evolved in Africa approximately 100,000 to 200,000 years ago and then spread and diversified throughout the rest of the world (Tishkoff et al., 1996; Zivellin et al., 1997). The ancestral population of Africans is characterized by the FV haplotypes of HR2 with the mutant alleles R2 and R3 and the FV-IVS16 polymorphism. We found these haplotypes in CR-Africans, who reached the Costa Rican area in the post-Columbian time, coming from the sub-Saharan African population (Ibarra, 2001). The similarity in the frequency of D2 and R2 in Africans and in Caucasoid subpopulations outside of Africa, including Europeans, Jews, Israeli Arabs and from India (Zivellin et al., 1997; Herrmann et al., 2001) is consistent with the migration of modern humans out of northeast Africa into the Middle East and Europe and out of southeast Africa to Asia, the Pacific Islands and the New World. Studies of both mitochondrial and nuclear DNA have suggested that the ancestral population leaving Africa towards the Southeast around 60,000 years ago was small (Tishkoff et al., 1996). The migration to Asia and the New World was accompanied by a further reduction of the rare D2 allele, probably by random genetic drift. This assumption provides a possible explanation for the absence or extremely low frequency of the D2 allele in the CR-Indians. Further studies of other populations descended from the Southeast migrators are needed in order to confirm this speculation.
Schröder et al. (2001) demostrated in German patients with deep venous thrombosis that FVL in Caucasians was always combined with the D2 allele. The investigation of 25 homozygous FVL thrombotic patients from Germany also showed homozygosity for D2D2, indicating that both mutations (FVL and D2) are localized as double mutations in the same allele (Herrmann et al., unpublished data). These results support a single origin hypothesis (Castoldi et al., 1997; Zivellin et al., 1997), indicating that the FVL mutation in European Caucasians has its ancestral origin in a D2 marked allele of the FV gene of a modern Caucasoid subpopulation, now widespread among the Indo-European group.
The FVL mutation is estimated to have arisen ca. 21,000 to 34,000 years ago, i.e. after the evolutionary divergence of Africans from non-Africans and of the Caucasoid from the Mongoloid subpopulation (Zivellin et al., 1997). The three FVL mutation carriers found in

CR-Africans are compound-heterozygous for FVL and D2 (D1D2, FVL/FVwt), and probably have a European/Caucasian origin caused through racial admixture in the past.

2.3 FVII gene: FVII IVS7, FVII R353Q and FVII IVS1a polymorphism

Epidemiological studies have shown that high blood levels of FVII are associated with an increased risk of ischaemic heart disease (Meade et al., 1986; Heinrich et al., 1994; Benardi et al., 1997). Environmental and biochemical factors influence the plasma level of FVII. Age, gender, BMI, insulin resistance and the use of oral contraceptives have been associated with FVII levels (Balleisen et al.,1985). Dietary fats and blood lipids are important determinants of FVII levels (Miller et al.,1991; Mennen et al.,1996). Several studies have demonstrated that three polymorphisms of the FVII gene can directly influence the FVII levels and also modulate its response to environmental stimuli (Lane et al., 1992; Humphries et al., 1994; Hong et al., 1999)

The Gln353 variant of the FVII gene has consistently been associated with lower levels of FVII in white Europeans (Humphries et al., 1994), Gujarati Indians (Lane et al., 1992), Afrocaribbean Britains (Lane et al., 1992; Temple et al., 1997) and Japanese (Kario et al., 1995). Individuals with the GlnGln genotype have a decreased risk for MI, and they have a lower level of FVII activity and FVII antigen in comparison to the ArgGln and homozygous Arg genotypes (Iacovello et al., 1998).

The Gln allele frequencies of the Arg353Gln polymorphism in NE Germany, CR-blood donors and CR-Africans were similar to those described in other studies (Bernardi et al., 1997; Di Castelnuovo et al., 1998). The Gln allele frequencies of the Arg353Gln polymorphism in NE Germany and various ethnic groups in Costa Rica ranged from 0.010 to 0.153 (Table 3). Significant differences in the allele frequencies in the Costa Rican groups were found. Among 627 CR-Indians, the homozygous GlnGln form was not found. The frequency of the mutant allele was lower in the CR-Indian groups (0.060) than in the North European populations (0.100) (Lane et al., 1992; de Maat et al., 1997). Smoking is a known risk for MI, but Iacoviello et al. (1999) and Niccoli et al. (2001) showed a decreased in the risk of MI in smokers subjects carrying the Gln353 allele.

Concerning the FVII IVS7 polymorphism, it is known that the 5 monomers genotypes are associated with the highest risk for MI, followed in descending order by the 66, 67 and 77 genotypes (Iacoviello et al., 1998; Niccoli et al., 2001). The frequency of the 7 allele was similar in German and CR-African population and slightly lower in CR-blood donors and CR-Indians. The prevalence of the 77 genotype was higher in the Chorotega (24.00%) and Bribri (17.82%) Indian groups, followed by CR-Africans (16.15%), in comparison with CR-blood donors (7.86%). In Chorotegas Indians, the potentially higher risk caused by the absence of the protective homozygous Gln353 genotype seems to be compensated by the high prevalence of the 77 genotype. The 5 monomers with a high risk for MI were only found in CR-groups. Moreover, the 4, 8 and 9 monomers were detected for first time in CR-ethnic groups.

The influence on FVII activity of the recently described polymorphism within the promotor region of the FVII, the G>A transition at nucleotide 73 in the intron 1a, is not yet known (Herrmann et al., 2000). In this study, we report the lowest frequency of the rare mutant allele in the CR- Indian group (0.058) and the highest in the CR-Africans (0.222). In the NE-Germans and the CR-blood donors, the frequency of the rare mutant allele was not significantly different.

2.4 FXII 46C>T

There are several reports of severe FXII deficiency in subjects with thrombotic events or MI, cohort as well as case control studies have reported an increased predisposition to vascular thrombosis, (Mannhalter et al., 1987; Halbmayer et al., 1994; Pandita et al., 1997). Other authors did not find a decrease of FXII to be a determinant of thrombosis (Lämmle et al., 1991; ; Koster et al., 1994) or CVD (Kelleher et al.,1992; Kohler et al., 1999).

The FXII 46 C>T mutation was found to be associated with diminished plasma FXII levels in homozygous and heterozygous carriers in comparison with normal individuals, principally in the homozygous form. These low plasma FXII levels were caused by the decreased translation efficiency of the mutant messenger RNA (Kanaji et al., 1998). The FXII 46C>T mutation exhibits an ethnic variability that might contribute to the racial differences observed in FXII plasma levels. In Orientals, the FXII level is lower than in Caucasians (Kanaji et al., 1998). The allele frequency of 46C/T was estimated to be 0.270/0.730 in Orientals and 0.800/0.200 in Caucasians. Franco et al. (1999) reported an allele 46T frequency of 0.250 in Whites and 0.320 in Blacks (n 19) and Mulattos (n15).

In the present study, the 46T allele frequency in NE Germany (0.186) was in the range of other Caucasians reports [(Kanaji et al., 1998, (0.200); Kohler et al., 1999, (0.280)]. In Costa Rica the frequency of the FXII 46T allele in CR- blood donors (0.300) was significantly higher than in the German population. The highest frequency was observed in the CR-African group (0.486) and more than 30 % of the CR-Africans from Limon were homozygotes for the T allele (Table 4). This is the highest rate reported in any population to date.

Among 1182 alleles, 734 T alleles were detected in the CR-Indians (allele frequency 0.620), but the frequency differed between the various tribes. the prevalence of the homozygous wild type and heterozygous genotypes was higher than expected. In the 591 CR-Indians, the prevalence of the TT genotype was significantly higher (15.23%) than in Germans (6.19%).

The role of this mutation as a risk factor in these populations is unclear and further studies are necessary. Franco et al. (1999) discussed that this mutation alone is probably not a major risk factor for venous thrombotic disease. Zeerleder et al. (1999) have shown that hereditary partial and probably severe FXII deficiency does not constitute a thrombophilic condition. The possibility of interactive effects of the FXII mutation with other genetic effects associated with vascular thrombosis and coronary artery disease need to be investigated.

2.5 FXIII Val34Leu

The FXIII Val34Leu was shown to confer protection for arterial and venous thrombosis and to predispose to intracerebreal hemorrhage (Kohler et al., 1998; Catto et al., 1998; Catto et al., 1999; Franco et al., 1999; Rosendaal et al., 1999). These findings support the hypothesis that the factor XIII Leu34 is involved in the production of weaker fibrin structures which might protect against clot formation (Kohler at al., 1998; Catto et al., 1999). The mechanism underlying this protective effect is still unclear. The FXIII Leu34 variant gives rise to increased FXIII specific transglutaminase activity. Anwar et al. (1999) and Rosendaal et al. (1999) reported activities for FXIII ValVal of 96%, FXIII ValLeu:131% and FXIII LeuLeu: 152% .

The factor XIII Val34Leu polymorphism was originally described in a Finnish population with a Leu34 allele frequency of 0.230 in 600 normal controls (Mikkola et al.,1994). A frequency from 0.245 to 0.288 was reported for other Caucasian populations from three continents (Balogh et al., 1999; Muszbek, 2000). In healthy South Asians, the Leu34 allele

frequency was less frequent (0.130) than in Whites (0.289) (McCormack et al.,1998; Kain et al., 1999). The allele frequency was also low in Brazilian Blacks (0.140) and African Blacks from Cameroon (0.118) and Angola (0.188) (Attie Castro et al., 2000). In the Japanese population the lowest frequency has been described (0.013) (Attie Castro et al., 2000).
In the CR-Indians with a Chibcha origin (Cabecar, Bribri, Guaymi and Guatuso), the Leu34 allele frequency (0.280) was similar to South Amerindians from Brazil and Peru (0.293) (Attie Castro et al., 2000). In contrast, the frequency of the mutant allele was lower (0.040) in the Chorotegas with Mesoamerican origin.
The mutant allele frequency in CR-Africans (0.244) was similar to Africans (0.243) from Zaire (Attie Castro et al., 2000).

2.6 MTHFR 677C>T

The 677C>T mutation in the MTHFR gene was very frequent in CR groups, particularly in the CR-Indians (Table 4). The mutant allele frequency of 0.822 and the prevalence of 70% homozygous subjects found in Guaymi Indians is the highest reported in the literature to date. For comparison, in Yupka Indians from western Venezuela an allele frequency of 0.45 (homozygosity 15%) was determined (Salazar-Sánchez et al., 1999; Vizcaino et al., 2001). In five Brazilian Amazonian tribes of Indians, Franco et al. (1998) found an allele frequency of 0.240 (homozygosity 7.8%). Arruda et al. (1998) described in Amazonian Tupy Indians a frequency of 0.114 (homozygosity 1.2%). It seems that intertribal heterogeneity exists, which might be caused by isolation of small subpopulations and a high degree of consanguinity, as well as by genetic drift (Zago et al., 1996). This might also be an explanation for the deviations from the Hardy-Weinberg equilibrium we found in Guaymi Indians and CR-Africans from Limon. The extremely high prevalence of the homozygous mutant allele (TT) in CR-Indians is remarkable, particularly considering that homozygosity has been discussed as a risk factor for cardiovascular diseases (CVD) caused by mild homocysteinemia.
The relationship between homocysteine, folate, vitamin B12 levels and the MTHFR 677C>T was studied in Indians from Western Venezuela by Vizcaino et al. (2001). An elevated homocysteine level was detected in the homozygous TT group which could be partially explained by the folate deficiency found in this group. The implication for an increased risk of thrombotic events in the Yupka Indians from Venezuela does not appear to be relevant since the life expectancy in this population is relatively short and a high incidence of coronary complicactions has not been described (Diez-Ewald et al., 1999; Salazar-Sanchez et al., 2006). Clinical studies are necessary to determine the influence of this genotype on the prevalence of CVD in different ethnic groups and the relation with different life styles, e.g. folate level or vitamin B12 intake.
In CR-Africans from Limon, the TT genotype and T allele frequency were similar to that of Caucasians. The higher frequencies of the T allele in the Guanacaste CR-Africans can probably be explained by admixture with Indians in this area since the $16^{th}/17^{th}$ century (Ibarra, 2001).

2.7 ACE

The frequency of the D allele of the ACE polymorphism and the prevalence of the DD genotype were lower in CR-Indians than in CR-blood donors, CR-Africans or Germans (Table 4). Foy et al. (1996) reported a similar low frequency of the D allele in Pima Indians. CR-Africans had the same frequencies of the ACE DD genotype or D allele as Caucasians.

This was also reported for individuals from Nigeria, Jamaica and the United States (Rotimi et al., 1996). However, it is still not clear and results are conflicting, whether there is an association between the I/D polymorphism of the ACE gene (Rotimi et al., 1996; Sagnella et al., 1999) and serum ACE activity in people of African descent (Bloem et al., 1996). All these results clearly suggest that ethnic origin should be carefully considered in association studies between ACE genotype and disease etiology.

Comparing the Indian tribes of this study, it appears that the Huetar Indians are a distinct group of CR-Indians. In Huetar Indians, the frequency of the FVL and ACE D-alleles was significantly higher and the R2-allele frequency of FV HR2 haplotype was lower than in the other tribes. These results are probably due to a higher degree of admixture with Europeans in the past, compared to other CR-Indian tribes (Barrantes et al., 1998; Ibarra, 2001). Concerning the frequencies of FV IVS16 and MTHFR polymorphisms, Chorotega Indians were different from Guatuso, Guaymi, Cabecar and Bribri, indicating their different origins. The similarity of the prevalence of the ACE polymorphism in the Chorotega and Bribri Indians is remarkable, but more markers should be studied before conclusions can be drawn. Note that in Chorotega Indians and CR-Africans from Guanacaste, ACE genotypes were not distributed as expected by the Hardy-Weinberg; the same although not significant tendency also occurred in Bribri Indians. One reason might be a higher degree of admixture with Caucasians, especially in the Chorotega, compared to the others tribes investigated in this study

In conclusion, the present study has shown that genetic polymporphisms may vary appreciably within and between racial groups. Clear differences in the prevalence of studied polymorphisms were found between the different subpopulations in Costa Rica. These results indicate the importance of considering more than one molecular risk factor for determination of the risk or predisposition for a given disease. It is necessary to analyze a panel of molecular factors to determine the genetic background of a subject or population in order to estimate the genetical predisposition to disease. It was demonstrated that the prevalence of some established risk factors was lower in CR Indians than in Caucasians (D allele of ACE) or absent (FVLeiden, FII 20210G>A polymorphisms). Concerning the FVII polymorphism the protective 77 genotype was frequent only in the Chorotegas Indians, but the protective homozygous Gln353 genotype was absent in all CR-Indian groups.

Knowledge of the prevalence of the studied polymorphisms in the Costa Rican populations provides the basis for follow studies of thrombosis in latinamerican populations.

3. Acknowledgment

This work was made possible by the support from the Faculty of Medicine, Ernst-Moritz-Arndt-University, Greifswald Germany; Deutscher Akademischer Austauschdienst (DAAD) and by Vicerrectoría de Investigación, University of Costa Rica (project No. 807-A3-903).

4. References

Agerholm-Larsen B, Nordestgaard BG, Tybjaerg-Hansen A. ACE gene polymorphism in cardiovascular disease: meta-analyses of small and large studies in whites. Arterioscler *Thromb Vasc Biol* 2000; 20: 484-492.

Anwar R, Gallivan L, Edmonds SD, Markham AF. Genotype/phenotype correlations for coagulations factor XIII: specific normal polymorphisms are associated with high or low factor XIII specific activity. *Blood* 1999; 93:897-905.

Arruda VR, Siqueira LH, Goncalves MS, Von Zuben PM, Soares MCP, Menezes R, Annichino Bizzacchi JM, Costa FF. Prevalence of the mutation C677T in the Methylene Tetrahydrofolate reductase gene among distinct ethnic groups in Brazil. *Am J Med Genet* 1998; 78:322-335.

Attié-Castro F, Zago AM, Lavinha J, Elion J, Rodriguez-Delfin L, Gerreiro JF, Franco R. Ethnic heterogeneity of the factor XIII Val34Leu polymorphism. *Thromb Haemost* 2000; 84: 601-603.

Balleisen L, Bailey J, Epping P-H, Schulte H, van de Loo J. Epidemiological study on factor VII, factor VIII and fibrinogen in an industrial population: I. baseline data on the relation to age, gender, body-weight, smoking, alcohol, pill-using, and menopause. *Thromb Haemost* 1985; 54: 475-479.

Balogh I, Póka R, Pfiegler G, Dékány M, Bereczky Z, Muszbek L. Prevalence of genetically determined major thrombosis risk factors in Eastern-Hungary. *Thromb Haemost* 1999; 82 (suppl) 667.

Barrantes R, Smouse PE, Mohrenweiser HW, Gershowitz H, Azofeifa J, Arias TD, Neel JV. Microevolution in Lower Central America: Genetic characterization of the Chibcha-speaking groups of Costa Rica and Panama, and a consensus taxonomy based on genetic and linguistic affinity. *Am J Hum Genet* 1990; 46: 63-84.

Barrantes R. Desarrollo y perspectivas de la genética humana en Costa Rica. *Acta Med Cost* 1998; 12: 87-94.

Bernardi F, Faioni EM, Castoldi E, Lunghi B, Castaman G, Sacchi E, Mannucci PM. A factor V genetic component differing from factor V R506Q contributes to the activated Protein C Resistance phenotype. *Blood* 1997; 90:1552-1557.

Bernardi F, Aricieri P, Bertina RM, Chiarotti F, Corral J, Pinotti M, Prydz H, Samama M, Sandset PM, Strom R, Vincente Garcia V, Mariani G. Contribution of factor VII genotype to activated FVII levels. Differences in genotype frequencies between Northern and Southern european populations. *Arterioscler Thromb Vasc Biol* 1997a; 17: 2548-2553.

Bloem LJ, Manatunga AK, Pratt JH. Racial difference in the relationship of an angiotensin I-converting enzyme gene polymorphism to serum angiotensin I-converting enzyme activity. *Hypertension* 1996; 27:62-66.

Castaman G, Ruggeri M, Tosetto A, Rodeghiero F. Heterogeneity of activated Protein C resistance phenotype in subjects with compound heterozygosity for HR2 haplotype and FV Leiden mutation (R506Q) in factor V gene. *Thromb Haemost* 2000; 84:357-358.

Castoldi E, Lunghi B, Mingozzi F, Ioannou I, Marchetti G, Bernardi F. New coagulation factor V gene polymorphisms define a single and infrequent haplotype underlying the Factor V Leiden mutation in mediterranean populations and indians. *Thromb Haemost* 1997; 78:1037-1041.

Castoldi E. Molecular bases of APC-resistance and factor V deficiency in thrombophilia. Ph.D thesis, University of Ferrara, Italy. 2000

Catto AJ, Kohler HP, Bannan S, Stickland M, Carter A, Grant PJ. Factor XIII Val34Leu. A novel association with primary intracerebral hemorrhage. *Stroke* 1998; 29: 813-816.

Catto AJ, Kohler HP, Coore J, Mansfield MW, Stickland MH, Grant PJ. Association of a common polymorphism in the factor XIII gene with venous thrombosis. *Blood* 1999; 93:906-908.

Della Valle CJ, Issack PS, Baitner A, Steiger DJ, Fang C, Di Cesare PE. The relationship of the factor V Leiden mutation or the deletion-deletion polymorphism of the angiotensin converting enzyme to postoperative thromboembolic evens following total joint arthroplasty. *BMC Musuloskelet Disord* 2001; 2:1.

de Maat MPM, Green F, de Knijff P, Jespersen G, Kluft C. Factor VII polymorphisms in populations with different risk of cardiovascular disease. *Arterioscler Thromb Vasc Biol* 1997; 17: 1918-1923.

de Visser MCH, Guasch JF, Kamphuisen PW, Vos HL, Rosendaal FR, Bertina RM. The HR2 haplotype of factor V: Effects on factor V levels, normalized activated protein C sensitivity ratios and the risk of venous thrombosis. *Thromb Haemost* 2000; 83: 577-582.

Di Castelnuovo A, D'Orazio A, Amore C, Falanga A, Kluft C, Donati MB, Iacoviello L. Genetic modulation of coagulation factor VII plasma levels: contribution of different polymorphism and gender-related effects. *Thromb Haemost* 1998; 80: 592-597.

Domenico G, Carla R, Ferraresi P, Olivieri O, Pinotti M, Friso S, Manzato F, Mazzucco A, Benardi F, Corrocher R. Polymorphisms in the factor VII gene and the risk of myocardial infarction in patients with coronary artery disease. *N Engl J Med* 2000; 343: 774-780.

Faioni EM, Franchi f, Bucciarelli P, Margaglione M, de Stefano V, Castaman G, Finazzi G, Casorelli I, Mannucci PM. The HR2 haplotype in the factor V gene confers an increased risk of venous thromboembolism to carriers of factor V R506Q. *Thromb Haemost* 1999; 82(suppl): 418.

Faioni EM. Factor V HR2: An ancient haplotype out of Africa - reasons for being interested. *Thromb Haemost* 2000; 83: 358-359.

Foy CA, McCormack LJ, Knowler WC, Barret JH, Catto A, Grant PJ. The angiotensin-I converting enzyme (ACE) gene I/D polymorphism and ACE levels in Pima Indians. *J Med Genet* 1996; 33: 336-337.

Franco RF, Reitsma PH, Lourenco D, Maffei FH, Morelli V, Tavella MH, Araújo AG, Piccinato CE, Zago MA. Factor XIII Val34Leu is a genetic factor involved in the aetiology of venous thrombosis. *Thromb Haemost* 1999; 81: 676-679.

Franco RF, Reitsma PH. Genetic risk factors of venous thrombosis. *Human Genet* 2001; 109: 369-384.

Frosst P, Blom HJ, Milos R, Goyette P, Sheppard CA, Matthews RG, Boers GJ, den Heijer M, Kluijmans LAJ, van den Heuvel LP, Rozen R. A candidate genetic risk factor for vascular diseases: a common mutation in methylenetetrahydrofolate reductase. *Nat Genet* 1995; 10: 111-113.

Green F, Kelleher C, Wilkes H, Temple A, Meade T, Humphries S. A common genetic polymorphism associated with lower coagulation factor VII level in healthy individuals. *Arterioscler Thromb* 1991; 11: 540-546.

Halbmayer WA, Haushofer A, Radek J, Schön R, Deutsch M, Fischer M. Prevalence of factor XII (Hageman Factor) deficiency among 426 patients with coronary heart disease awaiting cardiac surgery. *Coron Artery Dis* 1994; 5: 451-454.

Heinrich J, Balleisen L, Schulte H, Assmann G, van de Loo J. Fibrinogen and factor VII in the prediction of coronary risk. Results from the PROCAM study in healthy men. *Arterioscler Thromb* 1994; 14: 54-59.

Herrmann FH, Koesling M, Schröder W, Altman R. Jimenez Bonilla R, Lopaciuk S, Perez-Requejo JL, Singh JR. Prevalence of factor V Leiden mutation in various populations. *Genet Epidemiol* 1997; 14: 403-411.

Herrmann FH, Schröder W, Altman R, Jimenez Bonilla R, Perez-Requejo JL, Singh JR. Zur Prävalenz des G20210A-Prothrombin-Polymorphismus, der C677T-Mutation des MTHFR-Gens und der Faktor V-Leiden Mutation in Nordostdeutschland, Argentinien, Venezuela, Costa Rica und Indien. In: I. Scharrer/W. Schramm (Hrsg.) 28. Hämophilie-Symposium Hamburg 1997. Springer-Verlag Berlin Heidelberg 1999: 305-309.

Herrmann FH, Wulff K, Auberger K, Aumann V, Bergmann F, Bergmann K, Bratanof E, Franke D, Grundeis M, Kreuz W, Lenk H, Losonczy H, Maak B, Marx G, Mauz-Körholz C, Pollmann H, Serban M, Sutor A, Syrbe G, Vogel G, Weinstock N, Wenzel W, Wolf K. Molecular biology and clinical manifestation of hereditary factor VII deficiency. *Semin Thrombos Hemost* 2000; 26: 393-400.

Herrmann FH, Salazar-Sanchez L, Wulff K, Grimm R, Schuster G, Jimmez-Aru, Chavez M, Schröder W. Prevalence of common mutations and polymorphisms of the genes of FII, FV, FVII, FXIII, MTHFR and ACE. Identified as risk factors for venous and arterial thrombosis in Germany and different ethnic groups (Indians, Blacks) of Costa Rica. In: I. Scharrer/W. Schramm (Hrsg.) 30. Hämophilie-Symposium Hamburg 1999. Springer-Verlag Berlin Heidelberg 2001: 240-257.

Hoekema L, Castoldi E, Tans G, Manzato F, Bernardi F, Rosing J. Characterization of blood coagulation factor V (a) encoded by the R2-gene. *Thromb Haemost* 1999; 82 (Suppl.): 684.

Hoekema L, Castoldi E, Tans G, Girelli D, Gemmati D, Bernardi F, Rosing J. Funcitonal properties of factor V and factor Va encoded by the R2-gene. *Thromb Haemost* 2001; 85: 75-81.

Hong Y, Pedersen NL, Egberg N, de Faire U. Genetic effects for plasma factor VII levels independent of and in common with triglycerides. *Thromb. Haemost* 1999; 81: 382-386.

Humphries SE, Lane A, Green FR, Cooper J, Miller GJ. Factor VII coagulant activity and antigen levels in healthy men are determined by interaction between factor VII genotype and plasma triglyceride concentration. *Arterioscler Thromb Vasc Biol.* 1994; 14: 193-198.

Iacoviello L, Di Castelnuovo A, De Knijff P, D'Orazio A, Amore C, Arboretti R, Kluft C, Donati MB. Polymorphisms in the coagulation factor VII gene and the risk of myocardial infarction. *N Engl J Med* 1998; 338: 79-85.

Ibarra E. Fronteras étnicas en la conquista de Nicaragua y Nicoya. Entre la solidaridad y el conflicto 200 d.c.-1544. Editorial Universidad de Costa Rica. San José, Costa Rica. 2001.

Kain K, Catto A, Kohler HP, Grant PJ. Haemostatic risk factors in healthy white and south asian populations in U.K. *Thromb Haemost* 1999; 82 (suppl.) 185.

Kanaji T, Okamura T, Osaki K, Kuroiwa M, Shimoda K, Hamasaki N, Niho Y. A common genetic polymorphism (46C to T substitution) in the 5'-untranslated region of the coagulation factor XII gene is associated with low translation efficiency and decrease in plasma factor XII level. *Blood* 1998; 91: 2010-2014.

Kario K, Narita N, Matsuo T, Kayaba K, Tsutsumi A, Matuso M, Miyata T, Shimada K. Genetic determinants of plasma FVII activity in the Japanese. *Thromb Haemost* 1995; 73: 617-622.

Kelleher CC, Mitropoulos KA, Imeson J, Meade TW, Martin JC, Reeves BEA, Hughes LO. Hageman factor and risk of myocardial infarction in middle-aged men. *Atherosclerosis* 1992; 97: 67-73.

Khandanpour N, Willis G, Meyer FJ, Armon MP, Loke YK, Wright AJ, Finglas PM, Jennings BA. Peripheral arterial disease and methylenetetrahydrofolate reductase (MTHFR) C677T mutations: A case-control study and meta-analysis. J Vasc Surg. 2009 Mar;49(3):711-8.

Kluijtmans LAJ, Kastelein JJP, Lindemans J, Boers GHJ, Heil SG, Bruschke AVG, Jukema JW, van den Heuvel LPWJ, Trijbels JMF, Boerma GJM, Verheugt FWA, Willems F, Blom HJ. Thermolabile methylenetetrahydrofolate in coronary artery disease. *Circulation* 1997; 96: 2573-2577.

Kohler HP, Stickland MH, Ossei-Gerning N, Carter A, Mikkola H, Grant PJ. Association of a common polymorphism in the factor XIII gene with myocardial infarction. *Thromb Haemost* 1998; 79: 8-13.

Kohler HP, Futers TS, Grant PJ. FXII (46 C→T) polymorphism and in vivo generation of FXII activity. *Thromb Haemost* 1999; 81: 745-747.

Koster T, Rosendaal FR, Briet E, Vandenbroucke JP. John Hageman's factor and deep vein thrombosis: Leiden Thrombophilia Study. *Br J Haematol* 1994;87: 422-424.

Lämmle B, Wuillemin WA, Huber I, Krauskopf M, Zürcher C, Pflugshaupt R, Furlan M. Thromboembolism and bleeding tendency in congenital factor XII deficiency-A study on 74 subjects from 14 Swiss families. *Thromb Haemost* 1991; 65: 117-121.

Lane A, Cruickshank JK, Mitchell J, Henderson A, Humphries S, Green F. Genetic and environmental determinants of factor VII coagulant activity in ethnic group at differing risk of coronary heart disease. *Atherosclerosis* 1992; 94: 43-50.

Lane A, Green F, Scarabin PY, Nicaud V, Bara L, Humphries S, Evans A, Luc G, Cambou JP, Arveiler D, Cambie F. Factor VII Arg/Gln353 polymorphism determines factor VII coagulant activity in patients with myocardial infarction (MI) and control subjects in Belfast and France but is not a strong indicator of MI risk in the ECTIM study. *Artherosclerosis* 1996; 119: 119-127.

Lane DA, Grand PJ. Role of hemostatic gene polymorphisms in venous and arterial thrombotic disease. *Blood* 2000; 95: 1517-1532.

Lunghi B, Iacoviello L, Gemmati D, DiIasio MG, Castoldi E, Pinotti M, Castaman G, Redaelli R, Mariani G, Marchetti G, Bernardi F. Detection of new polymorphic markers in the factor V gene: Association with factor V levels in plasma. *Thromb Haemost* 1996; 75: 45-48.

Lunghi B, Castoldi E, Mingozzi F, Bernardi F. A new factor V gene polymorphism (His1254Arg) present in subjects of African origin mimics the R2 polymorphism (His1299Arg). *Blood* 1998; 91: 364-365.

Mannhalter C, Fischer M, Hopmeier P, Deutsch E. Factor XII activity and antigen concentrations in patients suffering from reccurrent thrombosis. *Fibrinolysis* 1987; 1: 259-263.

Marchetti G, Gemmati D, Patracchini P, Pinotti M, Bernardi F. PCR detection of a repeat polymorphism within the F7 gene. *Nucleic Acids Res* 1991; 19: 4570.

Marchetti G, Petracchini P, Papacchini M, Ferrati M, Bernardi F. A polymorphism in the 5′region of coagulation factor VII gene (F7) caused by an inserted decanucleotide. *Hum Genet* 1993; 90: 575-576.

Marchetti G, Ferraresi P, Quaglio S, Taddia C, Chiozzi A, Cataldi A, Bernardi F, Mascoli F. Study of FV genetic markers in carotid artery disease. *Thromb Haemost* 1999; 82 (suppl.): 450.

Margaglione M, D'Andrea G, d′Addedda M, Giuliani N, Cappucci G, Iannaccone L, Vecchione G, Grandone E, Brancaccio V, Di Minno G. The methylenetetrahydrofolate reductase TT677 genotype is associated with venous thrombosis independently of the coexistence of the FV Leiden and the prothrombin A^{20210} mutation. *Thromb Haemost* 1998; 79: 907-911.

Mariani G, Marchetti G, Arcieri P, Bernardi F. The role of factor VII gene polymorphism in determining FVII activity and antigen plasma level. *Blood* 1994; 84 (suppl)1: 86a .

Markus HS, Barley J, Lunt R, Bland JM, Jeffery S, Carter ND, Brown, MM. Angiotensin-converting enzyme gene deletion polymorphism - A new risk factor for lacunar stroke but not carotid atheroma. *Stroke* 1995; 26: 1329-1333.

McCormack LJ, Kain K, Catto AJ, Kohler HP, Stickland MH, Grant PJ. Prevalence of FXIII V34L in populations with different cardiovascular risk. *Thromb Haemost* 1998; 80: 523-524.

Meade TW, Brozovic M, Chakrabarti RR, Haines AP, Imeson JD, Mellows S, Miller GJ, North WRS, Stirling Y, Thompson SG. Haemostatic function and ischaemic heart disease: principal results of the Northwick Park Heart Study. *Lancet* 1986; 2: 533-537.

Meléndez C, Duncan Q. El Negro en Costa Rica durante la colonia. Editorial Costa Rica, San José, Costa Rica. 1989.

Mennen LJ, Schouten EG, Grobbee DE, Kluft C. Coagulation factor VII dietary fat and blood lipids: a review. *Thromb Haemost* 1996; 76: 492-499.

Mikkola H, Syrjälä M, Rasi V, Vahtera E, Hämäläinen E, Peltonen l, Paotie A. Deficiency in the A-subunit of coagulation faxtor XIII: two novel point mutations demonstrate different effects on transcript levels. *Blood* 1994; 84: 517-525.

Miller GJ, Martin JC, Mitropoulos KA, Reeves BE, Thompson RL, Meade TW, Cooper JA,Cruickshank JK. Plasma factor VII is activated by postprandial triglyceridemia, irrespective of dietary fat composition. *Atherosclerosis* 1991; 86: 163-171.

Morita H, Taguchi H, Kurihara H, Kitaoka M, Kaneda H, Kurihara Y, Maemura K, Shindo T, Minamino T, Ohno M,Yamaoki K, Ogasawara K, Aizawa T, Suzuki S, Yazaki Y. Genetic polymorphism of 5,10-methylenetetrahydrofolate reductase (MTHFR) as a risk factor for coronary artery disease. *Circulation* 1997; 95: 2032-2036.

Muszbek L. Deficiency causing mutations and common polymorphisms in the factor XIII-A gene. *Thromb Haemost* 2000; 84: 524-527.

Niccoli G, Iacovello L, Cianflone D, Crea F. Coronary risk factors: new perspectives. *Int J Epidemiol* 2001; 30: S41-S47.

Ozmen F, Ozmen MM, Ozalp N, Akar N. The prevalence of factor V (G1691A), MTHFR (C677T) and PT (G20210A) gene mutations in arterial thrombosis. Ulus Travma Acil Cerrahi Derg (Turkish J Trauma & Emergency Surgery) 15: 113-119, 2009

Palmer P. Wa'apin man: la historia de la costa talmanquena de Costa Rica, según sus protagonistas. 2ed. Editorial de la Universidad de Costa Rica, San José, Costa Rica. 2000: 13-110.

Pandita D, Steen P, Potti A. Risk factors for deep venous thrombosis of the upper extremities. *Ann Int Med* 1997; 127: 1129.

Philipp CS, Dilley A, Saidi P, Evatt B, Austin H, Zawadsky J, Harwood D, Ellingsen D, Barnhart E, Phillips DJ, Craig W. Deletion polymorphism in the angiotensin-converting enzyme gene as a thrombophilic risk factor after hip arthroplasty. *Thromb Haemost* 1998; 80: 869-873.

Pinotti M, Toso R, Girelli D, Bindini D, Ferraresi P, Papa ML, Corrocher R, Marcheti G, Bernadi F. Modulation of factor VII levels by intron 7 polymorphisms: population and in vitro studies. *Blood* 2000; 95: 3423-3428.

Rees DC, Cox M, Clegg JB. World distribution of factor V Leiden. *Lancet* 1995; 346:1133-1134.

Reiner A, Schwartz S, Frank M, Longstreth WT, Hindorff LA, Teramura G, Rosendaal FR, Gaur LK, Psaty BM, Siscovick D. Polymorphisms of coagulation factor XIII subunit A and risk of nonfatal hemorrhagic stroke in young white women. *Stroke* 2001a; 32: 2580-2587.

Rieder M, Scott LT, Clark AG, Nickerson DA. Sequence variation in the human angiotensin converting enzyme. *Nature Genetics* 1999; 22: 59-62.

Rosendaal FR, Doggen CJ, Zivelin A, Arruda VR, Aiach M, Sisovick DS, Hillarp A, Watzke HH, Bernardi F, Cumming AM, Preston FE, Reitsma PH. Geographic distribution of the 20210 G to A prothrombin variant. *Thromb Haemost* 1998; 79: 706-708.

Rosendaal FR, Grant PJ, Ariens RAS, Poort SR, Bertina RM. Factor XIII Val34Leu, factor XIII antigen and activity levels and risk of venous thrombosis. *Thromb Haemost* 1999; 82 (suppl.) 508.

Rotimi C, Puras A, Cooper R, McFarlane-Anderson N, Forrester T, Ogunbiyi O, Morrison L, Warld R. Polymorphisms of renin-angiotensin genes among Nigerians, Jamaicans, and African Americans. *Hypertension* 1996; 27: 558-563.

Sagnella GA, Rothwell MJ, Onipinla AK, Wicks PD, Cook DG, Cappuccio FP A population study of ethnic variations in the angiotensin-converting enzyme I/D polymorphism: relationships with gender, hypertension and impaired glucose metabolism. *J Hypertens* 1999; 17: 657-664.

Salazar-Sánchez L, Schröder W, Vizcaino G, Perez-Resquejo JL, Jiménez G, Grimm R, Herrmann FH The prevalence of three molecular risk factors (G20210A, Prothrombin, C677T MTHFR, factor V Leiden) in various ethnic groups in Costa Rica and Venezuela. *Thromb Haemost* 1999; 82 (suppl): 275.

Schröder W, Konrad H, Grimm R, Schuster G, Herrmann FH. Factor V variants- FV Leiden, FV R2 polymorphism (ex13), FV Dde-I polymorphism (Int 16). Risk factors for venous thrombosis? Results of a Pilot Study. 30th Hemophilia Symposium Hamburg 1999. Scharrer, Schramm (eds), Springer-Verlag, Berlin, 2001; 261-265.

Thiel BA. Monografia de la población de la República de Costa Rica en el siglo XIX, 2d Ed. Editorial Costa Rica, San José, Costa Rica. 1977; 15-72.

Thompson EA, Neel JV, Smouse PE, Barrantes R Microevolution of the Chibcha-speaking peoples of lower Central America: rare genes in an Amerindian complex. *Am J Hum Genet* 1992; 51: 609-626.

Tishkoff SA, Dietzsch E, Speed W, Pakstis AJ, Kidd JR, Cheung K, Bonné-Tamir B, Santachiara-Benerecetti AS, Moral P, Krings M, Pääbo S, Watson E, Risch N, Jenkins T, Kidd KK Global patterns of linkage disequilibrium at the CD4 Locus and modern human origins. *Science* 1996; 271: 1380-1387.

Torroni A, Neel JV, Barrantes R, Schurr TG, Wallace DC. Mitochondrial DNA "clock" for the Amerinds and its implications for timing their entry into North America. *Proc Natl Acad Sci USA* 1994; 91: 1158-1162.

Tug E, Aydin H, Kaplan E, Dogruer D. Frequency of genetic mutations associated with thromboembolism in the Western Black Sea Region. Intern Med. 2011;50(1):17-21.

Vizcaino G, Diez-Ewald M, Herrmann FH, Schuster G, Perez-Resquejo JL. Relationships between homocysteine, folate and vitamin B12 levels with the methylenetetrahydrofolate reductase polymorphism in Indians from Western Venezuela. *Thromb Haemost* 2001; 85: 186-187.

Zago MA, Silva Jr WA, Tavella MH, Santos SEB, Guerreiro JF, Figueiredo MS Interpopulational and intrapopulational genetic diversity of Amerindians as revealed by six VNTRs. *Human Hered* 1996; 46: 274-289.

Zeerleder S, Schloesser M, Redondo M, Wuillemin WA, Engel W, Furlan M, B Lämmle. Revaluation of the incidence of thromboembolic complications in congenital factor XII deficiency. *Thromb Haemost* 1999; 82: 1240-1246.

Zito F, Drummond F, Bujac S, Esnouf P, Morrissey J, Humphries SE, Miller GJ. Epidemiological and genetic associations of activated factor XII concentration with factor VII activity, fibrinopeptide A concentration, and risk of coronary heart disease in Men. *Circulation* 2000;102: 2058-2062.

Zivellin A, Griffin JH, Xu X, Pabinger I, Samama M, Conrad J, Brenner B, Eldor A, Seligsohn U. A single genetic origin for a common Caucasian risk factor for venous thrombosis. *Blood* 1997; 89: 397- 402.

4

Inherited Thrombophilia and the Risk of Vascular Events

Ivana Novaković, Dragana Cvetković and Nela Maksimović
Faculty of Medicine and Faculty of Biology, University of Belgrade, Belgrade, Serbia

1. Introduction

The definition of thrombophilia includes the impact of hereditary base in the tendency to develop thrombosis and its clinical manifestations. Prothrombotic phenotype results from the interaction of inherited disorders of coagulation and various "clinical" risk factors such as obesity, immobility, major and minor surgery, hormone therapy, malignancy, etc. According to the accepted multicausal model, inherited thrombophilia is a manifestation of mutual influence of gene-gene and gene-environmental factors. Inherited thrombophilia traits include a wide range of disorders. Deficits of some coagulation inhibitors are relatively rare, and their clinical significance is previously known. On the other hand, in genes which control the coagulation cascade, there are many variants that are widespread in the population. The practical significance of these variants, known as genetic polymorphisms, is different, and the subject of numerous epidemiological-genetic, clinical and health economic studies (Novaković et al, 2010; Krcunović et al., 2010; Pavlović et al., 2011).

In summary, the most common congenital disorders associated with thrombophilia are: a deficiency of antithrombin, protein C and protein S, variants of factor V Leiden and prothrombin 20210, and mild hyperhomocysteinemia (Table 1). Individually or in combination, these traits are present in about 40% of patients with venous thromboembolism (VTE), and in approximately the same percentage of women with disorders of pregnancy and puerperium, such as fetal loss, fetal growth restriction and preeclampsia (De Stefano et al, 2002).

1.1 Deficiency of natural coagulant inhibitors

Deficiency of antithrombin, protein C and protein S are rare disorders, the total present in about 1% of the general population. It is considered that holders of these properties have a 5-8 times greater risk of VTE, and VTE among patients with their representation is about 10-15%. They are usually associated with the action of environmental factors, and the first VTE event occurs before 45 years of age (De Stefano et al, 2002).

1.2 Factor V Leiden

It is determined that a variant of coagulation factor V, designated as factor V Leiden, is basically a genetic polymorphism. This is a SNP polymorphism in the 506th codon, which triplet CGA for arginine replaces the CAA triplet for glutamine. The prevalence of factor V

Leiden varies: is about 1-5% in North America, higher in North and Central Europe, while in the African and Asian population, this polymorphism is almost absent. It is estimated that this polymorphism originated 21- 24000 years ago. Under normal conditions, APC protein binds to factor V and cuts it into two inactive fragments. It is determined that the Leiden variant is resistant to APC protein, which prolongs the action of factor V. The result is a continuation of prothrombin activation and continuously maintain coagulation cascade (Robertson et al, 2005, Ho et al, 2006).

Hypercoagulable State	General Population (%)	Patients with Single VTE (%)	Thrombophilic Families (%)
Factor V Leiden	3-7	20	50
Prothrombin G20210A	1-3	6	18
Antithrombin deficiency	0.02	1	4-8
Protein C deficiency	0.2-0.4	3	6-8
Protein S deficiency	N/A	1-2	3-13
Hyperhomocysteinemia	5-10	10-25	N/A
Antiphospholipid antibodies	0-7	5-15	N/A

N/A, not readily available or unknown; VTE, venous thromboembolic event.

Table 1. Prevalence of major hypercoagulable states in different patient populations (after De Stefano et al, 2002).

Heterozygous for FVL have a 2-7 times greater risk of VTE event, while the homozygous risk increased even 40-80 times. The first event of VTE often occurs after 45 years of age. The risk is further multiplied in women during pregnancy, as well as due to the intake of oral contraceptives or hormone replacement therapy in menopause (Table 2). Thus, women heterozygous for factor V Leiden who take hormone preparations have 15.6 times higher risk of venous thrombosis, while pregnant women homozygous for this polymorphism show 34 times increased risk of thrombosis. The risk of spontaneous abortion is also increased (Robertson et al, 2005, Ho et al, 2006).

	Number of		% with factor in women who		Relative risk
Factor	Studies	Patients	Had VTE	Had no VTE	(95% CI)
Oral contraceptive use	7	2530	61	29	2.0 (1.8 to 2.2)
Factor V Leiden, no OC	6	1617	19	6	3.5 (2.5 to 4.9)
Oral contraceptive and Factor V Leiden	6	1612	27	2	12 (7.9 to 19)
Hormone replacement therapy	2	359	62	38	1.7 (1.4 to 2.1)
Factor V Leiden, no HRT	2	221	21	7	3.1 (1.4 to 6.7)
HRT and Factor V Leiden	2	218	27	3	9.2 (3.5 to 24)

Table 2. Results for association of venous thromboembolism with oral contraceptive or hormone replacement use, Factor V Leiden, or both (after Wu et al, 2006).

1.3 Prothrombin G20210A

The gene for prothrombin (coagulation factor II) also has a significant polymorphism 20210G> A. This polymorphism is located in the 3' untranslated region of gene, and is supposed to have a regulatory role. Its frequency in European populations is 1-5%, while it is very rare in people of African or Asiatic origin. 20210 allele leads to increased activity of prothrombin, and the hypercoagulation state (Robertson et al, 2005, Ho et al, 2006)
Meta analyzes show that the risk for the first thrombotic event increased 2-10 times in heterozygotes for factor V Leiden and 2-6 times in heterozygotes for allele 20210A. Combined heterozygous, possessing both polymorphisms, have as much as 20 times higher risk. These data are particularly important in situations that in themselves predispose thrombosis and thrombus-embolism, such as major orthopedic surgery or malignancy (Robertson et al, 2005, Ho et al, 2006).

1.4 Mild hyperhomocysteinemia

In relation to thrombophilia, the importance of some other polymorphisms should be emphasized, such as polymorphism in the gene for methylene-tetrahidrofolat-reductase, MTHFR 677C> T. This polymorphism leads to substitution of alanine to valine at position 222 in the polypeptide, which causes thermolable form of the enzyme with decreased activity. T allele frequency is highest in Asian populations, lower in white European and American, and the lowest in African populations. In Europe, the incidence of TT homozygosity is 5-15%. People with 677TT and 677CT genotype have only 30% and 50% MTHFR enzymatic activity, respectively. MTHFR catalyzes the development of methyl-tetrahidrofolate, which is the main donor of methyl group in the remethylation of homocysteine to methionine. That is why the MTHFR 677 polymorphism associated with hyperhomocysteinemia, which is considered to be an independent risk factor for thrombophilia, and other disorders, such as atherosclerosis, neural tube defects, etc (Robertson et al, 2005, Wu et al, 2006; Simić-Ogrizović et al. 2006; Todorović et al. 2006; Damnjanović et al. 2010).

- Patients with VTE, independently of the age of onset (</> 45 years), the circumstances of thrombosis (provoked /unprovoked), and the severity of the clinical manifestations.
- As a rule, patients with cancer may be excluded. Yet patients with hematologic neoplastic diseases and venous thromboembolism are potential candidates.
- Women with complications of a pregnancy other than VTE:
  - one or more episodes of late fetal loss
  - two or more episodes of early fetal loss
- Asymptomatic individuals who are first-degree relatives of a diagnosed carrier of a thrombophilic trait. This should be accompanied by accurate information and counseling.
- Potential candidates:
  - Women with pre-eclampsia, fetal growth retardation or abruptio placentae
  - Asymptomatic women with a family history of VTE, before use of oral contraceptives, hormone replacement therapy, or pregnancy.

Box 1. Candidates for screening for inherited thrombophilia (adapted from de Stefano et al, 2002 and Wu et al, 2006)

- Antithrombin heparin cofactor activity (amidolytic method)
- Protein C (clotting or amidolytic method)
- Protein S (total and free antigen fractions)
- APC-resistance plasma assay
- Factor V Leiden
- Prothrombin G20210A
- Homocysteine

Box 2. Screening for inherited thrombophilia (first line panel) (adapted from de Stefano et al, 2002 and Wu et al, 2006)

Oral anticoagulant prophylaxis for as long as in patients with a normal genotype:
- First unprovoked deep venous thrombosis with or without pulmonary embolism in patients with isolated heterozygosity for factor V Leiden or for the prothrombin G20210A or with moderate hyperhomocysteinemia.
- First provoked deep venous thrombosis with or without pulmonary embolism (all genotypes).

Oral anticoagulant prophylaxis for an indefinite duration:
- Two or more recurrent unprovoked episodes of deep venous thrombosis with or without pulmonary embolism (all genotypes).
- First unprovoked deep venous thrombosis with or without pulmonary embolism affecting individuals with severe thrombophilia (AT, PC, or PS deficiency, homozygosity for factor V Leiden, combined defects)
- First life-threatening thrombotic episode (massive pulmonary embolism, cerebral venous thrombosis, splanchnic venous thrombosis), in particular if unprovoked (all genotypes).

Uncertain indications for oral anticoagulant prophylaxis of indefinite duration to be given on an individual basis (all genotypes):
- Two or more recurrent unprovoked episodes of superficial thrombophlebitis
- Two or more recurrent provoked episodes of deep venous thrombosis with or without pulmonary embolism
- Two or more recurrent episodes of deep venous thrombosis with or without pulmonary embolism, of which only one unprovoked
- Diagnosis of severe thrombophilia in individuals with not recent occurrence of unprovoked deep venous thrombosis with or without pulmonary embolism.

Primary antithrombotic prophylaxis in asymptomatic relatives of proband patients with inherited thrombophilia:
- Contraindication to oral contraception or hormone replacement therapy (in par ticular for women with severe thrombophilia, i.e. AT, PC, or PS deficiency, homozygosity for factor V Leiden, combined defects)
- Prophylaxis:
  in the case of: surgery, bed immobilization, plastering of the arms or of the legs, long air journeys (more than 4 hours)
  in the puerperium (all genotypes)
  throughout the whole pregnancy (severe thrombophilia; the indication for primary antithrombotic prophylaxis with low molecular weight heparin throughout the pregnancy in women with isolated heterozygosity for factor V Leiden or for the prothrombin G20210A is not yet certain).

Box 3. Secondary prophylaxis with oral anticoagulants after VTE in patients with inherited thrombophilia (adapted from de Stefano et al, 2002 and Wu et al, 2006)

Results of extensive cost-benefit studies do not support universal polymorphism screening prior to the introduction of hormone therapy, during pregnancy or after major orthopedic surgery. Instead, selective testing of patients with a history previous thrombo-embolism is recommended. To prevent spontaneous abortions in women with thrombophilia, low-dose aspirin and heparin is recommended. There is no universal agreement on the need for preventive therapy in elective orthopedic surgery (Robertson et al, 2005, Ho et al, 2006, Wu et al, 2006).

2. New approaches and research strategies in inherited thrombophilia

Until recently, research aimed to elucidate the genetic component of the susceptibility to VTE was based on the traditional approach and employed primarily candidate gene studies; by this approach, the most significant and well-known polymorhisms of coagulation factors V and II (factor V Leiden and prothrombin 20210) were identified. Candidate genes are generally selected with respect to their known role in the traits and processes in interest. In relation to VTE, majority of studies have dealt with genes of coagulation/fibrinolysis cascade.

Thus, based on the known biology of clotting, Smith et al. (2007) investigated polymorphisms of 24 candidate genes coding for proteins affecting coagulation (factors II, V, VII, VIII, IX, X, XI, XII, XIIIa1, and XIIIb; fibrinogen α, β, and γ; and tissue factor), anticoagulation (antithrombin, proteins C and S, endothelial protein C receptor, thrombomodulin, and tissue factor pathway inhibitor [TFPI]), fibrinolysis (plasminogen and tissue-type plasminogen activator), and antifibrinolysis (PAI-1 and thrombin activatable fibrinolysis inhibitor [TAFI]).

Although candidate gene studies have yielded some significant results, selection of appropriate candidates may be difficult, and new approaches had to be employed. One of these modern, widely used and successful strategies for identification of new genetic variants associated with susceptibility to multifactorial diseases is GWAS (genome wide association studies). GWAS is based on testing the association of a complex phenotype with large numbers of SNPs in large samples of patients. Recent use of this and other modern strategies resulted in detection of a number of new genetic variants potentially associated with VTE, but further research is needed to elucidate their significance as general risk factors.

ABO locus variants were previously found to be associated with susceptibility to VTE: non-O blood group carriers were at higher risk, probably through higher levels of VWF and factor VIII, known risk factors for VTE (O'Donnell et al, 2002). This was confirmed by a recent study - Tregouet et al. (2009) conducted a GWAS on 317 000 SNPs in 453 VTE cases and 1327 controls, and found that 2 SNPs in ABO locus (rs505922 and rs657152) were significantly associated with VTE; carriers of O and A2 blood group were at lower risk.

Within the *FGB/FGA/FGG* gene cluster (coding for fibrinogen beta, alpha and gamma), several SNPs were associated with VTE: rs867186 located between FGB and FGA (Tregouet et al, 2009), rs6050 (Thr312Ala) in FGA (Gohil et al, 2009) and rs2066865 located in the 3'UTR of the FGG gene (Uitte de Willige et al, 2005).

Variation in gene encoding protein C (*PROC*) responsible for protein C deficiency was initially supposed to be strongly related to thrombosis, but this was not confirmed later (Dahlback, 2008). However, two polymorphisms within the promoter region (C/T at position -2405 and A/G at position -2418) were recently associated with increased risk of VT (Pomp et al. 2009). Carriers of CC/GG genotype, who showed the lowest protein C levels, were at higher risk of VT compared to carriers of the TT/AA genotype. Polymorphism at *CADM1*, encoding cell adhesion molecule 1, also expressed in endothelial cells, was recently identified as a probable risk factor for VTE in protein C-deficient kindreds (Hasstedt et al, 2009), but it is not clear whether it is a general risk factor also. In gene coding for protein C receptor (*PROCR* or *EPCR*) haplotype A3 (Gly219 allele of the Ser219Gly substitution) was associated with increased VTE risk (Qu et al, 2006; Tregouet et al, 2009), especially in high-risk groups of individuals, carriers of other mutations (Morange & Tregouet, 2010).

The association of gene *F12* (encoding coagulation factor FXII) variants with VTE has been subject to a long debate. Common *F12* variant has attracted much research interest, but the results were not unequivocal. *F12* C-46T variant (rs1801020) was reported to be associated with increased VTE risk (homozygous carriers of T allele compared to noncarriers; Tirado et al, 2004). This association was also observed in a number of other studies, e.g. in patients with cerebral VT (Reuner et al, 2008). However, some studies failed to confirm these findings, e.g. Grunbacher et al. (2005) found that F12 46-TT genotype was not associated with thrombosis risk, nor with age at first thrombosis. A metaanalysis by Johnson et al. (2011) led to conclusion that evidence for association of this *F12* variant with VTE was weak. By genomewide linkage analysis, Calafell et al. (2010) demonstrated that the F12 gene represents a quantitative trait locus (QTL) that influences factor XII levels, and showed that only the promoter -46C>T variant (rs1801020) accounted for the variance attributed to this QTL. The authors concluded that this variation is evolutionary neutral and that T allele appeared approximately 100,000 years ago, reaching high frequencies by genetic drift.

Buil et al. (2010) reported that a new locus, *C4BPB/C4BPA* (coding for C4-binding protein), is involved in susceptibility to VT through a still unknown, but protein S–independent mechanism. Bezemer et al. (2008) found SNPs significantly associated with VT in *CYP4V2/KLKB1/F11* gene cluster, as well as in the *GP6* and *SERPINC1* genes. Three SNPs were strongly associated with VT: rs13146272 in CYP4V2, rs2227589 in SERPINC1 and rs1613662 in GP6; 4 additional SNPs (in CYP4V2, KLKB1, and F11) were also associated with VT. The effect of CYP4V2 and GP6 loci polymorphisms (SNPs rs1613662 and rs13146272) was further confirmed by Tregouet et al. (2009), and the effect of F11 polymorphisms (SNPs rs2289252 and rs2036914) by Li et al. (2009). Recently, in a multi-stage multi-design study, Antoni et al. (2010) found evidence that *BAI3* locus (encoding brain specific angiogenesis inhibitor 3) is associated with early-onset VTE; rs9363864-AA genotype was associated with a lower risk for VTE and low levels of FVIII and VWF. Three variants were recently found to be associated with activated partial thromboplastin time: *F12* (rs2731672), *KNG1* (rs710446), and *HRG* (rs9898) (Houlihan et al. 2010); *KNG1* Ile581Thr was confirmed as a risk factor for VT (Morange et al., 2011).

Morange et al. (2010) in a follow-up study found another new locus involved in susceptibility to VT that was not a part of commonly studied coagulation/fibrinolysis pathway: *HIVEP1* (coding for human immunodeficiency virus type 1 enhancer-binding protein). Allele rs169713C was associated with an increased risk for VT.

Future research in relation to genetic basis of VTE is aimed to explore other possibilities as well (Morange & Tregouet 2010), such as the effects of CNVs (copy number variations) or changes in epigenetic mechanisms (e.g. DNA methylation patterns).

3. Molecular testing of inherited thrombophilia

Nowadays, direct molecular detection of thrombophilia risk factors including F2 G20210A, factor V Leiden and MTHFR C677T mutations is offered by many clinical diagnostic laboratories. It is possible to discriminate between individuals heterozygous and homozygous for factor V Leiden on the basis of the degree of APCR in functional clotting-based assays. Testing for APC resistance (using an accurate assay) can be helpful in assessing for the presence of FVL, whether used initially as a "screen" or if used in conjunction with molecular testing. Therefore the APCR test serves as a phenotypic marker for FVL. A normal modified APCR test excludes the presence of FVL, but if abnormal, the FVL genotype should be confirmed by genetic analysis. Although the presence of PT G20210A is associated with increased levels of prothrombin in plasma, there is no phenotypic screening test for PT G20210A, and detection is always by genotyping. In contrast, there are no analogous functional assays for the detection of the PT G20210A mutation because there is no simple distinction between measurable PT levels in those with and without the mutation. Similarly, although the MTHFR thermolabile variant may be associated with increased levels of homocysteine, there is no other direct functional measure of any effect upon in vitro clotting assays. Detection of thrombophilias by functional testing is associated with a degree of uncertainty because interpretation of results can be influenced by the accuracy of normal ranges and the influence of other factors (both genetic and environmental). Hence repeat testing is often required.

Many different DNA-based methods have been described. In every laboratory method is chosen based on required sensitivity, necessary equipment, number of samples and economical capacity. In contrast to functional analyses results obtained by DNA based methods are essentially absolute, provided the requisite controls are in place, such that repeat testing is not required. Most of the methods described rely on DNA amplification by polymerase chain reaction (PCR). Genomic DNA is required for genetic analysis, but quantity and quality of DNA preparation may vary, depending on the requirements of the assay. Most laboratories routinely purify DNA for the analysis, but where only one or two single nucleotide polymorphisms (SNP) are to be evaluated, avoidance of time consuming DNA preparation can be of benefit. PCR-based methods rely on different tools to detect the genotype of the amplified alleles, such as RED, amplification-refractory mutation system (ARMS), enzyme-linked immunosorbent assay (ELISA)-based primer extension assay and fluorescence resonance energy transfer (FRET) assay. Multiplexing allows single procedure to detect more than one mutation. However, when electrophoresis is used, there may be many fragments present and care must be taken to ensure that interpretation of genotypes is clear-cut and not prone to error. Rare mutations at, or very close to the SNP site of interest may suggest different genotypes, depending on methodology. For example, rare silent mutations within the F5 gene (A1692C, G1689A and A1696G) and rare sequence variations at or near the prothrombin (F2) G20210A mutation (C20209T, A20207C, A20218G and C20221T). These will influence genetic analysis in a manner dependent upon the test system used. However, when these sequence variations are rare in the population their influence on the assay may be considered negligible.

3.1 Restriction enzyme digestion

Original methods for detection of mutations are based on restriction fragment length polymorphism (RFLP). DNA fragment of interest is amplified by polymerase chain reaction

(PCR) and than subjected to digestion by specific restriction enzymes whose restriction site is either created or abolished by the presence of mutation. Fragments of different sizes, generated after digestion, are separated by agarose or polyacrylamide gel electrophoresis and visualized under ultraviolet light after staining with ethidium bromide. The number of bands allows the discrimination of possible genotypes. For the FVL mutation restriction enzyme MnlI is used. The fragment generated by PCR contains one restriction enzyme site which serves as a positive internal control. It ensures that the restriction enzyme has been added, and that the restriction digestion has occurred. The second restriction site for MnlI is created by FVL mutation (Bertina, 1994). In the method described for detection of the PT G20210A in the presence of the mutant allele an artificial HindIII restriction site had to be created by the mutagenic amplification primer (Poort et al, 1996). Improvement of the original method provides additional restriction site which serves as a control as in the case of FVL detection (Pecheniuk, 2000). The MTHFR C677T mutation is also easily detected by PCR and RFLP analysis since the mutation creates restriction enzyme site for HinfI enzyme (Frosst, 1995). The use of multiplex PCR prior to RFLP and the use of whole blood instead of isolated DNA largely improved the original RFLP analyses (Gomez, 1998).

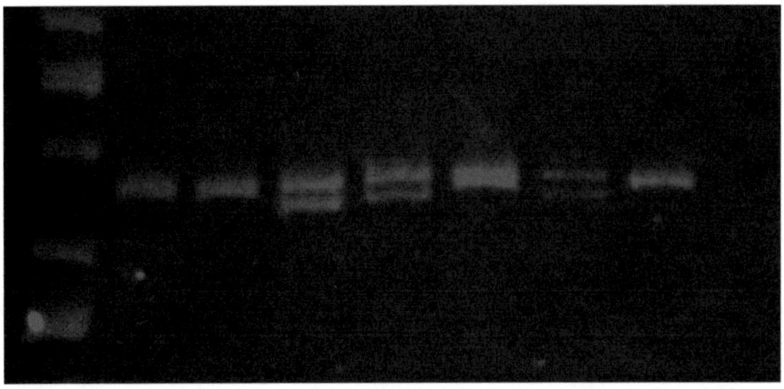

Fig. 1. Polyacrylamide gel electrophoresis of PCR-RFLP products for the FII polymorphism. Lane 1-molecular size marker; lane 2,3,6-normal patient; lane 4,5- heterozygous patient; lane7-heterozygous control; lane 8-normal control; lane 9-blank control

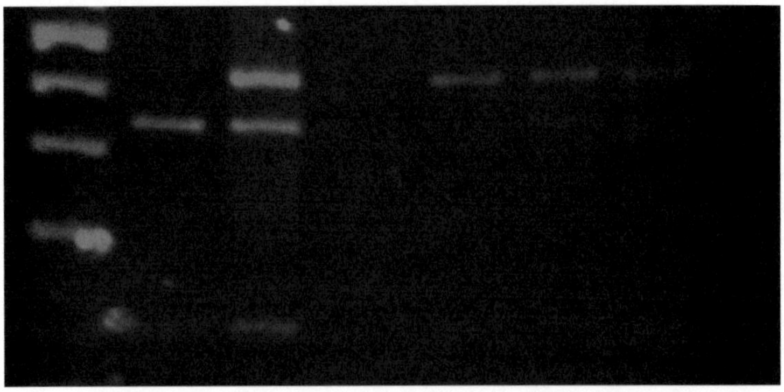

Fig. 2. Polyacrilamide gel elelctrophoresis of PCR-RFLP products for the FVL polymorphism Lane 1-molecular size marker; lane 2-normal control; lane 3-hetrozygous control; lane 5-homozygous mutant control, lane 6,7-heterozygous patients, lane 8-blank control

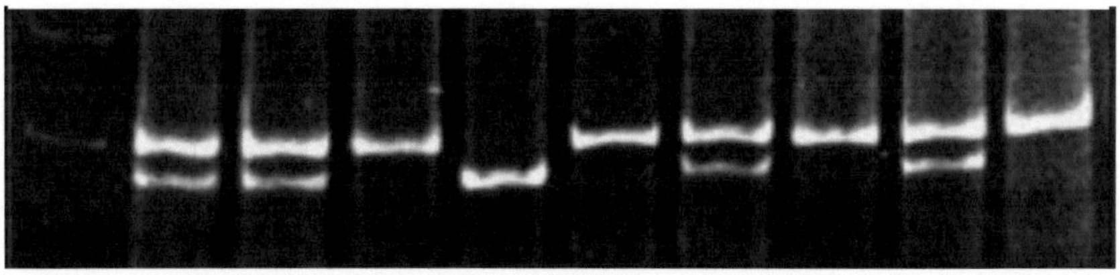

Fig. 3. Polyacrilamide gel electrophoresis of PCR-RFLP products for the MTHFR polymorphism Lane 1- molecular size marker; lane2,3,7,9-heterozygous patients; lane4,6,8,10-normal homozygous patients; lane 5-mutant homozygous patient

3.2 Amplification refractory mutation system (ARMS)

In order to simplify the procedure, increase the efficiency and reduce the costs by eliminating the use of restriction enzymes new methods have been developed. One of them is ARMS based on allele specific amplification of DNA sample. Standard procedure is performed in two separate reactions and with three different primers. In each reaction one of the primers is common (used in both reactions) and the other one is allele specific with 3'end complementary either to wild type allele or mutant allele. Results are obtained by analysis of PCR products on agarose or polyacrylamide gels. The presence or absence of PCR products represents the presence or absence of target alleles. Usually control primers are amplified in the same reaction with allele specific primers to ensure that the PCR reaction is working properly. Multiplex ARMS assay is also widely in use and it allows the analysis of two or more mutations. The Stagen kits for FVL and PT G20210A (Stago, Asnieres, France) amplify ß-2 microglobulin and an unconnected region of F5 (or F2) genes as controls, to ensure efficiency of the PCR reactions. Although this method is simple, efficient and cost effective the specificity of amplification relies highly on careful primer design, careful titration of primer concentrations, and stringent temperature cycling parameters (McGlennen, 2002).

3.3 Single strand conformational polymorphism

The other simple and fast method which avoids the need for restriction enzyme digestion is a single-strand conformation polymorphism (SSCP). It relies on the fact that denatured DNA molecules show different migration patterns on electrophoresis gels even when they differ in only one base. After PCR amplification DNA fragment of interest is denatured to single strands and analyzed by gel electrophoresis. Different alleles will form different 3D conformation and different migration patterns will be observed on gels. The advantage of this method is that it may identify rare mutations, such as the silent A1692C transition in the F5 gene, which is falsely identified as FVL when MnlI restriction enzyme is used (Keeney et al., 1999). These authors also described an SSCP multiplex assay to identify FVL and PT G20210A mutations in whole blood samples. Care must be taken on the interpretation of SSCP, as mutations may cause relatively small changes in electrophoretic mobility Cooper & Rezende (2007).

3.4 Enzyme-linked immunosorbent assays

ELISA-based methods generally hybridize a biotinylated PCR product to oligonucleotide bound to microtitre plate wells. Streptavidin-horseradish peroxidase conjugate then binds to the bound amplicon and finally, buffered hydrogen peroxide with chromophore detects the bound amplicon. Comparison of colour density generated by reactions with wild-type and mutant oligonucleotide probes determines the genotype. A variation of this test is a multiplex assay, where two separate PCR reactions utilize a common biotinylated primer and reverse primers specific for wild-type or the mutant allele, and PCR products hybridize onto an oligonucleotide probe in microtitre plate wells. The former assay design may be more robust, as a single amplification reaction amplifies DNA irrespective of genotype. An ELISA assay for FVL using a reverse allele-specific oligonucleotide hybridization was described by Kowalski et al. (2000). ELISA-based methods require the use of a thermocycler, but other specialist genotyping apparatus is not required. In comparison to gel technology, chemicals used are less hazardous. The StripA Assay (ViennaLab, Vienna, Austria) is an ELISA, which utilizes the reverse hybridization principle, binding reactants to a membrane strip rather than to microtitre plate wells. The target sequence of DNA is amplified in a single reaction which produces a biotin-labelled amplicon. The amplicon is selectively hybridized to wild-type and mutant oligonucleotide detector bands on an individual membrane strip, and detected by means of streptavidin–alkaline phosphatase with colour-forming substrate. Washing and hybridization steps can be automated. Control and test bands are examined by eye or scanned to determine genotype. StripA kits are available for the detection of FVL and PT G20210A mutations and as a multiplex assay.

3.5 Real-time PCR

Real time high resolution melting curve analysis (HRM) employs a new class of fluorescent dyes that intercalate with double-stranded DNA. The intercalating dye is incorporated in PCR reaction and the products are then heated to separate the two strands. Fluorescence levels decrease as the DNA strands dissociate and this melting profile depends on the PCR product size and sequence. HRM appears to be very sensitive and can be used for high throughput mutation screening. Melting temperatures of wild type and mutant allele differ and genotype can be easily interpreted. Whilst Tm values can be extremely useful and reliable in detecting wild-type and common mutations, they cannot be relied upon to characterize unusual mutations. Instrument is relatively expensive and prone to contamination. A multiplex assay for FVL and PT was developed by Van den Bergh et al. (2000). The authors considered their assay to be robust, reliable with high discrimination power. Interpretation of results is based on the presence or absence of peaks with a Tm that is specific for the wild-type or mutant allele. It helps to identify additional sequence variations. This approach is simple allowing the result to be obtained in approximately two hours. Although the instrument is relatively expensive and the method is prone to contamination it is robust and reliable for identification of mutation of interest.

3.6 Mutation detection using hydrolysis probes

Some systems use only a single fluorescently labeled oligonucleotide probe (TaqMan hydrolysis probes) that provide very sensitive and specific detection of DNA. For genotyping this technology uses a PCR primer pair and two allele specific hydrolysis probes, one designed to detect the mutated allele and the other wild-type allele. Both allele-specific hydrolysis probes have a quencher dye and different reporter dyes attached. During the extension phase of PCR amplification the probe is hydrolyzed by Taq polymerase, reporter and quencher dyes are separated which causes the increase in fluorescence. After

PCR amplification, an endpoint plate reading is performed using real time PCR system. Allelic discrimination is achieved by measuring of the fluorescence values based on the signals from each well (Spector, 2005).

3.7 Direct sequencing of DNA

The gold standard method of mutation detection (screening) is bidirectional sequencing. The advantage of this method is that unusual mutations which can cause analytical anomalies can be easily detected. Variation of the standard dideoxy sequencing is Pyrosequencing (Biotage AB, Uppsala, Sweden) which simplifies further the analysis and makes it possible to analyze a large number of PCR products quickly and with minimal effort.

3.8 DNA microarray technology

DNA microarray technology provides rapid simultaneous testing for large number of single point mutations. It is a method of choice for laboratories with large number of test requests (Schrijver, 2003). Custom designed oligonucleotide sequences complementary to the normal DNA sequence and known SNP are attached to a chip. The DNA sample screened for mutation is amplified by PCR, fluorescently labeled and hybridized with the oligonucleotides in the microarray. Computer analysis of the color pattern of the microarray generated after hybridization allows rapid automated mutation testing (Turnpeny & Ellard, 2007). Several commercial platforms which include factor V Leiden, PT G20210A and MTHFR C677T mutation are available. However, they are still expensive for most of the laboratories. Low-density arrays with 10 to 20 markers could be a good alternative. In a single test all thrombophilic markers identified through the human genome project could be analysed (McGlennen, 2002).

3.9 Invader assay

This assay, unlike most of the other DNA-based genotyping methods does not employ PCR. Analysis is performed with genomic DNA. The Invader technology is based on the generation of a fluorescent signal in the reaction solution following the cleavage of synthetic oligonucleotide probe assembled with a so called invader probe and the DNA template that contains either the normal or mutation nucleotide (McGlennen, 2002). The analysis is performed in microtiter well and the signal is detected by fluorescent plate reader.

The main advantages of the Invader assay are that it does not employ the PCR reaction, therefore, failures resulting from contamination are less likely to occur (Cooper & Rezende, 2007). There is only a requirement for heating block and a fluorometer, but no dedicated apparatus is required for this assay. Genotypes can be obtained reliably directly from genomic DNA. It suffers from two limitations. First it requires relatively large amounts of target DNA. Second, only one SNP can be genotyped per reaction (Olivier, 2005). Modifying of the technology to accommodate multiple SNPs and large numbers of samples simultaneously will significantly improve this assay .

4. Acknowledgement

This work was supported by Ministry of Science, Republic of Serbia (Grant No. 175091).

5. References

Antoni, G., Morange, P.E., Luo, Y., Saut, N., Burgos, G., Heath, S., Germain, M., Biron-Andreani, C., Schved, J.F., Pernod, G., Galan, P., Zelenika, D., Alessi, M.C., Drouet, L., Visvikis-Siest, S, Wells, P.S., Lathrop, M., Emmerich, J., Tregouet, D.A., Gagnon, F. (2010). A multi-stage multi-design strategy provides strong evidence that the BAI3 locus is associated with early-onset venous thromboembolism. *J Thromb Haemost* 8(12): 2671-9. ISSN 1538-7933

Bertina, R. (1994). Mutation in blood coagulation factor V associated with resistance to activated protein C. *Nature* 369 (6475): 64-67. ISSN 00280836

Bezemer, I.D., Bare, L.A., Doggen, C.J., Arellano, A.R., Tong, C., Rowland, C.M., Catanese, J., Young, B.A., Reitsma, P.H., Devlin, J.J., Rosendaal, F.R. (2008). Gene variants associated with deep vein thrombosis. *JAMA* 299: 1306–1314. ISSN 0098-7484

Buil, A., Trégouët, D.A., Souto, J.C., Saut, N., Germain, M., Rotival, M., Tiret, L., Cambien, F., Lathrop, M., Zeller, T., Alessi, M.C., Rodriguez de Cordoba, S., Münzel, T., Wild, P., Fontcuberta, J., Gagnon, F., Emmerich, J., Almasy, L., Blankenberg, S., Soria, J.M., Morange, P.E. (2010). C4BPB/C4BPA is a new susceptibility locus for venous thrombosis with unknown protein S-independent mechanism: results from genome-wide association and gene expression analyses followed by case-control studies. *Blood* 115(23): 4644–4650. ISSN 0006-4971

Calafell, F., Almasy, L., Sabater-Lleal, M., Buil, A., Mordillo, C., Ramirez-Soriano, A., Sikora, M., Souto, J. C., Blangero, J., Fontcuberta, J., Soria, J. M. (2010). Sequence variation and genetic evolution at the human F12 locus: mapping quantitative trait nucleotides that influence FXII plasma levels. *Hum Molec Genet* 19: 517-525, ISSN 0964-6906

Cooper, P., Rezende, S. (2007). An overview of methods for detection of factor V Leiden and the prothrombin G20210A mutations. *International Journal of Laboratory Hematology* 29 (3): 153-162. ISSN 1751-5521

Dahlback, B. (2008). Advances in understanding pathogenic mechanisms of thrombophilic disorders. *Blood* 112: 19-27. ISSN 0006-4971

Damnjanović T., Novković T., Jovičić O., Bunjevački V., Jekić B., Luković Lj., Novaković I., Redžić D., Milašin J. (2010). Association between the MTHFR 677 polymorphism and risk of acute lymphoblastic leukemia in Serbian children. *Journal of Pediatric Hematology Oncology* 32 (4): e148-150. ISSN: 1077-4114

De Stefano, V., Rossi, E., Paciaroni, K., Leone, G. (2002). Screening for inherited thrombophilia: indications and therapeutic implications. *Haematologica* 87: 1095-1108. ISSN 0390-6078

Frosst, P. (1995). A candidate genetic risk factor for vascular disease: a common mutation in methyleneterahydrofolate reductase. *Nature Genetics* 10 (1): 111-113. ISSN 1061-4136

Gohil, R., Peck, G. & Sharma, P. (2009). The genetics of venous thromboembolism. A meta-analysis involving 120,000 cases and 180,000 controls. *Thrombosis and Haemostasis* 102: 360–370. ISSN 0340-6245

Gomez, E. (1998). Rapid simultaneous screening of factor V Leiden and G20210A prothrombin variant by multiplex chain reaction on whole blood. *Blood* 91 (6): 2208-2211. ISSN 0006-4971

Grunbacher, G., Marx-Neuhold, E., Pilger, E., Koppel, H. & Renner, W. (2005). The functional -4C>T polymorphism of the coagulation factor XII gene is not associated with deep venous thrombosis. *Journal of Thrombosis and Haemostasis* 3: 2815–2817. ISSN 15387933

Hasstedt, S.J., Bezemer, I.D., Callas, P.W., Vossen, C.Y., Trotman, W., Hebbel, R.P., Demers, C., Rosendaal, F.R. & Bovill, E.G. (2009). Cell adhesion molecule 1 (CADM1): a novel risk factor for venous thrombosis. *Blood* 114: 3084–3091. ISSN 0006-4971

Ho, W.K., Hankey, G.J., Quinlan, D.J., Eikelboo, J.W. (2006) Risk of recurrent venous thromboembolism in patients with common thrombophilia. *Arch Intern Med* 166: 729-36. ISSN 0003-9926

Houlihan, L.M., Davies, G., Tenesa, A., Harris, S.E., Luciano, M., Gow, A.J., McGhee, K.A., Liewald, D.C., Porteous, D.J., Starr, J.M., Lowe, G.D., Visscher, P.M., Deary, I.J. (2010). Common variants of large effect in F12, KNG1, and HRG are associated with activated partial thromboplastin time. *Am J Hum Genet* 86(4): 626-31. ISSN 0002-9297

Johnson, C.Y., Tuite, A., Morange, P.E., Tregouet, D.A., Gagnon, F.(2011). The factor XII -4C>T variant and risk of common thrombotic disorders: A HuGE review and meta-analysis of evidence from observational studies. *Am J Epidemiol* 173(2): 136-44. ISSN 0002-9262

Keeney, S., Salden A., Hay, C., Cumming, A. (1999). A whole blood, multiplex PCR detection method for factor V Leiden and prothrombin G20210A variant. *Thrombosis and Haemostasis* 81 (3): 464-5. ISSN 0340-6245

Kowalski, A., Radu, D., Gold, B. (2000). Colorimetric Microwell Plate Detection of the Factor V Leiden Mutation. *Clinical Chemistry* 46: 1195-1198. ISSN 0009-9147

Krcunović Z., Novaković I., Maksimović N., Bukvić D., Simić-Ogrizović S., Janković S., Djukanović Lj., Cvetković D. (2010). Genetic clues to the etiology of Balkan endemic nephropathy: Investigating the role of ACE and AT1R polymorphisms. *Archives of Biological Sciences* 62(4): 957-965. ISSN: 03544664

Li, Y., Bezemer, I.D., Rowland, C.M., Tong, C.H., Arellano, A.R., Catanese, J.J., Devlin, J.J., Reitsma, P.H., Bare, L.A., Rosendaal, F.R. (2009). Genetic variants associated with deep vein thrombosis: the F11 locus. *J Thromb Haemost* 7(11): 1802-8. ISSN 1538-7933

McGlennen, R. (2002). Clinical and Laboratory Management of the Prothrombin G20210A Mutation. *Archives of Pathology and Laboratory Medicine* 126 (11): 1319-1325. ISSN 0003-9985

Morange, P.E., Tregouet, D.A. (2010). Deciphering the molecular basis of venous thromboembolism: where are we and where should we go? *Br J Haematol* 148(4): 495-506. ISSN 1365-2141

Morange, P.E., Bezemer, I., Saut, N., Bare, L., Burgos, G., Brocheton, J., Durand, H., Biron-Andreani, C., Schved, J.F., Pernod, G., Galan, P., Drouet, L., Zelenika, D., Germain, M., Nicaud, V., Heath, S., Ninio, E., Delluc, A., Munzel, T., Zeller, T., Brand-Herrmann, S.M., Alessi, M.C., Tiret, L., Lathrop, M., Cambien, F., Blankenberg, S., Emmerich, J., Tregouet, D.A., Rosendaal, F.R. (2010). A Follow-Up Study of a Genome-wide Association Scan Identifies a Susceptibility Locus for Venous Thrombosis on Chromosome 6p24.1. *Am J Hum Genet* 86(4): 592–595. ISSN 0002-9297

Morange, P.E., Oudot-Mellakh, T., Cohen, W., Germain, M., Saut, N., Antoni, G., Alessi, M.C., Bertrand, M., Dupuy, A.M., Letenneur, L., Lathrop, M., Lopez, L.M., Lambert, J.C., Emmerich, J., Amouyel, P., Trégouët, D.A (2011). KNG1 Ile581Thr and susceptibility to venous thrombosis. *Blood* 117(13): 3692-4. ISSN 0006-4971

Novaković, I., Maksimović, N., Cvetković, S., Cvetković, D. (2010). Gene polymorphisms as markers of disease susceptibility. (Review) *Journal of Medical Biochemistry* 29(3): 135-138. ISSN: 1452-8258

O'Donnell, J., Boulton, F.E., Manning, R.A. & Laffan, M.A. (2002). Amount of H antigen expressed on circulating von Willebrand factor is modified by ABO blood group genotype and is a major determinant of plasma von Willebrand factor antigen levels. *Arteriosclerosis Thrombosis and Vascular Biology* 22: 335–341. ISSN 1079-5642

Olivier M. (2005). The Invader assay for SNP genotyping. *Mutation Research,* 573 (12): 103-110. ISSN 0921-8262

Pavlović A., Pekmezović T., Obrenović R., Novaković I., Tomić G., Mijajlović M., Šternić N. (2011). Increased total homocysteine level is associated with clinical status and severity of white matter changes in symptomatic patients with subcortical small vessel disease. *Clin Neurol Neurosurg* [Epub ahead of print] ISSN: 0303-8467

Pecheniuk, N. (2000). DNA technology for detection of common genetic variants that predispose to thrombophilia. *Blood Coagulation and Fibrinolysis* 11 (8): 683-700. ISSN 0957-5235

Pomp, E.R., Doggen, C.J., Vos, H.L., Reitsma, P.H., Rosendaal, F.R. (2009). Polymorphisms in the protein C gene as risk factor for venous thrombosis. *Thromb Haemost* 101(1): 62-7. ISSN 0340-6245

Poort , S., Rosendaal F.R., Reitsma, P.H., Bertina, R.M. (1996). A common genetic variation in the 3′ untranslated region of the prothrombin gene is associated with elevated plasma prothrombin levels and increase in venous thrombosis. *Blood* 88 (10): 3698-3703. ISSN 0006-4971

Qu, D., Wang, Y., Song, Y., Esmon, N.L. & Esmon, C.T. (2006). The Ser219-->Gly dimorphism of the endothelial protein C receptor contributes to the higher soluble protein levels observed in individuals with the A3 haplotype. *Journal of Thrombosis and Haemostasis* 4: 229–235. ISSN 1538-7933

Reuner, K.H., Jenetzky, E., Aleu, A., Litfin, F., Mellado, P., Kloss, M., Juttler, E., Grau, A.J., Rickmann, H., Patscheke, H. & Lichy, C. (2008). Factor XII C46T gene polymorphism and the risk of cerebral venous thrombosis. *Neurology* 70: 129– 132. ISSN 0028-3878

Robertson, L., Wu, O., Langhorne, P., Twaddle, S., Clark, P., Lowe, G.D.O., et al. (2005). Thrombophilia in pregnancy: a systematic review. *Br J Haematol* 132: 171–196. ISSN 0007-1048

Schrijver, I. (2003). Diagnostic Single Nucleotide Polymorphism Analysis of Factor V Leiden and Prothrombin 20210G>A. *American Journal of Clinical Pathology* 119 (4): 490-496. ISSN 0002-9173

Simić-Ogrizović S., Stosović M., Novaković I., Pejanović S., Jemcov T., Radović M., Djukanovic Lj. (2006). Fuzzy role of hyperhomocysteinemia in hemodialysis patients' mortality. *Biomed Pharmacother* 60(4): 200-207. ISSN: 0753-3322

Smith, N.L., Hindorff, L.A., Heckbert, S.R., Lemaitre, R.N., Marciante, K.D., Rice, K., Lumley, T., Bis, J.C., Wiggins, K.L., Rosendaal, F.R. (2007). Association of genetic variations with nonfatal venous thrombosis in postmenopausal women. *JAMA* 297(5): 489-98. ISSN 0098-7484

Spector, E. (2005). Technical standards and guidelines: Venous thromboembolism (Factor V Leiden and prothrombin 20210G>A testing): A disease-specific supplement to the standards and guidelines for clinical genetics laboratories. *Genetics in Medicine* 7 (6): 444-453. ISSN 1098-3600

Tirado, I., Soria, J.M., Mateo, J., Oliver, A., Souto, J.C., Santamaria, A., Felices, R., Borrell, M. & Fontcuberta, J. (2004). Association after linkage analysis indicates that homozygosity for the 46C-->T polymorphism in the F12 gene is a genetic risk factor for venous thrombosis. *Thrombosis and Haemostasis* 91: 899–904. ISSN 0340-6245

Todorovic Z., Džoljić E., Novaković I., Mirković D., Stojanović R., Nešić Z., Krajinović M., Prostran M., Kostić V. (2006). Homocysteine serum levels and MTHFR C677T genotype in patients with Parkinson's disease, with and without levodopa therapy. *J Neurol Sci* 248(1-2): 56-61. ISSN: 0022-510X

Tregouet, D.A., Heath, S., Saut, N., Biron-Andreani, C., Schved, J.F., Pernod, G., Galan, P., Drouet, L., Zelenika, D., Juhan-Vague, I., Alessi, M.C., Tiret, L., Lathrop, M., Emmerich, J. & Morange, P.E. (2009). Common susceptibility alleles are unlikely to contribute as strongly as the FV and ABO loci to VTE risk: results from a GWAS approach. *Blood* 113: 5298–5303. ISSN 0006-4971

Turnpeny, P. & Ellard, S. (2007). *Emery's Elements of Medical Genetics* (13), Elsevier, Philadelphia, USA. ISBN 9780-7020-2917-2

Uitte de Willige, S., De Visser, M.C., Houwing-Duistermaat, J.J., Rosendaal, F.R., Vos, H.L. & Bertina, R.M. (2005). Genetic variation in the fibrinogen gamma gene increases the risk for deep venous thrombosis by reducing plasma fibrinogen gamma' levels. *Blood* 106: 4176–4183. ISSN 0006-4971 van den Bergh, F., van Oeveren-Dybicz, A., Bon, M. (2000). Rapid Single-Tube Genotyping of the Factor V Leiden and Prothrombin Mutations by Real-Time PCR Using Dual-Color Detection. *Clinical Chemistry* 46: 1191-1195. ISSN 0009-9147

Wu, O., Robertson, L., Twaddle, S., Lowe, G.D.O., Clark, P., Greaves, M., et al. (2006). Screening for thrombophilia in high-risk situations: systematic review and cost-effectiveness analysis. The Thrombosis: Risk and Economic Assessment of Thrombophilia Screening (TREATS) study. *Health Technology Assessment* 10: 1114 ISSN 1861-8863

5

APC Resistance

Gerry A.F. Nicolaes
Cardiovascular Research Institute Maastricht, Maastricht University
The Netherlands

1. Introduction

In order to secure the continued supply of oxygen to the tissues, the integrity of the vascular system is of prime importance for survival. Several systems therefore exist that safeguard the circulatory system and that include emergency- and repair systems. As a protective system, primary haemostasis and blood coagulation function in concert in order to prevent extensive loss of blood from the organism in the event of vascular damage (Dahlbäck, 2000). Not only humoral and cellular factors limit the loss of blood, a first-line-of-defense is formed by the physiological process of vasoconstriction which is initiated upon a breach of vascular integrity.

Being capable of converting the fluid-like medium blood into a gel-like blood clot within a very short span of time implies that the haemostatic system incorporates the intrinsic dangerous capacity of damaging the very system it is intended to protect. This is the reason why the haemostatic system is subject to strict regulation by several anticoagulant mechanisms, which together prevent the excessive or inappropriate deposition of blood clots within the vascular system.

Rather than being a dormant system that only responds to changes in the vasculature, it is generally accepted that the haemostatic response, as it occurs in healthy individuals, is instead the result of the upregulation of ongoing coagulation reactions. Under normal conditions, these coagulation reactions, as well as anticoagulation reactions proceed continuously at a low level and pro- and anticoagulant reactions balance each other in a dynamic equilibrium. The temporal upregulation of only procoagulant reactions will shift the balance to favor a procoagulant response, (Dahlbäck & Stenflo, 1994).

The maintenance of both pro- and anticoagulant reactions at a low but vigilant level, ensures that the haemostatic system is able to generate a swift response when needed, which can be achieved through up-regulation of either the pro- or anticoagulant processes. The initiation of procoagulant processes implicitly instigates the initiation of anticoagulation responses, as will be detailed below, by the activation of the proteolytic protein C anticoagulant pathway. The coupling of pro-and anticoagulant responses is of vital importance since whenever procoagulant reactions are not controlled by anticoagulant mechanisms, or when anticoagulant processes are defective, the formation of thrombin will become excessive and the risk for thrombosis will increase.

Despite considerable progress in their diagnosis and treatment, ischemic heart disease and cerebrovascular disease, remain to be the major cause of mortality worldwide, with over 80% of cardiovascular disease deaths now taking place in low-and middle-income countries

and occurring almost equally in men and women (Global Health Observatory (GHO), World Health Organisation [WHO], 2008).
Thromboembolic disease contributes to this overall mortality, as it is implicated in many manifestations of cardiovascular disease. The clinical manifestation of a thrombus is that of the pathological presence of an occlusion in a blood vessel or in the heart, which causes an obstruction of the physiological flow of blood through the circulatory system. Such occlusions can occur in either the venous or arterial part of the vessel tree and the condition is consequently classified as either venous or arterial thrombosis. Despite the fact that in both venous and arterial thrombosis the normal haemostatic balance is disturbed, the two types of thrombosis are considered distinct disease states that each have their own particular molecular pathology and underlying risk factors (Rosendaal, 1999, 2005).
The proper functioning of the anticoagulant protein C pathway is undisputedly required to prevent the occurrence of thrombosis, and in particular venous thromboses, as is most strikingly illustrated for protein C deficiency. Newborns who are homozygous protein C deficient can develop the life-threatening condition of acute onset "purpura fulminans" (Dreyfus et al, 1991, 1995) which can be treated by replacement therapy employing purified protein C concentrates.
Resistance to activated protein C (APC), or APC resistance, the subject of this chapter, has been implicated mostly in pathogenesis of venous thrombosis, despite the fact that the causative FV_{Leiden} mutation, which is present in a majority of cases, has been related to myocardial infarction and/or overall coronary disease (Rallidis et al.2003; Segev et al., 2005; Ye et al., 2006). Various clinical studies have been performed to identify the contribution of the anticoagulant protein C pathway to arterial thromboses and stroke and these have not been conclusive in providing clear evidence for the contribution of the protein C pathway to arterial thrombosis (e.g. Folsom, 1999; Hankey, 2001; Boekholdt, 2007). That there is a link between the hemostatic system and arterial thrombosis or atherosclerosis appears clear as it has been established that many complex diseases, such as atherosclerosis, show an extensive crosstalk between inflammation and coagulation, as was recently reviewed by Borisoff and coworkers (Borisoff et al, 2011).
Venous thrombosis (or venous thromboembolism, VTE) is a multifactorial disease (Seligsohn&Zivelin, 1997; Rosendaal, 1999) that affects one in 10,000 individuals under the age of 40 years annually and one in 1,000 individuals over 75 years of age, causing significant morbidity and mortality (Salzman & Hirsh, 1994; Anderson et al., 1991; Nordstrom et al. 1992). The multifactorial character of VTE implies that for the disease to occur often several circumstantial and genetic factors occur simultaneously. Together these factors are capable of tipping the natural haemostatic balance between pro- and anticoagulant forces. Important to note is that environmental and acquired factors are able to modulate the existing genetic risk factors for thrombosis in an individual and these acquired factors, which may be very diverse by nature, are consequently directly involved in the pathogenesis of thrombosis. Thrombosis will develop then when the combined risk factors interact such that the threshold for thrombosis is surpassed. Upon passing of the threshold, the anticoagulant mechanisms are no longer able to counteract the procoagulant forces. Consequently a thrombotic event can occur (Rosendaal, 1999).
Of the inherited risk factors for venous thrombotic disease, most are found in the protein C anticoagulant system which will be detailed below. Examples of these are resistance to activated protein C (APC) caused by the FV_{Leiden} mutation (FV R506Q) and the deficiencies of the cofactor, protein S, and deficiency of protein C itself (Segers et al., 2007). Of the

acquired risk factors, use of oral contraceptives, pregnancy/puerperium, the presence of antiphospholipid antibodies, immobilization, surgery, malignancies and trauma are amongst the most studied. Furthermore, age and sex are recognized as independent contributing factors in the pathogenesis of venous thrombosis (Bertina, 2001).
In this chapter resistance to APC, the central protein of the protein C anticoagulant pathway, will be discussed, both for genetically determined forms of APC resistance and acquired types of APC resistance. Particular attention will be given to the molecular events that occur during the APC-catalyzed down-regulation of thrombin formation in normal individuals, since knowledge of these processes is pivotal in our understanding of the causative role of APC resistance in the occurrence of thromboembolic disease.

2. Protein C anticoagulant pathway

During homeostasis several anticoagulant systems balance the procoagulant forces that act in human blood, thereby preventing excessive platelet and fibrin depositions. A major inhibitory buffer is formed by the circulating inhibitors, which include antithrombin, alpha-2-macroglobulin, antitrypsin or tissue factor pathway inhibitor (TFPI) which provide the necessary negative feedback to procoagulant forces. These circulating inhibitors target the activated forms of the serine proteases from the coagulation cascade like thrombin and FXa and act by complex formation with their target proteases, resulting in a loss of proteolytic activity and clearance of the active protease from circulation.
Key regulators in the amplification of thrombin formation are however the non-enzymatic cofactor proteins factor V (FV) and factor VIII (FVIII) and by virtue of the absolute requirement of their activity for normal thrombogenesis, they are obvious targets for the attenuation of thrombin formation. Given that these molecules lack proteolytic activity, they cannot be inactivated via complex formation but instead they are targeted by proteolytic inactivation, resulting in disintegration of the protein structure and concomittant loss of cofactor activity. The main proteolytic enzyme responsible for the inactivation of activated FV (FVa) and FVIII (FVIIIa) is the activated form of protein C.
Low levels of activated protein C circulate, but for a sufficient anticoagulant response to occur, an upregulation of protein C is required through a specific set of molecular events, which together are described as the protein C anticoagulant pathway. The main player in this pathway is protein C. Protein C is a vitamin K dependent zymogen belonging to the class of chymotrypsin-like serine proteases (Stenflo, 1976). Being a zymogen, protein C circulates at a plasma concentration of ~65 nM in humans as an inactive pro-enzyme which requires processing in order to obtain its enzymatic activity. A pivotal role in the initiation of the protein C pathway is the formation of a complex between thrombin and thrombomodulin (Fuentes-Prior et al, 2000), see Fig. 1 below. Note that it is thrombin, the very enzyme that ultimately needs to be downregulated, that initiates its own attenuation. Thrombomodulin is a transmembrane protein that is present on the undamaged endothelium, in particular the endothelium of the smaller blood vessels. The membrane-bound thrombomodulin is able to capture thrombin by binding to the exosite I of thrombin upon which the thrombin-thrombomodulin complex is formed. The exosite I of thrombin is primarily involved in procoagulant interactions of the enzyme, namely in the recognition and activation of fibrinogen, FV and FVIII (Lane & Caso, 1989). After binding of thrombomodulin to the thrombin exosite I the procoagulant properties of any thrombin molecules that have migrated from a site of ongoing coagulation and are transported into

the microvasculature, are lost, thereby thrombomodulin is anticoagulant in itself. However, not only are the procoagulant properties of thrombin inhibited, given the fact that the active site of thrombin is still available, a conformational change that is accompanied by the binding to thrombomodulin causes the local active site structure of thrombin to change. This structural change alters the substrate specificity of thrombin (Fuentes-Prior et al, 2000; Dahlbäck & Villoutreix, 2005) such that thrombin is transformed from a procoagulant into an anticoagulant protein. In the anticoagulant state, thrombin is able to efficiently activate protein C by removal of a 12 amino acid activation fragment from the serine protease domain of protein C. For optimal activation of protein C by thrombin furthermore the presence of the endothelial cell protein C receptor (EPCR) is required.

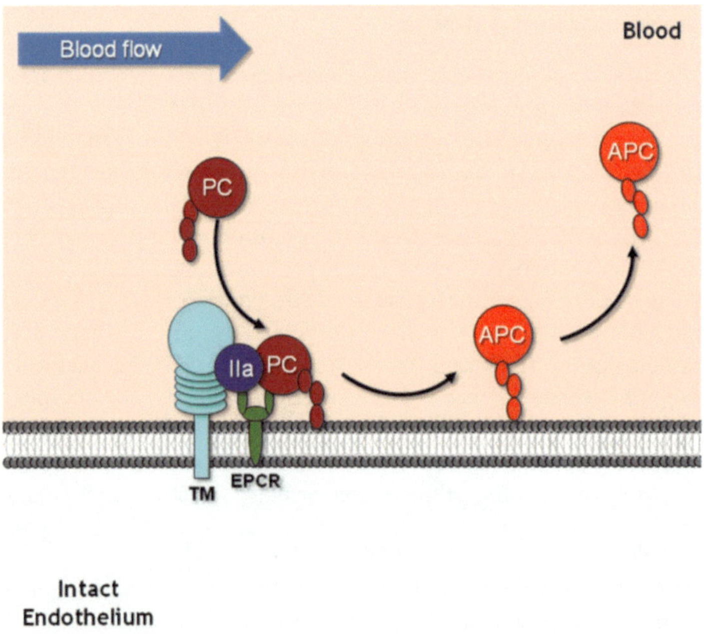

Fig. 1. Activation of protein C by thrombin. When bound to thrombomodulin (TM), in the presence of the endothelial cell protein C receptor (EPCR), thrombin (IIa) is able to activate protein C (PC) to activated protein C (APC).

The physiological requirement for the presence of both thrombomodulin and EPCR is most strikingly evidenced by the early embryonic lethal phenotypes being associated with deficiency of either of the two proteins in mice (Fukudome & Esmon, 1994; Esmon, 2001).
In the protein C pathway, a number of factors are important for the full expression of APC anticoagulant properties. These include the presence of the cofactor proteins, protein S and coagulation factor V (FV) and in addition a suitable membrane surface onto which both APC and its substrates can assemble in the presence of calcium.
Like protein C, protein S is also a vitamin K dependent coagulation factor, which however is devoid of enzymatic activity as it does not contain a catalytic domain. FV, the procofactor protein, has a dual function in coagulation and has been described as a "Janus faced" protein (Nicolaes & Dahlbäck, 2002), with properties in both the pro- and anticoagulant

pathways. In the APC-catalyzed inactivation of FVIIIa (see also below) FV acts in synergy with protein S as a cofactor to APC (Shen & Dahlbäck, 1994; Varadi et al, 1995). Somewhat conflicting results were obtained whether or not FV is also a cofactor in the inactivation of FVa. Though extremely difficult to study in purified reaction systems, this issue was recently addressed (Cramer et al, 2010) and it was concluded that FV expresses activity in FVa inactivation.

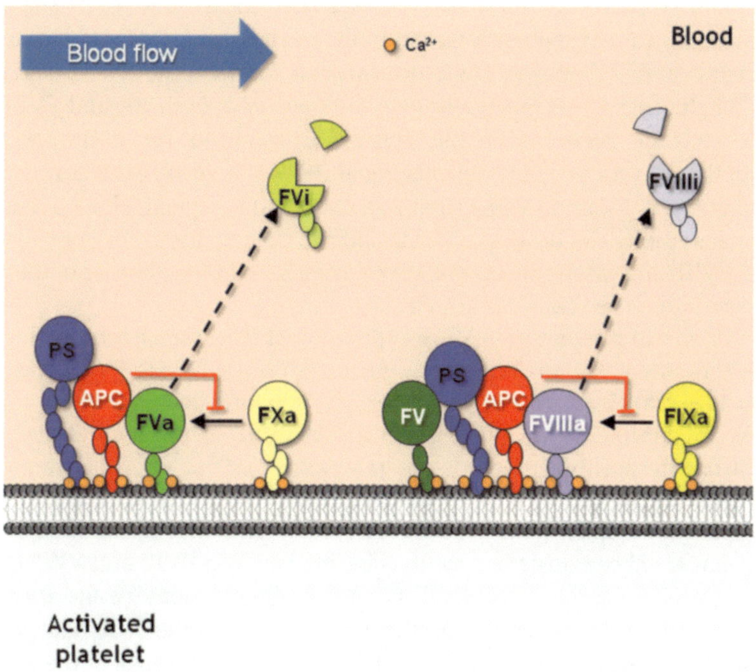

Fig. 2. APC catalyzed inactivation of FVa and FVIIIa. Left: APC, together with its cofactor protein S (PS) proteolytically inactivates factor Va (FVa) resulting in a loss of protein integrity and concomitant loss of cofactor activity. As a result, complex formation between FVa and factor Xa (FXa) is not possible, leading to lowered conversion of prothrombin by FXa. Right: analogous to regulation of FVa activity, factor VIIIa (FVIIIa) is leaved by APC, resulting in dissociation of FVIIIa units and loss of activity. Factor V, FV. Factor IXa, FIXa.

In the absence of protein C, individuals are at high risk for the development of thrombosis, such as in the case of the classical homozygous protein C deficiencies that are seen in neonates where purpura fulminans develop (Dreyfus et al, 1991, 1995). This indicates the important function that the protein C pathway has, in particular in the microcirculation. Not only the deficiencies of the zymogen protein C, also those of the cofactor protein S are associated with a prothrombotic state. Deficiency of the other APC cofactor, FV, is by itself not associated with thrombosis, which indicates that, particularly at low FV levels, the procoagulant properties of this coagulation protein are dominant (Govers-Riemslag et al, 2002; Duckers et al, 2009). There are however reports in literature in which cases were described where individuals who developed autoantibodies against FV have suffered from thrombosis rather than from bleeding problems (Ortel, 1999). It was hypothesized that in these cases antibodies may specifically target the anticoagulant properties of FV.

3. Structure and function of coagulations factors V and VIII

FV and FVIII are large plasma glycoproteins, primarily synthesized in hepatocytes, with relative molecular masses of ~330 kDa that share a common architecture. Both proteins have a mosaic domain structure of A1-A2-B-A3-C1-C2 (Fig. 3). FV and FVIII share a common ancestral gene and are consequently structurally related, with 40% amino acid sequence identity in their A and C domains. The B-domain that connects the A1-A2 heavy chains and the A3-C1-C2 light chains are much less (~15%) conserved. Both FV and FVIII are heavily glycosylated, and the presence of the glycans is required for a proper folding and functioning of the cofactor proteins (Nicolaes et al, 1999; Yamazaki et al, 2010).

The activated forms of FV and FVIII, called FVa and FVIIIa respectively, are required for full expression of activity by the prothrombinase and intrinsic tenase complexes respectively. In fact, FVa and FVIIIa are essential non-enzymatic cofactors: in the absence of the cofactors the prothrombinase and tenase complex are virtually inactive.

To protect FVIII and to prevent premature expression of its cofactor activity, FVIII circulates in plasma in complex with von Willebrand factor (VWF), whereas FV in plasma is in free form (Weiss, 1977). In thrombocytes however, FV is bound to multimerin 1 (MMRN1), a large protein much like VWF, that protects FV from expression of its activity and presumably from intracellular degradation (Hayward, 1995). Upon activation of FV, the binding affinity of multimerin for FVa is decreased slightly, which will allow dissociation of the multimerin-FVa complex (Jeimy, 2008). A similar mechanism, modification of affinity by activation, has also been described for the binding between FVIII and VWF (Lollar, 1988).

The circulating procofactors FV and FVIII possess negligible activity and for them to gain activity, they need to be proteolyzed. During activation, the large B-domain will be excised from the molecule. In fact it has been shown for FV that the presence of the B-domain itself is the reason that the cofactor is not active and that proteolysis is needed to eliminate steric and/or conformational restraints that are imposed on the cofactor by the B-domain. A lifting of these restraints by removal of the B-domain allows the availability of discrete binding interactions between FVa and its binding partners FXa and prothrombin (Kane, 1990; Keller 1995; Toso, 2004). Activation of FV and FVIII is essentially a positive feedback reaction since the potential activators are alpha-thrombin (Kane et al, 1981; Suzuki et al, 1982), meizothrombin (Tans et al, 1994), FXa (Monkovic & Tracy, 1990), FXIa (Whelihan et al, 2010) and tissue factor-FVIIa (Safa et al, 1999). Of these, activation by alpha-thrombin, the very enzyme that is produced by the prothrombinase complex, is regarded as most important.

The cleavages by thrombin and FXa are indicated in Fig 3. For both cofactors these result in the release of the B-domain, a process that is accompanied by expression of cofactor activity. The molecular weight of the FVa light chain is not unique due to incomplete N-glycosylation at Asn2181 in the C2 domain (Nicolaes et al, 1999; Kim et al, 1999). As a result of this variable glycosylation, two different forms of FV are present in human blood. These two glycoisoforms express different activities in both pro- and anticoagulation pathways (Váradi et al 1996, Hoekema et al, 1997) and glycosylation of the FVa light chain, more precisely the N-linked glycosylation at Asn2181, has been implicated in the pathogenesis of venous thrombosis (Yamazaki et al, 2002, 2010).

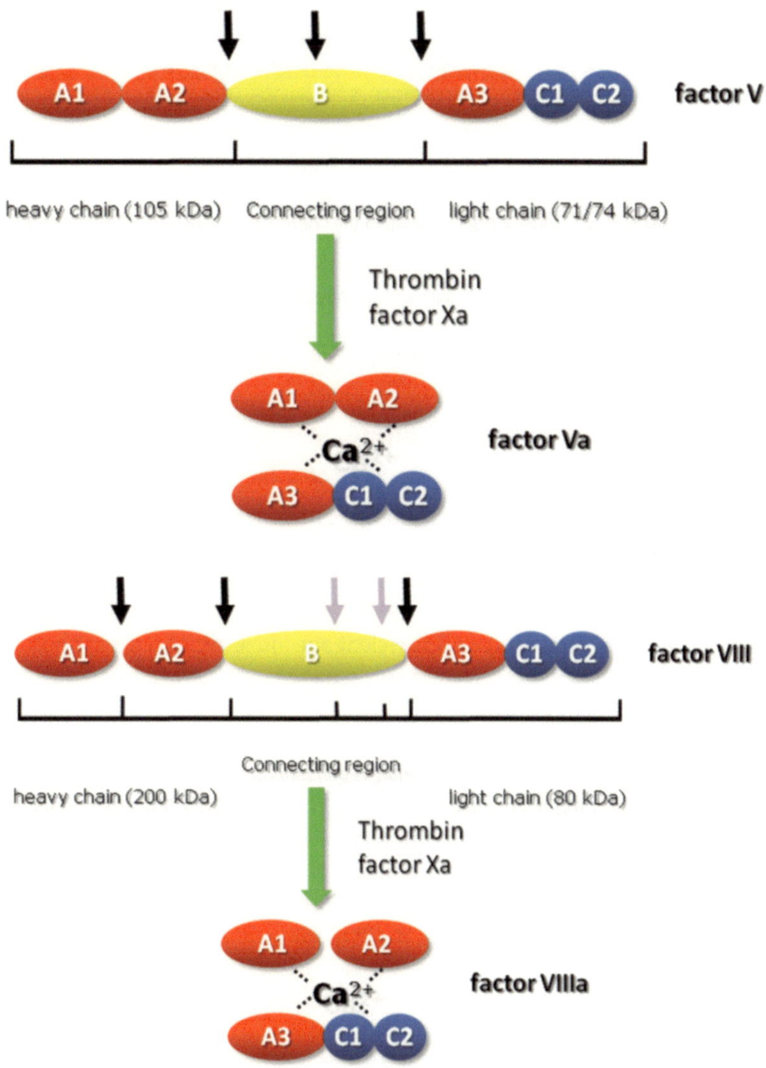

Fig. 3. Activation of FV and FVIII. The domain structures of FV (top) and FVIII (bottom) are indicated. FV is activated by thrombin or FXa at Arg709, Arg1018, and Arg1545, as indicated by the black arrows. The active cofactor is formed by the association of the A1-A2 heavy chain with the A3-C1-C2 light chain via calcium-dependent noncovalent bonding. FVIII is cleaved at residues Arg1313 and Arg1648 (upper arrows in purple) upon secretion from the cell, yielding a 200-kDa fragment (also referred to as the heavy chain, consisting of the A1, A2 and part of the B-domain) and an 80-kDa light chain. FVIII thus circulates as a dimer. Activation of FVIII by thrombin or FXa occurs through proteolytic cleavage at Arg372, Arg740, and Arg1689 (black arrows), yielding the heterotrimeric FVIIIa, consisting of a 50-kDa A1 domain–derived polypeptide, a 43-kDa A2 domain–derived polypeptide, and the 73-kDa A3-C1-C2–derived light chain, which are noncovalently associated via divalent metal ions.

The function of the cofactors FVa and FVIIIa is, like their structure, very similar. Both proteins express their cofactor activities when assembled in a membrane-bound complex that furthermore comprises a serine protease (FXa and FIXa respectively) and a zymogen-substrate (prothrombin and FX respectively). A functional complex is only formed in the presence of calcium. Calcium is needed for the Gla-domains of the vitamin K dependent proteins involved to reach their calcium-induced active conformation (Huang et al, 2004) and furthermore for the occupation of the single calcium binding sites in FVa and FVIIIa, which are necessary for expression of cofactor activity.

Involvement of the cofactor protein Va and VIIIa increases the Vmax of the prothrombinase and tenase complex respectively, by several orders of magnitude. This implies that the presence of FVa or FVIIIa is essential for the formation of thrombin or FXa under physiological conditions (Nesheim et al, 1979; Rosing et al, 1980, van Diejjen, 1981).

4. Regulation of FVa and FVIIIa activities

Given their potency and essential character, it is of prime importance for homeostasis that the activities of FVa and FVIIIa are tightly regulated. As mentioned above, the main proteolytic process responsible for FVa/FVIIIa regulation is limited proteolysis by the serine protease activated protein C (APC).

The inactivation process occurs much in analogy to the activation described before: APC targets its substrates at multiple but specific cleavage sites, provided that both the substrate and the enzyme are bound to a membrane surface (Kalafatis et al, 1994; Nicolaes et al, 1995, Egan et al, 1997, Barhoover & Kalafatis, 2011). In the absence of a lipid surface, reactions occur too slowly to be physiologically relevant (Bakker et al., 1992; Nicolaes et al, 1995). Cleavage at each of the cleavage sites is characterized by its own kinetic parameters and since there is no specific order of cleavages, the rates of the cleavage reactions are being determined mostly by the local concentrations of FVa, APC and any cofactors or modifiers present. Though cleavages are random, the reaction products formed after cleavage at each of the single cleavage sites express different residual cofactor activities. For FVa this means that where cleavage at Arg306 results in a complete loss of protein integrity, cleavage at Arg506 results in a reaction product that has considerable remaining cofactor activity, an activity which will depend on the concentrations of other reactants present (e.g. FXa, Nicolaes et al., 1995).

At a concentration around or lower than the plasma concentration of FV (21 nM) the cleavage at Arg506 is the preferred cleavage however, being ~20 fold faster than cleavage at Arg306. The inactivation of FVa is enhanced by the presence of protein S which selectively appears to stimulate the slower cleavage at Arg306 by a factor of 20 (Walker, 1981; Rosing et al, 1995), the dominant cleavage at Arg506 is only stimulated 2-fold by protein S (Rosing et al, 1995; Norstrom et al, 2006). Interesting to note in this respect is a recent finding that protein S, which circulates in both a free form and in complex with C4b binding protein (C4BP) has different effects on APC- catalyzed FVa inactivation, depending on whether it is free or not. Whereas it had prior been deemed that only free protein S is active as a cofactor to APC, it was shown that also the protein S-C4BP complex is able to stimulate the Arg306 cleavage in FVa more than 10-fold, while cleavage at Arg506 is inhibited 3- to 4-fold (Maurissen et al, 2008). In the absence of protein S, FVa when incorporated in the prothrombinase complex, is protected from inactivation by APC. FXa specifically protects FVa from cleavage at Arg506 (Rosing et al, 1995; Norstrom et al, 2006), whereas prothrombin has no preferred protection and attenuates the cleavage at both Arg306 and Arg506 (Rosing et al, 1995; Smirnov et al, 1999; Tran et al, 2008).

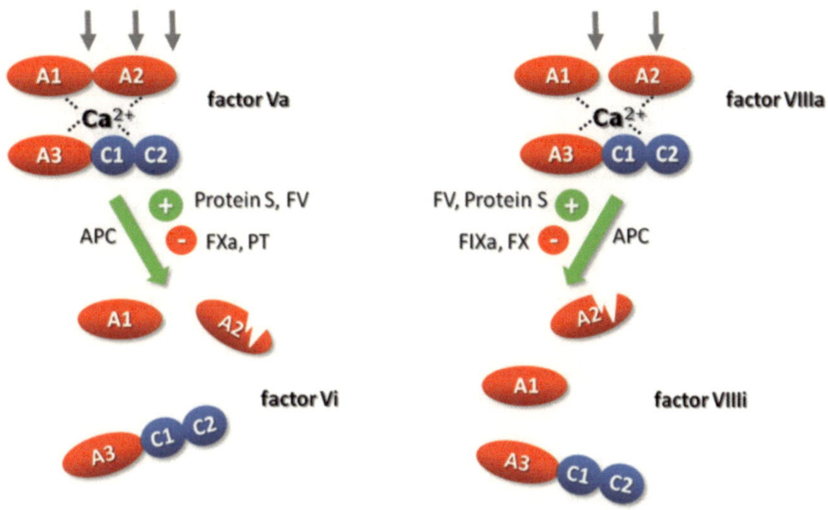

Fig. 4. APC-catalyzed inactivation of FVa and FVIIIa. FVa Inactivation proceeds primarily via cleavages after residues Arg306 and Arg506 and to a lesser extent at Arg679 in the heavy chain domain (Kalafatis et al, 1994; Nicolaes et al, 1995) (upper grey arrows). In FVIIIa, APC targets the peptides bonds after Arg336 and Arg562(Fay et al, 1991), (upper grey arrows). For FVa, cleavage at Arg506 is preferred over that at Arg306. Full loss of activity requires cleavage at Arg306. Complete cleavage by APC then results in a loss of protein integrity, generating inactivated FVa, FVi, and inactivated FVIIIa, FVIIIi. The disintegration is accompanied by a loss of protein activity. Cofactors that influence the reactions are indicated: protein S and FV are able to enhance the cleavages in both FVa and FVIIIa, whereas FXa and prothrombin (PT) are able to protect FVa from inactivation by APC. Likewise, FIXa and FX are protective for FVIIIa.

A quantitative explanation for the protection by FXa has recently been given, since both APC and FXa bind with similar affinity to similar/overlapping binding regions on the surface of FVa and thus are in direct competition for complex formation with FVa (Nicolaes et al, 2010). Interesting in this respect is the observation that APC, when bound to FVa can completely but reversibly inhibit the activity of FVa, even in the absence of irreversible cleavage of FVa by APC (Nicolaes et al, 2010).

APC-mediated cleavages in FVIIIa occur at Arg336-Met337 and Arg562-Gly563 (Fay et al, 1991) and are, like is the case for FVa, not ordered but rather determined by kinetic parameters and local concentrations of FVIIIa, APC and other proteins that may modify the reaction kinetics (Fig. 4, upper grey arrows). This means that Arg336 is usually cleaved first and, very similar to FVa, a secondary cleavage at Arg562 is required for a complete loss of activity (Varfaj et al, 2006; Gale et al., 2008). The relevance of APC-catalyzed inactivation of FVIIIa is not undisputed since, in contrast to FVa, FVIIIa is not stable and its activity is subject to rapid decay caused by dissociation of the A2 domain from the rest of the molecule. Note that FVIIIa is a heterotrimer, with the A1 domain being separated from the

A2 domain. It has been estimated that the majority of FVIIIa activity (70-80%) is lost spontaneously (Lollar et al, 1990).
Moreover, the affinity of APC for FVIIIa was estimated to be ~100-fold lower than the affinity of APC for FVa (Nicolaes et al, 2010), which may indicate the lesser importance of APC-catalyzed FVIIIa inactivation, especially if the 100-fold lower plasma concentration of FVIII, as compared to FV, is taken into account. When FVIIIa is incorporated in the tenase complex however, FVIIIa is much more stable and a role for FVIIIa regulation by APC becomes more evident. Like is the case for FVa, when incorporated in the prothrombinase complex, FVIIIa is protected from APC-catalyzed inactivation not only by increased stability of the FVIIIa heavy chain, FIXa and FX have been reported to selectively protect FVIIIa from cleavage at Arg336 and Arg562 (O'Brien et al, 2000).
APC-catalyzed FVIIIa inactivation is specifically enhanced by the synergistic cofactors protein S and FV. In FVIIIa, cleavage at Arg562 is most pronouncedly enhanced in the presence of protein S, though FV and protein S stimulate both APC cleavage sites in FVIIIa (Shen & Dahlbäck, 1994; Varadi et al, 1996; Lu et al, 1996; Gale et al, 2008). Resultingly, when both protein S and FV are present, cleavage at Arg336 and Arg562 occurs at similar rates in FVIIIa (Gale et al., 2008).

5. APC resistance: First observations

In 1993, a first report (Dahlbäck et al, 1993) was published in which three different families were described that presented an abnormal anticoagulant response to APC when the plasma of family members was tested in a classical activated partial thromboplastin time (APTT) . In the plasma of normal individuals a prolongation of the APTT will occur when APC is added. However, for certain family members of the families studied, this prolongation was observed to be much less than for other family members or normal controls. The plasmas showed a poor response to APC and the term "APC resistance" was coined. APC resistance was found to be an inheritable trait that was hypothesized to be caused by a defective function of a hitherto unknown cofactor to APC (Dahlbäck & Hildebrand, 1994). A surprisingly large proportion of thrombophilic patients, vz. 20-60%, proofed to be resistant to APC and thus the new discovery attracted broad scientific interest (Griffin et al, 1993; Koster et al, 1993; Svensson & Dahlbäck, 1994; Halbmayer et al, 1994).
To discover a molecular mechanism for APC resistance, attempts were made to isolate the unknown cofactor from normal plasma and this revealed that this factor was FV (Dahlbäck & Hildebrand, 1994). Addition of FV to an APC resistant plasma sample could normalize the response to APC. This was the first evidence that FV is not only a procoagulant protein, but these experiments established FV as well as an anticoagulant protein. Soon after, the involvement of the FV gene was confirmed. In 1994 several research groups succeeded simultaneously in the identification of the molecular cause for APC resistance by a thorough study of the FV gene of APC resistant individuals. The cause was identified as a single nucleotide polymorphism (SNP) at position 1691 which codes for a missense mutation at Arg506, replacing the arginine by glutamine, exactly at one of the APC cleavage sites in FVa. The FV gene containing the Arg506 mutation was since then described as FVLeiden, FVR506Q or FV:Q506. (Bertina et al, 1994; Zöller et al, 1994; Voorberg et al, 1994; Greengard et al, 1994).
With a genetic cause unveiled and relatively easy DNA sequencing technologies becoming increasingly available, the allelic frequencies of the FVLeiden mutation was studied in

various patient and ethnic populations. The FVLeiden mutation was found in ~95% of families with APC resistance, which makes FVLeiden the major cause of hereditary APC resistance (Zöller et al, 1994). The FVLeiden mutation is very common in general populations though it is found exclusively in populations of Caucasian descent (~5% of Europeans are carrier of the mutation) and the high prevalence implied that, at the time, inherited APC resistance was 10 times more prevalent than the sum of all other hereditary causes of thrombophilia known (Rees et al, 1995, 1996). The FVLeiden mutation is known as the most common hereditary causal factor for thrombosis, by virtue of the APC resistance it causes in its carriers.

6. The molecular basis of FVLeiden related APC resistance

The role that the FVLeiden mutation, i.e. the replacement of arginine by a glutamine at position 506, has in the etiology of APC resistance been well studied. Several mechanisms contribute to the explanation of the prothrombotic tendency that is present in carriers of the mutation. First, given that the mutation abrogates the preferred mutation at Arg506, this means that one of the prime APC cleavage sites is lost in FVaLeiden. The absence of a cleavage site will impair efficient downregulation of procoagulant FVa activity (Kalafatis et al, 1994, Nicolaes et al, 1995). Second, it was discovered that for FV to act as a cofactor in the APC-catalyzed inactivation of FVIIIa, it must not be cleaved by thrombin (more precisely, the C-terminal region of the B domain must be intact) and furthermore, FV should be cleavable at Arg506 (Thorelli et al, 1998, 1999). This implies that FVLeiden, is not a cofactor in the inactivation of FVIIIa by APC, since it cannot be transformed into an anticoagulant molecule (Varadi et al, 1996). Third, it was found that APC also possesses a proteolysis-independent anticoagulant activity (Gale et al, 1997; Nicolaes et al, 2010). By virtue of its binding to FVa, thereby effectively competing with FXa for prothrombinase complex formation, APC is able to down-regulate thrombin formation in the absence of FVa cleavage. It was estimated that the non-enzymatic anticoagulant effect accounts for ~6% of the overall APC activity. In the case of FVaLeiden however, APC is not able to bind to the FVa region around the most favored cleavage site at Arg506 and consequently APC cannot regulate the activity of FVaLeiden via the proteolysis-independent mechanism.

Taken together, the FVLeiden mutation has an effect both on the inactivation of FVa and of FVIIIa, the two cofactors that are essential to thrombin formation, and the inactivation of which was shown to be both contributing to APC resistance in the plasma of FVLeiden carriers (Castoldi et al, 2004).

The *in vivo* effects of FVLeiden are perhaps most strikingly illustrated in the APC resistance phenotype that is observed in the plasma of so-called pseudo-homozygous APC resistant individuals. The individuals are genotyped as heterozygous FVLeiden carriers. However, their phenotype is that of a homozygous FVLeiden carrier. Due to a null-mutation in their normal FV allele, the normal FV is lacking in these individuals and only the FVLeiden allele is expressed (at ~50% of a normal FV level). The associated thrombosis risk in pseudo-homozygotes is in the same range as that of homozygous carriers of the FVLeiden mutation (50- to 80-fold increased). When purified FV is however added to pseudohomozygous plasma, the response to APC is corrected such that it will reach the same range as that of heterozygous carriers of the FVLeiden mutation. Heterozygous carriers however have an associated risk of thrombosis that is ~5-fold higher than normals. The increased risk of thrombosis in homozygous and pseudohomozygous carriers of the FVLeiden mutation therefore appears not so much to be caused by a defect in the FVLeiden that is present, more likely it illustrates the absence of the anticoagulant normal FV (Simioni et al, 1996, 2005; Castoldi et al., 2004; Brugge et al, 2005).

7. Modifiers of the APC resistance phenotype

The discovery of the FVLeiden mutation boosted the research into APC resistance and APC resistance as such was established as an indepent risk factor for thrombosis (de Visser et al, 1999) even when the FVLeiden mutation was not present. Research showed that in 10-15% of individuals who are APC resistant (as determined via an APTT-based assay), the FVLeiden mutation is not present (Taralunga et al, 2004; Tosetto et al, 2004). This implies that besides FVLeiden, other factors exist that may modify the outcome of an APC resistance assay. These modifying factors of the APC resistance phenotype can be roughly divided into genetic and acquired factors and of the genetic factors, those that originate from the FV gene have been best studied.

Important to mention is the fact that, since APC resistance is diagnosed according to the function of APC in plasma, the very test that is used to determine the presence of APC resistance is of influence as to whether a certain individual is described as APC resistant or normal. This is illustrated by the observation that in the endogenous thrombin potential (ETP) -based APC resistance assay (Nicolaes et al, 1997), most of the non-FVLeiden APC resistant samples are caused by an abnormal female hormonal status (as in pregnancy, hormone replacement therapy or oral contraceptive (OC) use) (Rosing et al, 1997; Curvers et al, 2002). In the APTT-based APC resistance assays other factors besides OC use and pregnancy were found to be prevalent among cases on non-FVLeiden APC resistance. These include high FVIII levels, elevated prothrombin levels, malignancy and the presence of lupus anticoagulants (Henkens et al, 1995; Cumming et al, 1995; Laffan & Manning, 1996; Aznar et al, 1997; Tosetto et al, 1997; de Visser et al, 1999; Castaman et al, 2001; Tosetto et al, 2004; Taralunga et al, 2004; Sarig et al, 2005).

Several allelic variants of the FV gene have been described that contribute to the APC resistance phenotype and to venous thrombosis. FV Cambridge (Williamson et al, 1998) and FV Hong Kong (Chan et al, 1998) were both discovered in thrombosis patients. One of the predominant APC cleavage sites, at Arg306, is replaced in both these FV variants as a result of a missense mutation in the FV gene. In FV Cambridge Arg306 is replaced by Thr, and in FV Hong Kong Arg306 is replaced by a Gly residue. Interestingly, whereas FV Cambridge was discovered in the plasma of an individual with unexplained APC resistance, FV Hong Kong was not associated with APC resistance. This phenotypic difference has thus far not been explained. Investigations with recombinant FV variants that mimic FV Hong Kong and FV Cambridge have shown that both recombinant FV variants have only a slightly decreased APC response in a plasma system with an *in vitro* APC resistance phenotype being intermediate between those of normal FV and FVLeiden (Norstrom et al, 2002). Epidemiological studies have shown that FV Hong Kong is not a risk factor for venous thrombosis whereas more data on the rare FV Cambridge condition are needed to establish whether or not this FV genotype is associated with venous thrombosis.

The FV2 haplotype is characterized by several linked mutations (both missense and silent) in exons 4,8,13, 16, and 25 of the gene for FV associated with slightly reduced FV levels. It has a high incidence in the general population (10-15%) (Bernardi et al, 1997; de Visser et al, 2000). Especially when present in combination with FVLeiden, R2 FV may enhance the APC resistance phenotype (the majority of circulating FV will be FVLeiden) and increase the risk of thrombosis (Faioni et al, 1999) Moreover, carriers of the R2 allele seem to have increased amounts of FV1 in their plasma (Castoldi et al, 2000; Hoekema et al, 2001). FV1 is a glycosylation isoform of FV that may be more thrombogenic than the other isoform, FV2 (Hoekema et al, 1997). Where the reduced FV levels in R2 FV carriers can be attributed to the Asp2194Gly mutation (Yamazaki et al, 2002, 2010) it remains questionable whether the R2 FV molecule itself is APC resistant.

Another FV-related cause for APC resistance is the so-called FVLiverpool. In this variant, which was found in two related individuals with severe thrombosis at a young age, Ile359 has been replaced by Thr (Mumford et al, 2003; Steen et al, 2004). This missense mutation introduces a novel site for N-linked glycosylation at Asn357. Due to the presence of an extra glycan structure, APC-catalyzed inactivation at Arg306 is hampered by steric hindrance. Like in the case of FVLeiden, FVLiverpool is not active as a cofactor to APC in the APC-catalyzed inactivation of FVIIIa such that the mutation affects both inactivation of FVa and FVIIIa.

Besides these mentioned mutated FV variants, also autoantibodies have been reported to be associated with APC resistance. In three cases, these antibodies were directed against FV (Ortel, 1999), however also antibodies against protein S (Nojima et al, 2009) and APC (Zivelin et al, 1999) have been described in this context. An exact causal mechanism for the thrombosis in these cases is not known, but may involve the broader context of an anti-phospholipid syndrome. In addition, the coverage of epitopes on the surface of FV, that are in particular important for the FV anticoagulant functions, have been suggested.

Given that APC resistance is diagnosed from plasma samples and knowing that human plasma contains many proteins that contribute to the functional assay outcome, it will be conceivable that APC resistance as such cannot be attributable to a single cause. Whether or not acquired factors such as pregnancy, malignancy, oral contraceptives or hormone replacement are involved, a final outcome of the interaction of genetic and acquired factors is the potential change of several important coagulation factors. A change in the level of these coagulation factors, and in particular, prothrombin, protein S, FVIII or tissue factor pathway inhibitor (TFPI) may influence assay outcome and render a plasma sample APC resistant (de Visser et al, 2005).

8. Genetic and acquired interactions determine thrombosis risks

Given that thrombosis is a multi-factorial disease, several factors can work in concert so as to disturb the haemostatic balance (Seligsohn & Zivelin, 1997; Rosendaal, 1999). Whether or not the presence of APC resistance, with its high prevalence in the general population, will result in a thrombosis, is dependent on the interplay between the various factors that influence the haemostatic balance in an individual (Martinelli, 2001). The contribution of inherited risk factors to the total risk for thrombosis development was estimated over 60%, and of these, the FVleiden mutation is considered the most important by virtue of its very high prevalence.

Risk factors may show synergism in the events that cause a thromboembolic episode as was concluded from several studies where it was found that the prevalence of the FVLeiden mutation was much higher in thrombotic families with antithrombin, protein C or protein S deficiencies or with the HR2 haplotype or the prothrombin G20210A mutation, than in the general population. Not only is the prevalence of the FVLeiden mutation higher than

expected, also the combined risks for thrombosis in these families are much higher than what would be concluded from the sum of the risks associated with the single thrombophilic defects present (Koeleman et al, 1995; Gandrille et al, 1995; van Boven et al, 1999; Faioni et al, 1999; Salomon et al, 1999).
Not only gene-gene, also gene-environment (which is interpreted as interactions between a genetically determined risk factor and an acquired risk factor) contribute significantly to the overall risk for thrombosis. This type of interaction includes interactions between FVLeiden and the antiphospholipid syndrome (Simantov et al, 1996), or those between FVLeiden and long-distance travel or immobilization (Cannegieter et al, 2006; Schreijer et al, 2010).

group		**Risk***	**RR**
FVLeiden	OC use		
no	no	0.8	1.0
no	yes	3.0	3.7
yes	no	5.7	6.9
yes	yes	28.5	34.7

*Indicated are annual thrombosis risks (Risk) per 10,000 individuals and the related relative risk (RR) the data were obtained from Vandenbroucke et al, 1994

Table 1. Interaction between carriership of the FVLeiden mutation and OC use

The most studied interaction however, in this respect, is that between carriership of the FVLeiden mutation and the use of oral contraceptives (OC) (Vandenbroucke et al, 1994, 2001; Wu et al, 2005; van Hylckama Vlieg, 2009). Given the world-wide use of OC, this is an interaction of great importance. As is illustrated by Table 1, the relative risk for thrombosis is ~ 5 fold higher in FVLeiden carriers who use OC than in those who do not use OC. Interaction between the risk factors, both having effects on the protein C anticoagulant system, is the likely cause for the overall multiplicative risk which is higher than the sum of the individual risks. This is illustrated by the various changes in coagulation parameters that have been associated to the use of OC or pregnancy: lowering of protein S, rise in prothrombin levels, lowering of FV levels, rise in FVIII levels, a rise in the levels of FIX and FX and a decrease in the TFPI levels. Each of these changes can have an effect on the coagulability of the blood (Tchaikovsky & Rosing, 2010), which overall changes the APC resistance phenotype.

9. Conclusion

The protein C pathway is vital for a normal haemostatic balance in that it down-regulates thrombin formation by inactivation of the non-enzymatic cofactor molecules of the prothrombinase en tenase complex. Resistance to APC, or "APC resistance", is a functional defect of the protein C anticoagulant pathway, characterized by a reduced responsiveness of plasma to the addition of APC. Several factors, both genetic or acquired, can act in concert and result in an APC resistant phenotype. In a great majority of cases, the presence of the FVLeiden, a widespread hereditary variation of the gene product of FV, is involved. FVLeiden contributes to APC resistance in multiple ways, affecting both the inactivation of FVa and of FVIIIa. Given its high penetrance in the general population, the simultaneous occurrence of FVLeiden and other risk factors for thrombosis is common. Knowledge about the interactions between various risk factors and the underlying mechanisms that result in the onset of thrombosis is vital to our understanding, diagnosis and treatment of thrombosis.

10. References

Anderson, FA, Jr., HB Wheeler, RJ Goldberg, DW Hosmer, NA Patwardhan, B Jovanovic, A Forcier, and JE Dalen. (1991) A population-based perspective of the hospital incidence and case- fatality rates of deep vein thrombosis and pulmonary embolism. The Worcester DVT Study. *Arch Intern Med,* 151(5): p. 933-8

Aznar J, Villa P, España F, Estellés A, Grancha S, Falcó C. (1997) APC resistance phenotype in patients with antiphospholipid antibodies *J Lab Clin Med,* 130(2):202-8

Bakker HM, Tans G, Janssen-Claessen T, Thomassen MC, Hemker HC, Griffin JH, Rosing J. (1992) The effect of phospholipids, calcium ions and protein S on rate constants of human FVa inactivation by activated human protein C. *Eur J Biochem,* 208(1):171-8

Barhoover MA, Kalafatis M. (2011) Cleavage at both Arg306 and Arg506 is required and sufficient for timely and efficient inactivation of factor Va by activated protein C. *Blood Coagul Fibrinolysis,* 22(4):317-24

Bernardi F, Faioni EM, Castoldi E, Lunghi B, Castaman G, Sacchi E, Mannucci PM. (1997) A factor V genetic component differing from factor V R506Q contributes to the activated protein C resistance phenotype. *Blood,*90(4):1552-7

Bertina, RM, BPC. Koeleman, T Koster, FR Rosendaal, RJ Dirven, H De Ronde, PA Van der Velden, and PH Reitsma. (1994) Mutation in blood coagulation factor V associated with resistance to activated protein C. *Nature,* 369: p. 64-67

Bertina, RM. (2001) Genetic aspects of venous thrombosis. *Eur J Obstet Gynecol Reprod Biol.* 95(2): p. 189-92

Boekholdt SM, Kramer MH. (2007) Arterial thrombosis and the role of thrombophilia, *Semin Thromb Hemost,* 33(6):588-96

Borissoff JI, Spronk HM, ten Cate H (2011) The hemostatic system as a modulator of atherosclerosis. *N Engl J Med,* 364(18):1746-60

van Boven HH, Vandenbroucke JP, Briet E, Rosendaal FR. (1999) Gene-gene and gene-environment interactions determine risk of thrombosis in families with inherited antithrombin deficiency. *Blood,* 94(8):2590-2594

O'Brien LM, Mastri M, Fay PJ. (2000) Regulation of FVIIIa by human activated protein C and protein S: inactivation of cofactor in the intrinsic factor Xase, *Blood,* 95(5):1714-20

Brugge JM, Simioni P, Bernardi F, Tormene D, Lunghi B, Tans G, Pagnan A, Rosing J, Castoldi E. (2005) Expression of the normal FV allele modulates the APC resistance phenotype in heterozygous carriers of the FV Leiden mutation, *J Thromb Haemost,* 3(12):2695-702

Cannegieter SC, Doggen CJ, van Houwelingen HC, Rosendaal FR. (2006) Travel-related venous thrombosis: results from a large population-based case control study (MEGA study), *PLoS Med,* 3(8):e307

Castaman G, Tosetto A, Simioni M, Ruggeri M, Madeo D, Rodeghiero F. (2001) Phenotypic APC resistance in carriers of the A20210 prothrombin mutation is associated with an increased risk of venous thrombosis, *Thromb Haemost,* 86(3):804-8

Castoldi E, Rosing J, Girelli D, Hoekema L, Lunghi B, Mingozzi F, Ferraresi P, Friso S, Corrocher R, Tans G, Bernardi F. (2000) Mutations in the R2 FV gene affect the ratio between the two FV isoforms in plasma. *Thromb Haemost*, 83:362–365

Castoldi E, Brugge JM, Nicolaes GAF, Girelli D, Tans G, Rosing J. (2004) Impaired APC cofactor activity of factor V plays a major role in the APC resistance associated with the factor V Leiden (R506Q) and R2 (H1299R) mutations. *Blood*, 103(11):4173-9

Chan WP, Lee CK, Kwong YL, Lam CK, Liang R. (1998) A novel mutation of Arg306 of factor V gene in Hong Kong Chinese. *Blood*, 91:1135–1139

Cramer TJ, Griffin JH, Gale AJ. (2010) Factor V is an anticoagulant cofactor for activated protein C during inactivation of factor Va, *Pathophysiol Haemost Thromb*, 37(1):17-23

Cumming AM, Tait RC, Fildes S, Yoong A, Keeney S, Hay CR. (1995) Development of resistance to activated protein C during pregnancy. *Br J Haematol*, 90(3):725-7

Curvers J, Thomassen MC, Rimmer J, Hamulyak K, van der Meer J, Tans G, Preston FE, Rosing J. (2002) Effects of hereditary and acquired risk factors of venous thrombosis on a thrombin generation-based APC resistance test. *Thromb Haemost*, 88(1):5-11

Dahlbäck, B., M. Carlsson, and P.J. Svensson. (1993) Familial thrombophilia due to a previously unrecognized mechanism characterized by poor anticoagulant response to activated protein C: Prediction of a cofactor to activated protein C. *Proc.Natl.Acad.Sci.USA*, 90: p. 1004-1008

Dahlbäck, B and B Hildebrand. (1994) Inherited resistance to activated protein C is corrected by anticoagulant cofactor activity found to be a property of factor V. *Proc.Natl.Acad.Sci.USA*, 91: p. 1396-1400

Dahlbäck, B and J Stenflo. (1994) A natural anticoagulant pathway: protein C,S, C4b-binding protein and thrombomodulin, in *Haemostasis and Thrombosis*, A.L. Bloom, et al., Editors. 1994, Tokyo. p. 671-698, Churchill Livingstone: Edinburgh

Dahlbäck, B. (2000) Blood coagulation. *Lancet*, 355(9215): p. 1627-32

Dahlbäck B, Villoutreix BO. (2005) Regulation of blood coagulation by the protein C anticoagulant pathway: novel insights into structure-function relationships and molecular recognition. *Arterioscler Thromb Vasc Biol*, 25(7):1311-1320

van Dieijen, G, G Tans, J Rosing, and HC Hemker. (1981) The role of phospholipid and factor VIIIa in the activation of bovine factor X. *J Biol Chem*, 256(7): p. 3433-42

Dreyfus, M, JF Magny, F Bridey, HP Schwarz, C Planche, M Dehan, and G Tchernia. (1991) Treatment of homozygous protein C deficiency and neonatal purpura fulminans with a purified protein C concentrate. *N Engl J Med*, 325(22): p. 1565-8

Dreyfus, M, M Masterson, M David, GE Rivard, FM Muller, W Kreuz, T Beeg, A Minford, J Allgrove, JD Cohen, and et al., (1995) Replacement therapy with a monoclonal antibody purified protein C concentrate in newborns with severe congenital protein C deficiency. *Semin Thromb Hemost*, 21(4): p. 371-81

Duckers C, Simioni P, Rosing J, Castoldi E (2009) Advances in understanding the bleeding diathesis in factor V deficiency. *Br J Haematol*, 146(1):17-26

Egan, JO, M Kalafatis, and KG Mann. (1997) The Effect Of Arg(306)] Ala And Arg(506)] Gln Substitutions In The Inactivation Of Recombinant Human Factor Va By Activated Protein C And Protein S. *Protein Science*, 6(9): p. 2016-2027

Esmon, C.T. (2001) Role of coagulation inhibitors in inflammation. *Thromb Haemost*, 86(1): p. 51-6

Faioni EM, Franchi F, Bucciarelli P, Margaglione M, De Stefano V, Castaman G, Finazzi G, Mannucci PM. (1999) Coinheritance of the HR2 haplotype in the factor V gene confers an increased risk of venous thromboembolism to carriers of factor V R506Q (factor V Leiden). *Blood*, 94:3062–3066

Fay, PJ, Coumans JV, and Walker FJ. (1991) von Willebrand factor mediates protection of factor VIII from activated protein C-catalyzed inactivation. *J Biol Chem*, 266(4): 2172-7

Folsom AR, Rosamond WD, Shahar E, Cooper LS, Aleksic N, Nieto FJ, Rasmussen ML, Wu KK. (1999) Prospective study of markers of hemostatic function with risk of ischemic stroke. The Atherosclerosis Risk in Communities (ARIC) Study Investigators. *Circulation*, 100(7):736-42

Fuentes-Prior P, Iwanaga Y, Huber R, Pagila R, Rumennik G, Seto M, Morser J, Light DR, Bode W. (2000) Structural basis for the anticoagulant activity of the thrombin-thrombomodulin complex. *Nature*, 404(6777):518-525

Fukudome, K and CT Esmon (1994) Identification, cloning, and regulation of a novel endothelial cell protein C/activated protein C receptor. *J Biol Chem*, 269: p. 26486-26491

Gale AJ, Sun X, Heeb MJ, Griffin JH. (1997) Nonenzymatic anticoagulant activity of the mutant serine protease Ser360Ala-activated protein C mediated by factor Va. *Protein Sci*. 6(1):132-40.

Gale AJ, Cramer TJ, Rozenshteyn D, Cruz JR. (2008) Detailed mechanisms of the inactivation of factor VIIIa by activated protein C in the presence of its cofactors, protein S and factor V. *J Biol Chem*, 283(24):16355-62

Gandrille S, Greengard JS, Alhenc-Gelas M, Juhan-Vague I, Abgrall JF, Jude B, Griffin JH, Aiach M. (1995) Incidence of activated protein C resistance caused by the ARG 506 GLN mutation in factor V in 113 unrelated symptomatic protein C-deficient patients. The French Network on the behalf of INSERM. *Blood*, 86(1):219-224

Govers-Riemslag JW, Castoldi E, Nicolaes GAF, Tans G, Rosing J. Thromb Haemost. 2002 Sep;88(3):444-9. Reduced factor V concentration and altered FV1/FV2 ratio do not fully explain R2-associated APC-resistance

Greengard, JS, X Sun, X Xu, JA Fernández, JH Griffin, and B Evatt. (1994) Activated protein C resistance caused by Arg506Gln mutation in factor Va. *Lancet*, 343: p. 1361-1362

Griffin, JH, B Evatt, C Wideman, and JA Fernandez. (1993) Anticoagulant protein C pathway defective in majority of thrombophilic patients. *Blood*, 82(7): p. 1989-1993

Halbmayer, WM, A Haushofer, R Schon, and M Fischer. (1994) The prevalence of poor anticoagulant response to activated protein C (APC resistance) among patients suffering from stroke or venous thrombosis and among healthy subjects. *Blood Coagul Fibrinolysis*, 5(1): p. 51-7

Hankey GJ, Eikelboom JW, van Bockxmeer FM, Lofthouse E, Staples N, Baker RI. (2001) Inherited thrombophilia in ischemic stroke and its pathogenic subtypes. *Stroke*, 32(8):1793-9

Hayward CP, Furmaniak-Kazmierczak E, Cieutat AM, Moore JC, Bainton DF, Nesheim ME, Kelton JG, Côté G. (1995) Factor V is complexed with multimerin in resting platelet lysates and colocalizes with multimerin in platelet alpha-granules. *J Biol Chem*. 270(33):19217-24

Henkens CM, Bom VJ, Seinen AJ, van der Meer J. (1995) Sensitivity to activated protein C; influence of oral contraceptives and sex. *Thromb Haemost*. 73(3):402-4

Hoekema, L, GAF Nicolaes, HC Hemker, G Tans, and J Rosing. (1997) Human Factor Va1 and Factor Va2: Properties in the procoagulant and anticoagulant pathways. *Biochemistry*, 36(11): p. 3331-3335

Hoekema L, Castoldi E,Tans G, Girelli D, Gemmati D, Bernardi F, Rosing J. (2001) Functional properties of factor V and factor Va encoded by the R2-gene. *Thromb Haemost* 85:75–81 85

Huang M, Furie BC, Furie B. (2004) Crystal structure of the calcium-stabilized human factor IX Gla domain bound to a conformation-specific anti-factor IX antibody. *J Biol Chem*. 279(14):14338-46

van Hylckama Vlieg A, Helmerhorst FM, Vandenbroucke JP, Doggen CJ, Rosendaal FR. (2009) The venous thrombotic risk of oral contraceptives, effects of oestrogen dose and progestogen type: results of the MEGA case-control study. *BMJ*. 339:b2921

Jeimy SB, Fuller N, Tasneem S, Segers K, Stafford AR, Weitz JI, Camire RM, Nicolaes GAF, Hayward CP. (2008) Multimerin 1 binds factor V and activated factor V with high affinity and inhibits thrombin generation, *Thromb Haemost*, 100(6):1058-67

Kalafatis, M, MD Rand, and KG Mann. (1994) The mechanism of inactivation of human factor V and human factor Va by activated protein C. *J Biol Chem*, 269: p. 31869-31880

Kane, WH and PW Majerus. (1981) Purification and characterization of human coagulation factor V. *J Biol Chem*, 256: p. 1002-1007

Kane WH, Devore-Carter D, Ortel TL. (1990) Expression and characterization of recombinant human factor V and a mutant lacking a major portion of the connecting region. *Biochemistry*, 29:6762–8

Keller FG, Ortel TL, Quinn-Allen MA, Kane WH. (1995) Thrombin-catalyzed activation of recombinant human factor V. *Biochemistry*, 34:4118–24

Kim, SW, TL Ortel, MA Quinn-Allen, L Yoo, L Worfolk, X Zhai, BR Lentz, and WH Kane. (1999) Partial glycosylation at asparagine-2181 of the second C-type domain of human factor V modulates assembly of the prothrombinase complex. *Biochemistry*, 38(35): p. 11448-54

Koeleman BP, van Rumpt D, Hamulyak K, Reitsma PH, Bertina RM. (1995) Factor V Leiden: an additional risk factor for thrombosis in protein S deficient families? *Thromb Haemost*, 74(2):580-583

Koster, T, FR Rosendaal, H De Ronde, E Briët, JP Vandenbroucke, and RM Bertina. (1993) Venous thrombosis due to a poor anticoagulant response to activated protein C: Leiden Thrombophilia Study. *Lancet*, 342: p. 1503-1506

Laffan MA, Manning R. (1996) The influence of factor VIII on measurement of activated protein C resistance. *Blood Coagul Fibrinolysis*, 7(8):761-5

Lane DA, Caso R. (1989) Antithrombin: structure, genomic organization, function and inherited deficiency. *Baillieres Clin Haematol*, 2(4):961-998

Lollar P, Hill-Eubanks DC, Parker CG. (1988) Association of the factor VIII light chain with von Willebrand factor. *J Biol Chem*, 263(21):10451-5

Lollar, P and CG Parker. (1990) pH-dependent denaturation of thrombin-activated porcine factor VIII. *J Biol Chem*, 265(3): p. 1688-92

Lu D, Kalafatis M, Mann KG, Long GL. (1996) Comparison of activated protein C/protein S-mediated inactivation of human factor VIII and factor V. *Blood*, 87(11):4708-17

Martinelli I. (2001) Risk factors in venous thromboembolism. *Thromb Haemost*, 86(1):395-403

Maurissen LF, Thomassen MC, Nicolaes GAF, Dahlbäck B, Tans G, Rosing J, Hackeng TM. (2008) Re-evaluation of the role of the protein S-C4b binding protein complex in activated protein C-catalyzed factor Va-inactivation. *Blood*, 111(6):3034-41

Monkovic, D and P Tracy. (1990) Activation of Human Factor V by Factor Xa and Thrombin. *Biochemistry*, 29: p. 1118-1128

Mumford AD, McVey JH, Morse CV, Gomez K, Steen M, Norstrom EA, Tuddenham EG, Dahlbäck B, Bolton-Maggs PH. (2003) Factor V I359T: a novel mutation associated with thrombosis and resistance to activated protein C. *Br J Haematol*, 123(3):496-501

Nesheim, ME, JB Taswell, and KG Mann. (1979) The contribution of bovine Factor V and Factor Va to the activity of prothrombinase. *J Biol Chem*, 254(21): p. 10952-62

Nicolaes GAF, Tans G, Thomassen MC, Hemker HC, Pabinger I, Varadi K, Schwarz HP, Rosing J. (1995) Peptide bond cleavages and loss of functional activity during inactivation of FVa and FVaR506Q by APC. *J Biol Chem*, 270(36):21158-66

Nicolaes GAF, Thomassen MC, Tans G, Rosing J, Hemker HC. (1997) Effect of activated protein C on thrombin generation and on the thrombin potential in plasma of normal and APC-resistant individuals. *Blood Coagul Fibrinolysis*, 8(1):28-38

Nicolaes GAF, Villoutreix BO, Dahlbäck B. (1999) Partial glycosylation of Asn2181 in human factor V as a cause of molecular and functional heterogeneity. Modulation of glycosylation efficiency by mutagenesis of the consensus sequence for N-linked glycosylation. *Biochemistry*, 38(41):13584-91

Nicolaes GAF, Dahlbäck B. (2002) Factor V and thrombotic disease: description of a Janus-faced protein. *Arterioscler Thromb Vasc Biol*, 22(4):530-8

Nicolaes GAF, Bock PE, Segers K, Wildhagen KC, Dahlbäck B, Rosing J. (2010) Inhibition of thrombin formation by active site mutated (S360A) activated protein C. *J Biol Chem*, 23;285(30):22890-900

Nojima J, Iwatani Y, Ichihara K, Tsuneoka H, Ishikawa T, Yanagihara M, Takano T, Hidaka Y. (2009) Acquired APC resistance is associated with IgG antibodies to protein S in patients with systemic lupus erythematosus. *Thromb Res*, 124(1):127-31

Nordstrom, M., B. Lindblad, D. Bergqvist, and T. Kjellstrom. (1992) A prospective study of the incidence of deep-vein thrombosis within a defined urban population. *J Intern Med*, 232(2): p. 155-60

Norstrøm E, Thorelli E, Dahlbäck B. (2002) Functional characterization of recombinant FV Hong Kong and FV Cambridge. *Blood*, 100(2):524-530

Norstrøm EA, Tran S, Steen M, Dahlbäck B. (2006) Effects of factor Xa and protein S on the individual activated protein C-mediated cleavages of coagulation factor Va. *J Biol Chem*. 281(42):31486-94

Ortel, T.L. (1999) Clinical and laboratory manifestations of anti-factor V antibodies. *J Lab Clin Med*, 133(4): p. 326-34

Rallidis LS, Belesi CI, Manioudaki HS, Chatziioakimidis VK, Fakitsa VC, Sinos LE, Laoutaris NP, Apostolou TS. (2003) Myocardial infarction under the age of 36: prevalence of thrombophilic disorders.*Thromb Haemost*, 90(2):272-8

Rees, DC, MJ Cox, and JB Clegg. (1995) World distribution of FV Leiden. *Lancet*, 346: 1133-34

Rees DC. (1996)The population genetics of FV Leiden *Br J Haematol*. 95(4):579-86

Rosendaal, F.R. (1999) Venous thrombosis: a multicausal disease. *Lancet*, 353(9159): 1167-73

Rosendaal FR. (2005) Venous thrombosis: the role of genes, environment, and behavior. *Hematology Am Soc Hematol Educ Program*,1-12

Rosing, J, G Tans, JWP Govers-Riemslag, RFA Zwaal, and HC Hemker. (1980) The role of phospholipids and FVa in the prothrombinase complex. *J Biol Chem* , 255: p. 274-283

Rosing J, Hoekema L, Nicolaes GAF, Thomassen MC, Hemker HC, Varadi K, Schwarz HP, Tans G. (1995) Effects of protein S and FXa on peptide bond cleavages during inactivation of FVa and FVaR506Q by APC. *J Biol Chem.* 270(46):27852-8

Rosing J, Tans G, Nicolaes GAF, Thomassen MC, van Oerle R, van der Ploeg PM, Heijnen P, Hamulyak K, Hemker HC. (1997) Oral contraceptives and venous thrombosis: different sensitivities to activated protein C in women using second- and third-generation oral contraceptives. *Br J Haematol*, 97(1):233-8

Safa, O, JH Morrissey, CT Esmon, and NL Esmon. (1999) Factor VIIa/tissue factor generates a form of FV with unchanged specific activity, resistance to activation by thrombin, and increased sensitivity to activated protein C. *Biochemistry*, 38(6): p. 1829-37

Salomon O, Steinberg DM, Zivelin A, Gitel S, Dardik R, Rosenberg N, Berliner S, Inbal A, Many A, Lubetsky A, Varon D, Martinowitz U, Seligsohn U. (1999) Single and combined prothrombotic factors in patients with idiopathic venous thromboembolism: prevalence and risk assessment. *Arterioscler Thromb Vasc Biol*, 19(3):511-518

Salzman, EW and J Hirsh. (1994) The epidemiology, pathogenesis and natural history of venous thrombosis., in *Hemostasis and Thrombosis*. Basic Principles and Clinical Practice., R.W. Colman, et al., Editors., p. 1275-961994, JB Lippincott: Philadelphia

Sarig G, Michaeli Y, Lanir N, Brenner B, Haim N. Mechanisms for acquired activated protein C resistance in cancer patients. *J Thromb Haemost*. 2005 Mar;3(3):589-90

Schreijer AJ, Hoylaerts MF, Meijers JC, Lijnen HR, Middeldorp S, Büller HR, Reitsma PH, Rosendaal FR, Cannegieter SC. (2010) Explanations for coagulation activation after air travel. *J Thromb Haemost*, 8(5):971-8

Segers K, Dahlbäck B, Nicolaes GAF (2007) Coagulation factor V and thrombophilia: Background and mechanisms, *Thromb Haemost*, 98(3), 530-542

Segev A, Ellis MH, Segev F, Friedman Z, Reshef T, Sparkes JD, Tetro J, Pauzner H, David D. (2005) High prevalence of thrombophilia among young patients with myocardial infarction and few conventional risk factors, *Int J Cardiol*. 28;98(3):421-4

Seligsohn, U and A Zivelin. (1997) Thrombophilia as a multigenic disorder. *Thromb Haemost*, 78(1): p. 297-301

Shen, L and B Dahlbäck. (1994) Factor V and protein S as synergistic cofactors to activated protein C in degradation of factor VIIIa. *J Biol Chem*, 269: p. 18735-18738

Simantov R, Lo SK, Salmon JE, Sammaritano LR, Silverstein RL. (1996) Factor V Leiden increases the risk of thrombosis in patients with antiphospholipid antibodies. *Thromb Res*; 84(5):361-365

Simioni P, Scudeller A, Radossi P, Gavasso S, Girolami B, Tormene D, Girolami A. (1996) "Pseudo homozygous" APC resistance due to double heterozygous FV defects (FV Leiden mutation and type I quantitative FV defect) associated with thrombosis. *Thromb Haemost*, 75(3):422-6

Simioni P, Castoldi E, Lunghi B, Tormene D, Rosing J, Bernardi F. (2005) An underestimated combination of opposites resulting in enhanced thrombotic tendency. *Blood*. 106(7):2363-5

Smirnov MD, Safa O, Esmon NL, Esmon CT. (1999) Inhibition of activated protein C anticoagulant activity by prothrombin. *Blood*, 94(11):3839-46

Steen M, Norstrøm EA, Tholander AL, Bolton-Maggs PH, Mumford A, McVey JH, Tuddenham EG, Dahlbäck B. (2004) Functional characterization of factor V-Ile359Thr: a novel mutation associated with thrombosis. *Blood*, 103(9):3381-7

Stenflo, J. (1976) A new vitamin K-dependent protein. Purification from bovine plasma and preliminary characterization. *J Biol Chem*, 251(2): p. 355-63

Suzuki, K., B. Dahlbäck, and J. Stenflo. (1982) Thrombin-Catalyzed Activation of Human Coagulation Factor V. *J Biol Chem*, 257-11: p. 6556-6564

Svensson, PJ and B Dahlbäck (1994) Resistance to activated protein C as a basis for venous thrombosis. *N Engl J Med*, 330(8): p. 517-522

Tans, G, GAF Nicolaes, MCLGD Thomassen, HC Hemker, A-J Van Zonneveld, H Pannekoek, and J Rosing. (1994) Activation of human factor V by meizothrombin. *J Biol Chem*, 269: p. 15969-15972

Taralunga C, Gueguen R, Visvikis S, Regnault V, Sass C, Siest G, Lecompte T, Wahl D. (2004) Phenotypic sensitivity to activated protein C in healthy families: importance of genetic components and environmental factors. *Br J Haematol*, 126(3):392-7

Tchaikovski SN, Rosing J. (2010) Mechanisms of estrogen-induced venous thromboembolism. *Thromb Res*, 126(1):5-11

Thorelli E, Kaufman RJ, Dahlbäck B. (1998) The C-terminal region of the factor V B-domain is crucial for the anticoagulant activity of factor V. *J Biol Chem*, 273(26):16140-5

Thorelli E, Kaufman RJ, Dahlbäck B. (1999) Cleavage of FV at Arg 506 by activated protein C and the expression of anticoagulant activity of FV. *Blood*, 93(8):2552-8

Tosetto A, Missiaglia E, Gatto E, Rodeghiero F. (1997) The VITA project: phenotypic resistance to activated protein C and FV Leiden mutation in the general population. Vicenza Thrombophilia and Atherosclerosis. *Thromb Haemost*. 78(2):859-63

Tosetto A, Simioni M, Madeo D, Rodeghiero F. (2004) Intraindividual consistency of the activated protein C resistance phenotype. *Br J Haematol*. 126(3):405-9

Toso R, Camire RM. (2004) Removal of B-domain sequences from FV rather than specific proteolysis underlies the mechanism by which cofactor function is realized. *J Biol Chem*, 279:21643–50

Tran S, Norstrøm E, Dahlbäck B. (2008) Effects of prothrombin on the individual activated protein C-mediated cleavages of coagulation factor Va. *J Biol Chem*, 283(11):6648-55

Vandenbroucke JP, Koster T, Briet E, Reitsma PH, Bertina RM, Rosendaal FR. (1994) Increased risk of venous thrombosis in oral-contraceptive users who are carriers of factor V Leiden mutation. *Lancet*, 344(8935):1453-1457

Vandenbroucke JP, Rosing J, Bloemenkamp KW, Middeldorp S, Helmerhorst FM, Bouma BN, Rosendaal FR. (2001) Oral contraceptives and the risk of venous thrombosis. *N Engl J Med*, 344(20):1527-1535

Váradi, K., J. Rosing, G. Tans, and H.P. Schwarz. (1995) Influence of factor V and factor Va on APC-induced cleavage of human factor VIII. *Thromb.Haemost*, 73(4): p. 730-731

Váradi, K., J. Rosing, G. Tans, I. Pabinger, B. Keil, and H.P. Schwarz (1996) FV enhances the cofactor function of protein S in the APC-mediated inactivation of FVIII: influence of the FVR506Q mutation. *Thromb.Haemostas*, 76(2): p. 208-214

Varfaj F, Neuberg J, Jenkins PV, Wakabayashi H, Fay PJ. (2006) Role of P1 residues Arg336 and Arg562 in the activated-Protein-C-catalysed inactivation of Factor VIIIa. *Biochem J*, 396(2):355-62 de Visser MC, Rosendaal FR, Bertina RM. A reduced sensitivity for APC in the absence of FV Leiden increases the risk of venous thrombosis. *Blood* 1999;93(4):1271-1276

de Visser MC, Guasch JF, Kamphuisen PW, Vos HL, Rosendaal FR, Bertina RM. (2000) The HR2 haplotype of factor V: effects on factor V levels, normalized activated protein C sensitivity ratios and the risk of venous thrombosis. *Thromb Haemost.* 83(4):577-82

de Visser MC, van Hylckama Vlieg A, Tans G, Rosing J, Dahm AE, Sandset PM, Rosendaal FR, Bertina RM. (2005) Determinants of the APTT- and ETP-based APC sensitivity tests. *J Thromb Haemost*, 3(7):1488-94

Voorberg, J, JC Roelse, R Koopman, HR Büller, F Berends, JW Ten Cate, K Mertens, and JA Van Mourik. (1994) Association of idiopathic venous thromboembolism with single point-mutation at Arg506 of factor V. *Lancet*, 343: p. 1535-1536

Walker FJ. (1981) Regulation of activated protein C by protein S. The role of phospholipid in factor Va inactivation. *J Biol Chem*, 256(21):11128-31

Weiss, HJ, Sussman, II, and LW Hoyer. (1977) Stabilization of factor VIII in plasma by the von Willebrand factor. Studies on posttransfusion and dissociated factor VIII and in patients with von Willebrand's disease. *J Clin Invest*, 60(2): p. 390-404

Whelihan MF, Orfeo T, Gissel MT, Mann KG. (2010) Coagulation procofactor activation by factor XIa, *J Thromb Haemost*, 8(7):1532-9

Williamson D, Brown K, Luddington R, Baglin C, Baglin T. (1998) Factor V Cambridge: a new mutation (Arg306-->Thr) associated with resistance to activated protein C. *Blood*, 91(4):1140-4

Wu O, Robertson L, Langhorne P, Twaddle S, Lowe GD, Clark P, Greaves M, Walker ID, Brenkel I, Regan L, Greer IA. (2005) Oral contraceptives, hormone replacement therapy, thrombophilias and risk of venous thromboembolism: a systematic review. The Thrombosis: Risk and Economic Assessment of Thrombophilia Screening (TREATS) Study. *Thromb Haemost*, 94(1):17-25

World Health Organisation, Global Health Observatory 2008, Available from: http://www.who.int/gho/mortality_burden_disease/causes_death_2008/en/index.html

Yamazaki T, Nicolaes GAF, Sørensen KW, Dahlbäck B. (2002) Molecular basis of quantitative factor V deficiency associated with factor V R2 haplotype. *Blood.* 100(7):2515-21

Yamazaki T, Okada H, Balling KW, Dahlbäck B, Nicolaes GAF. (2010) The D2194G mutation is responsible for increased levels of FV1 in carriers of the factor V R2 haplotype. *Thromb Haemost.* 104(4):860-1

Ye Z, Liu EH, Higgins JP, Keavney BD, Lowe GD, Collins R, Danesh J. (2006) Seven haemostatic gene polymorphisms in coronary disease: meta-analysis of 66,155 cases and 91,307 controls. *Lancet*, 367(9511):651-8

Zivelin A, Gitel S, Griffin JH, Xu X, Fernandez JA, Martinowitz U, Cohen Y, Halkin H, Seligsohn U, Inbal A. (1999) Extensive venous and arterial thrombosis associated with an inhibitor to activated protein C. *Blood.* 94(3):895-901

Zöller B, Svensson PJ, He X, Dahlbäck B. (1994) Identification of the same factor V gene mutation in 47 out of 50 thrombosis-prone families with inherited resistance to activated protein C. *J Clin Invest*, 94(6):2521-4

Part 2

Thrombophilia and Pregnancy

6

Inherited and Acquired Thrombophilia in Pregnancy

Feroza Dawood
University of Liverpool, Liverpool Women's Hospital, United Kingdom

1. Introduction

The thrombophilia represent a spectrum of coagulation disorders associated with a predisposition for thrombotic events (deep vein thrombosis (DVT) and pulmonary embolism (PE)) (Kaandorp et al, 2009). Inherited thrombophilia include a single-point mutation on the Factor V gene (factor V Leiden (FVL), prothrombin (PT) G20210A gene mutation, deficiencies in protein C and protein S as well as antithrombin (AT) deficiency. The most entrenched acquired thrombophilia is the antiphospholipid syndrome (APS). APS is a non-inflammatory auto-immune disease characterised by thrombosis or pregnancy complications in the presence of antiphospholipid antibodies (Urbanus et al, 2008). Recognized obstetric complications include fetal loss, recurrent miscarriage, intrauterine growth restriction (IUGR), pre-eclampsia and preterm labour (Lassere and Empson, 2004). The association between the diverse group of thrombophilias and adverse pregnancy outcome has been studied for over 40 years with numerous studies identifying varying coagulation defects. A meta-analysis assessing the impact of thrombophilia and fetal loss described varying outcomes and concluded that positive or negative associations were dependent on the type of thrombophilia (Rey et al, 2003). This chapter will focus on inherited and acquired thrombophilia in pregnancy, except for the antiphospholipid syndrome, which is extensively described in other chapters.

2. Coagulation changes in normal pregnancy

During the course of normal pregnancy dramatic changes occur in the haemostatic system. Coagulation factors increase physiologically in pregnancy and this is thought to be an evolutionary mechanism to prevent excessive blood loss at childbirth (Lindqvist, 1999). Furthermore, venous stasis, venous damage, decreased fibrinolysis and decreasing concentrations of some natural anticoagulants synergistically induce a state of hypercoagulation in pregnancy. However these physiological mechanisms also increase the risk of thrombo-embolism and this risk of thrombosis is aggravated in the presence of pathological conditions that cause hypercoagulation (Stirling et al, 1984). A study of the changes in the concentrations of haemostatic components in normal pregnancy demonstrated an increase in von Willebrand factor, factors V, VII, and factor X (Clark et al, 1998). The greatest increase is usually observed in factor VIIIC, although increases in the levels of fibrinogen factors II, VII, X and XII may also be as high as 20-200%. In contrast,

endogenous anticoagulant levels increase minimally. While levels of antithrombin III and protein C remain constant there is a fall in the free and total protein S antigen.
The fibrinolytic system too, undergoes major changes to meet the haemostatic challenges during pregnancy. An increase in the levels of plasminogen, plasminogen activator antigen, and tissue plasminogen activator is evident as well (Lockwood, 2002). Simultaneously the concentration and activity of plasminogen activator-inhibitor (PAI-1) increases five-fold and an additional plasminogen activator-inhibitor (PAI-2), not generally detectable in the non-pregnant state, is produced by the plasma. These plasminogen activators ensure successive depression of fibrinolytic activity (Walker et al, 1998).

3. Thrombophilia and pregnancy

The term thrombophilia is an umbrella term for a diverse group of blood clotting disorders of the haemostatic mechanisms. The term was coined in 1965 following a Norwegian familial study of venous thrombosis (Egeberg, 1965). Simmons (1997) described thrombophilia as a disorder in which there is a predisposition to thrombosis due to abnormally, enhanced coagulation and elsewhere they are described as disorders of the coagulation systems that are likely to predispose to thrombosis (Walker et al, 2001).
Thrombophilias may be hereditary or acquired or sometimes mixed (as a result of exogenous factors for example with oestrogen use in combined oral contraceptives or hormone replacement therapy) superimposed on a genetic predisposition. It is now becoming clear that there are many genetic abnormalities that impart an increased risk for thrombophilia, and that the presence of more than one abnormality results in a further increased risk of thrombosis (Bertina R M, 1999; Rosendaal FR, 1999). Individuals who have an identifiable thrombophilic defect on laboratory testing as well as a family history of proven venous thrombosis are at greater risk of thrombosis than individuals who have a thrombophilic defect with a negative personal or family history of venous thrombosis (Lensen et al, 1996). Some genetic variants have been proven to be independent risk factors for venous thrombo-embolism. Amongst these, are Activated Protein C Resistance (APCR), protein S deficiency, protein C deficiency, prothrombin mutation (G20210A), antithrombin III deficiency, and hyperhomocysteinaemia (methylenetetrahydrofolate reductase mutation, C677T MTHFR). Patients who exhibit combinations of thrombophilias seem to be at additional risk of venous thromboembolism (Zoller et al, 1995; Van Boven et al, 1996)).

3.1 Thrombophilia and pregnancy

A successful pregnancy is dependent on the development of an adequate feto-maternal circulation, relying on adequate placental circulation. In pregnancy the pre-existence of a thrombophilic disorder may exaggerate the physiologically induced state of hypercoagulation and therefore potentiate the thrombotic risk. It has been hypothesised that thrombophilia may be associated with serious obstetric complications such as placental abruption, stillbirth, preeclampsia and recurrent miscarriage as a result of microthrombi in the placental circulation resulting in decreased uteroplacental perfusion (Gharavi et al, 2001; Dizon-Townson et al, 1997; Kupferminc et al, 1999; Coumans et al, 1999).
However, the mechanisms by which adverse pregnancy outcomes are influenced by the presence of a thrombophilia are varied and obscure. Indeed, the complex nature and pathogenesis of thrombophilia-associated pregnancy loss is poorly understood. Whilst several studies have expounded the prothrombotic theory, placental thrombosis has not

been a universal feature in several cases of pregnancy loss (Mousa et al, 2000;Sikkima et al, 2002). There is further emerging evidence that the adverse obstetric outcome may not be solely secondary to a thrombotic state, but that other pathogenetic mechanisms may aggravate the existing hypercoagulable state. Inhibition of extravillous trophoblast differentiation has been described in the presence of antiphospholipid antibodies (Quenby et al, 2005). Furthermore some invitro studies have described impaired signal transduction controlling endometrial decidualisation and impaired trophoblastic invasion (Sebire et al, 2003;Mak et al, 2003;Di Simone et al, 1999). Genetic polymorphisms and inflammatory mechanisms associated with thrombosis may also be implicated (Sebire etal, 2002).

4. Inherited thrombophilia and pregnancy

Hereditary thrombophilias may be categorised into abnormalities of the natural anticoagulant system or elevated levels of plasma activated coagulation factors.

4.1 Prothrombin gene mutation

The prothrombin gene mutation (PT) is signalled by a defect in clotting factor II at position G20210A. This mutation occurs as a result of the G→ A transition at nucleotide 20210 in the prothrombin gene. The reported prevalence in Europe is around 2 %to 6% and the risk of venous thrombosis to heterozygous carriers is three times the normal population (Poort et al, 1996). This risk may be increased during pregnancy and in the postpartum period. The PT mutation was found to be present in 17% of pregnant women who have suffered a VTE (Gerhardt et al, 2000). Women with a prior history of VTE have an increased recurrence risk during pregnancy although recurrence rates range from 0% to 15% among published studies. The risk is likely higher in women with a prior unprovoked episode and/or coexisting genetic or acquired risk factors (Kujovic, 2011).

As far as its association with pregnancy loss is concerned, several small studies reported similar frequencies in women with recurrent miscarriage compared to controls, but some documented studies have reported a statistically significant increased frequency. One of these studies report a frequency of 9% in women with recurrent miscarriage while a frequency of 2 % occurred in the control group ($p < 0.05$) (Foka et al, 2000). A second study reported a frequency of 6.7% compared to 0.8% in the control group ($p < 0.05$) (Pihusch et al, 2001). Many et al (2002), found a frequency as high as 71 % in women with fetal loss while a 30% frequency in controls.

Pooled data from seven other small studies indicate a significant association between the prothrombin gene mutation and recurrent fetal loss (Kujovic, 2004). One systematic review reported an odds ratio (OR) of 2.70 (95% CI 1.37-5.34) for recurrent miscarriage with women who were positive for the prothrombin gene mutation compared with those without (Robertson et al, 2006). The NOHA (Nîmes Obstetricians and Haematologists) first study, a large case-control study nested in a cohort of nearly 32,700 women, of whom 18% had pregnancy loss with their first gestation found on multivariate analysis a clear association between unexplained first pregnancy loss between 10 and 39 weeks gestation and heterozygosity for the prothrombin gene mutation (OR 2.60; 95% CI, 1.86–3.64 (Lissalde-Lavigne et al, 2005; Bates, 2010).

More recently, two European case-control studies found no correlation between the prothrombin gene mutation and recurrent miscarriage (Altintas et al, 2007; Serrano et al, 2010). A recent prospective cohort study of more than 4000 women concurred that there is no correlation (Silver et al, 2010). Furthermore, a meta-analyses of prospective cohort studies with a cumulative sample size of 9225 women reported a prevalence of the prothrombin gene mutation of 2.9%. A pooled odds ratio estimate of 1.13 and wide 95 % Confidence Interval of 0.64-2.01 for the association for the prothrombin gene mutation and pregnancy loss was reported. The mutation was found to have no association with pre-eclampsia (OR = 1.25, 95% CI 0.79–1.99) or for neonates deemed small for gestational age (OR 1.25, 95% CI 0.92–1.70)(Rodger et al, 2010).

4.2 Antithrombin deficiency

The antithrombin glycoprotein is synthesized in the liver and is the most important physiological inhibitor of thrombin and of the activated clotting factors of the intrinsic coagulation system. It possesses two important functional regions, namely, a heparin-binding domain and a thrombin -binding domain. Antithrombin deficiency was the first of the inherited thrombophilias to be described and is the most thrombogenic. Antithrombin I deficiency refers to a quantitative reduction in functionally normal antithrombin while type II antithrombin deficiency describes the production of a qualitatively abnormal protein. The clinical relevance of a distinction between antithrombin I and antithrombin II deficiency lies in the higher risk of thrombosis associated with the type I variety. The prevalence of type I mutations in the general population is of the order of 0.02% (Tait et al, 1993). The relative risk of venous thromboembolism is around 25 to 50 -fold for individuals with type I antithrombin deficiency (Rosendaal et al, 1999). Indeed the relative risk for venous thrombo-embolism during pregnancy in individuals who have this heritable thrombophilia is as high as 4.1(Rosendaal et al, 1999).

One study reported a significant increase in miscarriage in association with antithrombin deficiency compared to controls (22.3% versus 11.4% in controls)(Miletich, 1987). Another study demonstrated a fetal loss of between 28 to 32% in women with antithrombin III deficiency compared with 23 % in unaffected controls (Sanson et al, 1996). However no significant association between antithrombin deficiency and recurrent loss was found in other studies (Hatzis et al, 1999; Roque et al, 2004; Folkeringa et al, 2007). A Spanish retrospective study found 56% of women with antithrombin deficiency had an adverse pregnancy outcome (Robertson et al, 2006). Two women suffered a spontaneous miscarriage however no cases of recurrent pregnancy loss were observed.

Thus far there is insufficient evidence to comment positively or negatively on the relationship between antithrombin deficiency and pregnancy loss, but as it is the rarest thrombophilia, it is unlikely that it will play a major factor in adverse pregnancy outcome.

4.3 Protein C deficiency

Protein C is a naturally occurring vitamin K dependent protein that is produced in the liver. It is a key component of the protein C system. Upon activation by thrombin, a complex is formed between thrombin, thrombomodulin, protein C and protein S. Protein S functions as an important cofactor in the inhibitory effect of protein C.

The prevalence of hereditary protein C deficiency in the general population is approximately 0.2 to 0.3 % (Miletich et al, 1987). The risk of venous thrombo-embolism is increased seven to ten fold in patients with this deficiency. Two studies that examined the association between protein C deficiency and fetal loss, showed a non-significant association (Raziel et al, 2001; Gris et al, 1999).

4.4 Protein S deficiency

Protein S deficiency has a prevalence in the general population of between 0 to 0.2% (Gris et al, 1999). In a meta-analysis, protein S deficiency conferred an overall 15-fold increased risk of recurrent pregnancy loss and a 7-fold higher risk of late fetal loss (Rey et al, 2003).

4.5 Methylenetetrahydrofolate reductase deficiency and hyperhomocystinaemia

Homocysteine is metabolised by either the transsulfaration pathway (excess homocysteine is converted to methionine) or the remethylation pathway (recycling of homocysteine to form methionine). Increased homocysteine is an independent risk factor for venous thrombo-embolism (Perry, 1999). The 667 C → T MTHFR mutation results in a thermolabile enzyme with reduced activity for the remethylation of homocysteine. The homozygous form of the mutation induces a state of hyperhomocysteinaemia (Kujovic, 2004).

Hyperhomocysteinaemia has a reported prevalence of around 5 % to 16 % in the general population (Kumar et al, 2003; Raziel et al, 2001). A meta-analysis reported a 3- to 4-fold increased risk of recurrent early pregnancy loss in women with hyperhomocysteinaemia (Nelen et al, 2000(a)). Other studies have also described a high prevalence of hyperhomocysteinaemia in women with recurrent pregnancy loss (Quere et al, 1998;Nelen et al (b), 2000; Coumans et al, 1999).

4.6 Activated protein C resistance

Activated protein C resistance (APCR) is an important thrombophilic disorder. The first description of resistance to the effect of activated protein C, added to plasma from patients with a history of deep-vein thrombosis, was reported by Amer et al (1990). APCR refers to the inability to mount an effective anticoagulant response. As described previously, the clotting cascade is a complex system regulating a balance of procoagulation and anticoagulation. APCR causes prolongation of the activated partial thromboplastin time by interfering with the protein C pathway. Protein C and its cofactor substrate, protein S, are integral key components of the anticoagulation pathway. Protein C is a natural anticoagulant and limits the conversion of fibrinogen to fibrin through the degradation of factors Va and VIIIa (Dahlback, 1995; Koster et al, 1993) and activated protein C adopts a major role in the coagulation cascade.

Activated protein C normally degrades factors Va and VIIIa by proteolytic cleavage at specific arginine residues. Activated protein C is only effective when bound to its cofactor protein S. Protein S is available as a cofactor for protein C only when it is bound to C - binding protein. In the basal state, approximately forty percent of protein S is free (unbound) and thereby is available to serve as a cofactor for activated protein C. In the clotting pathway, the activated protein C/protein S complex degrades factors Va and factor VIIIa, and their loss is associated with a decrease in fibrin formation and hence a reduced ability to form a fibrin clot (Tait et al, 1993). The activated form of factor V enhances the activation of prothrombin by several thousand-fold (Nesheim et al, 1979; Rosing et al, 1980).

Blood coagulation Factor V is a large glycoprotein synthesized by the liver hepatocytes (Wilson et al 1984; Mazzorana et al, 1989) and megakaryocytes (Gerwitz et al, 1992). It has a molecular weight of 330-kd and circulates in plasma as an asymmetrical single chain. Factor V is also partially stored in platelets (Tracey et al, 1982). The gene for human factor V has been localised to chromosome 1q21-25 and spans approximately 80 kilobases of DNA and consists of 25 exons and 24 introns.

The complete complementary DNA and derived amino acid sequence of the factor V gene have already been determined (Jenny et al, 1997). Analysis of factor V cDNA has demonstrated that the protein is multidomain and contains two types of internal repeats with the following domain structure: A1-A2-B-C1-C2 (Vehar, 1984; Toole, 1984). The gene is composed of 3 homologous A-type domains, 2 smaller homologous C-type domains and a heavily glycosylated B domain that connects the N-terminal A1-A2 region with the light chain and the C-terminal A3-C1-C2 region (Rosing et al, 1997; Ajzner et al, 1999). Most changes are located in the heavily glycosylated B domain (Pittman et al, 1994). B -domain fragments derived from the activated protein C-mediated cleavage of intact factor V, have been directly implicated in the protein C anticoagulant pathway (Lu et al, 1996). Cleavage of the internal B domain occurs via limited proteolysis by thrombin, the physiological activator of factor V (Dahlback, 1980). Although Factor V and factor VIII share homologous A and C domains, the B domain of factor V is not homologous to that in factor VIII. Cleavage of the B domain from factor V results in an inert factor V. This suggests that the B domain is of vital importance in activated protein C cofactor activity, and that mutations in this domain may contribute to an impaired activated protein C response (Kostka, 2000).

Activated factor V (factor Va) is a cofactor protein in the prothrombinase complex that, together with the serine protease factor Xa, is responsible for conversion of prothrombin to the active enzyme thrombin. Activated protein C regulates the functionality of the complex by proteolytic degradation of factor Va at critical cleavage sites. Factor V itself also acts as a cofactor for activated protein C/protein S in the degradation of factor VIIIa. By degrading activated clotting factors Va and VIIIa, activated protein C functions as one of the major inhibitors of the coagulation system. When factor Va is resistant to degradation by activated protein C the anticoagulation pathway defaults, increasing the risk of thrombosis. It was later discovered that activated protein C resistance may present as a hereditary or acquired phenomenon.

4.6.1 Hereditary APCR

The first description of hereditary APCR was derived from a familial study of thrombosis in Leiden in 1993 (Dahlback et al, 1993). Dahlback and his co-workers recognised that prolongation of the activated partial thromboplastin time (APTT), by activated protein C was reported to be considerably less in a large group of patients with venous thrombosis than in a control group of healthy individuals. They termed this previously unknown thrombophilia activated protein C resistance. Subsequently a hereditary defect for activated protein C resistance was described. The molecular basis for this defect was shown to be a point mutation in the factor V gene located on chromosome 1 (1691 G→A) (Bertina et al, 1994; Greengard et al, 1994; Voorberg et al, 1994; Zoller and Dahlback, 1994). This mutation has been coined the factor V Leiden mutation (Aparicio and Dahlback, 1996; Heeb et al, 1995; Nicolaes et al, 1996).

The mutant factor V gene causes the replacement of an amino acid arginine by glycine Arg → Gln at a critical cleavage site 506, the site of the first molecular cleavage of factor Va by APC. This substitution results in diminished APC cleavage of factor Va and continued formation of thrombin by the prothrombinase complex, rendering the activated form of factor V, factor Va, less susceptible to proteolysis by activated protein C. Cleavage of this site by activated protein C is necessary for the exposure of the two additional cleavage sites needed for inactivation. The rate of inactivation is therefore slower than that of normal factor V. Thus far, the factor V Leiden mutation has been the only genetic defect for which a causal relationship to APCR has been clearly demonstrated. The existence of APCR in the absence of this mutation and the variability of the APCR phenotype in heterozygotes for the R506Q mutation suggested the possibility that alternative gene variations may be responsible for or contribute to APCR. Two other rare, low frequency factor V mutations at other arginine cleavage sites have also been identified, the factor V Hong Kong (Arg 306 Gln) (Chan et al, 1998) and the factor V Cambridge (Arg 306 Thr) (Hooper et al, 1996). Although factor V Cambridge may cause activated protein C resistance, no association exists with factor V Hong Kong. These mutations may result in APCR but the clinical association with thrombosis is less clear.

A HR 2 haplotype has been described in association with APCR. The R2 haplotype has been associated with mild APCR (both in the presence and the absence of FVL). However not all studies have been convincing regarding the role of the haplotype in clinical disease (Luddington et al, 2000). The polymorphic sites within the HR2 haplotype do not explain why the haploptype should alter APCR. The two amino acid substitutions coded by the haplotype, 1299His→Arg and 1736 Met→ Val also appear to be neutral (Soria et al, 2003). Some data suggest that the R2 allele represent a marker in linkage with an unknown defect rather than a functional polymorphism (Lunghi et al, 1996).

4.6.2 The factor V Leiden mutation

The factor V Leiden mutation has a different prevalence in distinct populations with, a founder effect about 20 000 to 34 000 years ago after the divergence of non-Africans from Africans and after the more recent divergence of Caucasians and Mongolians (Seligsohn,1997). Thus among the endogenous populations of Africa and Eastern Asia the incidence of the polymorphism is very low (Ozawa et al, 1996; Ridker et al, 1997). Chan et al,1996 reported a frequency of about 3 % to 5% in the general Caucasian population. A tabulation of the prevalence of the factor V Leiden mutation in various populations, range from 0 % to 32 % (Finan et al, 2002; Villareal et al, 2002). Other sources reveal a frequency as high as 15 % in whites (Rees et al, 1995). The mutation has a high incidence in Jews of approximately 31.2%. Perhaps the most important clinical determinant of factor V Leiden expression is the genotype (heterozygous or homozygous). This confers an approximately three to ten-fold increased risk of venous thrombosis in heterozygotes and an eighty to hundred -fold increased risk in homozygosity (Rosendaal et al, 1995). The risk of recurrent thrombosis is not yet clear. A small retrospective study found that there was no difference in the probability of recurrent thrombosis in heterozygotes compared with controls, but the risk was higher among homozygotes (Rintelen et al 1996). The thrombotic risk also increases with age, and a few studies suggest that among individuals with the factor V Leiden mutation, those with type O blood may have less risk for thrombosis than individuals with type A, B or AB blood (Gonzales et al, 1999; Robert et al, 2000). Among the population of individuals who have a family history of thrombophilia, approximately fifty percent have the factor V Leiden mutation (Griffin et al, 1993; Svensson et al, 1994). Thus, this particular mutation accounts for a significant percentage of people with a thrombotic event or a family history of thrombosis. Indeed activated protein C resistance has emerged as the commonest risk factor for venous thrombosis (Griffin et al, 1993; Koster et al, 1993; Rosendaal et al, 1995; Svensson and Dahlback, 1994).

4.6.3 Hereditary APCR (factor V Leiden) and pregnancy loss

There are several studies that have elucidated the association between hereditary APCR and pregnancy loss. Grandone et al (1997) reported a 31.2% prevalence of factor V Leiden in women with second trimester fetal losses compared to 4.2 % in matched controls. These findings were further supported by Younis et al (2000) who described a significantly higher incidence of factor V Leiden in women with first trimester and second trimester losses compared to a control group; 16%; 22% and 6% respectively. Reznikoff- Etievant et al (2001) also found a higher incidence of factor V Leiden; 10.38% (27/260) compared to a control group (4.7 % (11/240)).

Fouka et al (2000) described a significant difference in the prevalence of factor V Leiden APCR in their study of women with recurrent miscarriage. Similarly a 15.4% prevalence of the mutation was described by Wramsby et al (2000) in their study group whereas a prevalence of only 2.89 % was present in the control group. Sarig et al (2002) found an incidence of factor V Leiden of 25% (36/145) in women with fetal losses compared to 7.6% (11/145) in controls.

In a case control study limited to first trimester losses only, Balasch et al (1997) could not demonstrate any clear association with hereditary APCR. This finding was echoed by Dizon-Townson et al (1997), who did not find hereditary APCR in any of the participating women with idiopathic recurrent miscarriage. Preston et al (1996), in a retrospective study, could not elicit a link between hereditary APCR and first and second-trimester losses either. In a larger study, Rai et al (2001), found a similar prevalence of factor V Leiden in patients with first and second trimester losses compared to a control group of parous women.

A composite study of the association between the known thrombophilias and fetal loss demonstrated that fetal loss occurred among 10 of 48 women with thrombophilia (21%), and among 10 of 60 control women (17%). There was a similar risk of fetal loss in women with the factor V Leiden mutation compared to those without (Vossen et al, 2003).

The prevalence of factor V Leiden among women with recurrent miscarriage has revealed discordant results. Some studies have espoused a link between the two, while other studies have refuted any association. There appears to be a degree of polarisation in the findings.

The incongruity of the composite results regarding hereditary APCR, is not surprising, as there is a wide variation in patient numbers, inherent differences in study design, and lack of uniformity regarding pregnancy classification.

With regard to other obstetric morbidity parameters, there appears to be a significant increase in rates of stillbirth, pre-eclampsia and abruption concurring, in this respect, with the EPCOT study which found an increased risk of stillbirth (OddsRatio = 3.6 CI= 1.4 to 9.4) among carriers of the factor V mutation (Preston et al, 1996). The EPCOT study defined miscarriage as a pregnancy loss less than 28 weeks and could not detect an increased risk for fetal loss, however the focus of this study was on heritable thrombophilias, and thus excluded acquired ACPR. The association between stillbirth, abruption, and pre-ecclampsia, with acquired activated protein C resistance, needed further exploration to draw a definite conclusion, as the limitation of this study, is the small numbers in these groups.

The NOHA (Nîmes Obstetricians and Haematologists) first study, a large case-control study nested in a cohort of nearly 32,700 women, of whom 18% had pregnancy loss with their first gestation found on multivariate analysis a clear association between unexplained first pregnancy loss between 10 and 39 weeks gestation and heterozygosity for factor V Leiden (OR 3.46; 95% CI, 2.53–4.72) (Lissalde-Lavigne et al,2005).

A recent meta-analysis (Rodger et al, 2010) found that the odds of pregnancy loss in women with FVL appears to be 52% higher as compared with women without FVL, however these results are influenced by statistical and clinical heterogeneity in the analysis. Overall the absolute event rate for pregnancy loss is low (4.2%) and only appears slightly higher than the rate of pregnancy loss in women without FVL (3.2%) (Rodger et al, 2010).

5. Acquired thrombophilias

The antiphospholipid syndrome, described in great detail elsewhere in this book, is an acquired thrombophilia with a well-established role in the aetiology of adverse pregnancy outcomes.

5.1 Acquired activated protein C resistance

As described above, APCR is the most prevalent risk factor for thrombosis. The presence of the factor V Leiden mutation produces a protein that is intrinsically resistant to activated protein C, causing the pathological phenotype. The factor V Leiden mutation accounts for approximately ninety-five percent of cases of activated protein C resistance (Bertina et al, 1994). However in vitro resistance to activated protein C (causing APCR) may occur in the absence of the factor V Leiden mutation. The term used to describe this phenomenon is acquired activated protein C resistance (Clark et al, 2001).

The presence of non-factor V Leiden APCR or acquired APCR may be influenced by many variables. It is evident from the complexity of the coagulation cascade that perturbations in the levels of coagulation levels that play a key role in activating protein C, will affect resistance to activating protein C. Acquired APCR may be demonstrated in protein S deficiency (de Ronde & Bertina, 1994), increased antithrombin levels (Freyburger et al, 1997) and with increased levels of factor VIIIc (Koster et al, 1995; Kraaijenhagen et al, 2000). A modification of resistance to APC has also been demonstrated with the use of exogenous oestrogen as in the combined oral contraceptive pill (Henkens et al, 1995; Rosing et al, 1997) and in hormone replacement therapy (Lowe, et al 1999). The various physiological alterations to the clotting factors during pregnancy may also potentiate the development of acquired APCR (Clark et al, 1998). Lupus anticoagulants and anticardiolipin antibodies are also known to exert their influence on APCR (Oosting et al, 1993; Bokarewa et al, 1994; Martinuzzo et al, 1996). Despite the numerous confounding factors that may potentiate APCR, several studies have been able to demonstrate APCR as an independent factor for thrombosis (Kiehl et al, 1999; de Visser et al, 1999).

5.2 Acquired APCR and pregnancy loss

The majority of documented studies do not explore the entity of acquired activated protein C resistance. However, in those studies that do address this, none of them dispute the definite association between acquired APCR and recurrent pregnancy loss. Younis et al (2000) were intrigued with their finding of a higher prevalence of acquired as opposed to hereditary activated protein C resistance in the second trimester. Rai et al (2000), also reported a significantly higher incidence of acquired APCR in women with recurrent first trimester and second trimester losses 8.8% (80/904) and 8.7%(18/207), compared to a control group of parous women 3.3%(5/150).

Sarig et al (2002) point out that non-factor V Leiden APCR is one of the most common thrombophilic defects associated with recurrent pregnancy loss. They report an incidence of

9% (13/145) in women with fetal losses, but a complete absence of acquired APCR in women in their control group. The reported prevalence of acquired activated protein C resistance from studies so far, ranges from 9% to 26.8% in women with first, second and third trimester losses. It would be interesting to ascertain the converse relationship with greater emphasis on the type of pregnancy loss in women with acquired APCR. Ostensibly, it appears that the entity of acquired activated protein C resistance in the pregnancy loss setting cannot be ignored and is indeed gaining importance. There is a physiologically induced increased level of APCR in pregnancy. The mechanism of recurrent pregnancy loss associated with activated protein C resistance may be due to an exaggeration of the insult in the presence of pre-existing APCR.

Several studies of pregnancy loss and APCR have revealed discrepant results, with some demonstrating a convincing association whereas others nullifying any link between the two. However, most published studies have focused exclusively on hereditary APCR leaving the entity of acquired APCR inadequately explored. In a historical case-control study relating pregnancy loss and APCR, Brenner et al (1997) described a 50 % first trimester loss rate, 17% second trimester loss rate and a 47 % intrauterine fetal death rate. However, this study only included a select group of patients attending a specialist haemostasis unit and had a limited number of patients, with only 9 of the 39 patients having acquired APCR.

Balasch et al (1997), could not demonstrate a higher incidence of APCR in a study group of 55 women with first trimester pregnancy loss (1.8%, n=1/55) compared to a control group of 50 women 2% (1/50). This study was confined to hereditary APCR. Another case control study which lacked pregnancy loss classification, showed that the incidence of factor V Leiden was significantly higher among women with recurrent miscarriage (cases 8.0% (n=9/113) versus controls 3.7% (n=16/437) (Ridker et al, 1998), again, not examining acquired APCR. A further case-control study (Younis et al, 2000), showed a significantly higher prevalence of both congenital 19% (n=15/78) and acquired activated protein C resistance 19% (n=15/78), compared to controls 6% (8/139) and 2% (3/139) respectively. Although, this study ventured a pregnancy loss classification, there were only 15 patients with acquired APCR. In another study, van Dunne et al (2005) has supported the theory that APCR is associated with fetal losses. They determined that women with the factor V Leiden mutation had fewer embryo losses than matched controls.

A more convincing association between pregnancy loss and acquired APCR, which included a classification of pregnancy loss, was described in a small case control study of 7 patients (Tal et al, 1998). However, this study deviated from the definition of recurrent miscarriage and included patients with just one first or a single second trimester loss, and consequently, there was only one patient who had recurrent miscarriage and acquired APCR. More recently, a larger case control study found acquired activated protein C resistance to be significantly higher in women with recurrent early miscarriage 8.8% (80/904) as well as late miscarriage 8.7% (18/207) compared with controls 3.3% (5/150) (Rai et al, 2001). Rai et al clearly distinguished between hereditary and acquired activated protein C resistance, and indeed emphasised the importance of the latter in pregnancy loss, but used a more general classification of pregnancy loss. Another case control study described a fetal loss rate of 75% in women suffering with recurrent miscarriage and who also demonstrated the presence of acquired activated protein C resistance (Dawood et al, 2003).

The thrombophilia activated protein C resistance (APCR) has emerged as the commonest risk factor for venous thrombosis. APCR has also been implicated in increasing the propensity for placental thrombosis and subsequent recurrent fetal losses. Despite extensive research within the field of thrombophilia, the specific cause of many thrombotic episodes remains an enigma. The hypothesis of alternative polymorphisms on the factor V gene was explored by Dawood et al (2007) to elucidate the existence of acquired APCR. Fifty- one women with recurrent pregnancy loss and acquired APCR were recruited and their factor V gene was intensely analysed to identify single-nucleotide polymorphisms (SNP's). Samples were compared with controls and results showed there was a significantly increased number of particular SNP's in the acquired APCR cohort. This study also explored the theory of whether some SNP's increase the risk of pregnancy loss in women with acquired APCR (Dawood et al, 2007).

More recent work from mouse models has suggested a role for maternal carriage of the factor V Leiden mutation in causing fetal losses in the absence of placental thombosis. It is suggested that the mutation caused fetal losses in mice by a disruption to the materno-fetal interaction controlling the protein C anticoagulant pathway on the surface of the trophoblast, which led to poor placental development (Sood et al, 2007). Furthermore, there is emerging evidence from knockout mice embryos that the fetal genotype exerts an important procoagulative effect on placental trophoblasts (Sood et al, 2007). Human placenta is known to express the same factors that control the protein C anticoagulant pathway as that in mice; thrombomodulin (a membrane glycoprotein that activates protein is localized to the apical membranes of syncytiotrophoblast), a variant of tissue factor protein that was identified in the syncytiotrophoblast cells, and annexin V (an anticoagulant that binds to negative membrane phospholipids) is abundant on normal placentas (Lanir et al, 2003). Inactivation of the gene for protein C and endothelial protein C receptor gene deletion are (Li et al, 2005) also associated with mice embryo death. In vitro observations suggest that the presence of activated coagulation factors results in cell-type specific changes in trophoblast gene expression (Bates et al, 2010).

5.3 Acquired hyperhomocystinaemia

Hyperhomocystinaemia may be acquired secondary to dietary and lifestyle factors such as a reduced intake of folate, vitamin B6 or vitamin B12, excessive caffeine consumption and excessive coffee intake. The acquired form of hyperhomocystinaemia may also result from certain medical conditions such as hypothyroidism or renal impairment. The Homocysteine Lowering Trial Collaboration (Clark et al, 2007) has suggested that endothelial dysfunction, alteration of platelet reactivity and disruption of prostacyclin pathways, may be some of the mechanisms responsible for the reported venous thrombosis risk as well as the theoretical risk of pregnancy loss. A meta-analysis of ten studies concluded that acquired hyperhomocysteinaemia is a risk factor for recurrent pregnancy loss (Nelen et al, 2000).

6. Treatment options in thrombophilia

6.1 Prevention of venous thrombo-embolism

The optimal management for the prevention of venous thrombo-embolism in pregnancy in asymptomatic women has not been fully elucidated by high-grade evidence. Influencing factors include the absolute risk of venous thrombo-embolism and other risk factors such as obesity, older maternal age and smoking. Where the risk of venous thrombo-embolism is increased by other attenuating factors, consideration for antepartum thrombophylaxis is justified. The risk of thrombosis is considerably higher in the puerperium so prophylaxis is generally recommended (Bates, 2008).

Few studies have looked at the optimal management of women who have sustained a previous venous thrombo-embolic episode with a thrombophilic disorder. One prospective study described a higher recurrence risk in all trimesters, so the administration of anticoagulant thromboprophylaxis should be seriously considered (Brill-Edwards et al, 2000).

6.2 Prevention of adverse pregnancy outcome

This is an area that is subject to great debate. Although there is a paucity of data supporting the use of antithrombotics to prevent adverse obstetric outcome in women with thrombophilic disorders, the incongruity largely lies in inherent differences in study designs and definitions. While the American College of Chest Physicians recommends both aspirin and heparin for treatment in women with antiphospholipid antibodies and recurrent miscarriage, the European Society of Human Reproduction recommends aspirin with or without heparin and the British Committee for Standards in Haematology has recently recommended against antithrombotic therapy.

One of the first proponents for the use of antithrombotic prophylaxis was a study that treated 61 pregnancies in 50 women with recurrent pregnancy loss and thrombophilia with enoxaparin (Low Molecular Weight Heparin) throughout pregnancy and 4–6 weeks into the postpartum period. Forty-six of the 61 pregnancies (75%) resulted in live birth compared to a success rate of 20% in previous pregnancies without antithrombotic therapy (Brenner et al, 2003). Subsequently a randomised controlled trial was published; the LIVE-ENOX study comparing varying does of enoxaparin (Brenner et al, 2005). Results of the trial demonstrated an increase in live birth rate and a decrease in the incidence of complications in thrombophilic women. Doses of 40 mg day and 80 mg day led to similar clinical results (Brenner et al, 2005). Another study treated selected patients with heritable thrombophilia and recurrent pregnancy loss with enoxaparin and results exhibited a higher live birth rate, 26/37 (70.2%) compared to 21/48 (43.8%) in untreated patients (Carp et al, 2003).

Proponents in favour of treatment in the form of low dose aspirin and heparin tend to acquire results from small observational studies (Gris et al, 2005). Not all studies use a randomization technique and therefore present the problem of confounding variables. The strength of association between subgroups of inherited thrombophilia (i.e. AT III, FVL) and pregnancy loss does fluctuate. A large dedicated recurrent miscarriage clinic coordinated a prospective study comparing pregnancy outcome in 25 women whose screening blood tests were positive for the heterozygous form of the factor V Leiden mutation with a control group. Participants in the control group also had suffered at least 3 consecutive miscarriages. The live birth rate was lower in women positive for factor V Leiden (38%) compared to the control group (49%). The authors suggested the use of thromboprophylaxis in future pregnancies (Lindqvist et al, 2006). Prospective observational studies analyzed 37 women positive for antithrombin defiency, protein C deficiency or protein S deficiency and were followed through the index pregnancy. Thromboprophylactic treatment included low molecular weight heparin, unfractionated heparin and vitamin K antagonists. Twenty-six women (70%) received treatment and no fetal losses occurred. This compares with a 45% fetal loss rate (5/11) in women with no treatment intervention. When comparing fetal loss rates in women without thromboprophylaxis, the presence was the highest with antithrombin deficiency (63%) followed by protein C deficiency (50%). The authors state that thromboprophylaxis reduces the fetal loss rate in women with such inherited thrombophilia by 15% (Folkeringa et al, 2007); however small numbers limits this study. It is of upmost importance to state that women were identified and recruited with reference to a large family cohort study and not due to previous recurrent miscarriage. In addition, 81% (21/26) of patients receiving thromboprophylaxis in pregnancy had suffered a previous thromboembolic event. A more recent descriptive retrospective study assessed the pregnancy outcomes for 9 women diagnosed with antithrombin deficiency (Sabadell et al, 2010). Out of a total of 18 pregnancies, 67% (12) received low molecular weight heparin, as antithrombin defiency had not been diagnosed in the other participants at the time. Miscarriage occurred in 11 %(2) of patients, one case of pre-eclampsia was diagnosed and 2 women suffered a stillbirth. Three episodes of venous thromboembolism occurred in women without thromboprophylaxis. A significant observation was that no cases of recurrent miscarriage transpired (Sabadell et al, 2010).

Well- designed trials are the solid basis for evidence-based practice. The description of a 'before and after' study design, used in publications to assess the evidence for inherited thrombophilia and recurrent miscarriage has been explored. A population based prospective cohort study of 2480 women to assess the pregnancy outcome of women with the factor V Leiden mutation with a prior fetal loss showed a substantial 'regression towards the mean,' as those with previous low birth weight consequently increased to a high live birth rate (Lindqvist et al, 1999). Those with no treatment intervention had in fact the highest current birth rate in the study. Evidence such as this supports the argument that antithrombotic prophylaxis is not required for hereditary thrombophilia in the RM setting. No pharmacological therapy, especially in pregnancy should be allowed prior to robust evidence from comprehensive clinical trials. Low molecular weight heparin administration can be laborious with daily subcuticular injections, often associated with bruising and skin reactions. A Danish study (Lund et al, 2010) reviewed pregnancy outcome in 35 women with either the factor V Leiden or prothrombin gene mutation compared to a control group. Every participant had suffered a minimum of three pregnancy losses and no anticoagulation therapy was prescribed. The adjusted odds ratio for live birth with the factor V Leiden or prothrombin gene mutation was 0.48(95% CI=0.23-1.01), P=0.05 and therefore results did not reach a statistical significance.

The role of anticoagulation therapy in the treatment of recurrent miscarriage patients with hereditary thrombophilia remains to be accurately assessed. Historical study design and small participant numbers limits the impact found in published data. Recruitment criteria varies significantly even in randomised controlled trials and so conclusions cannot be assumed to represent the recurrent miscarriage setting. Limited numbers of studies incorporate women with at least three consecutive miscarriages as their inclusion criteria and therefore results have to be treated with caution. There is a dearth of well-structured placebo controlled trials in the literature. Patients should be counselled and reassured that there is a good prognosis for subsequent pregnancy however if appropriate, they could potentially be included in high quality research to ascertain a more reliable evidence base for prevention of adverse pregnancy outcomes with thrombophilia.

More recently a case control study not only elicited an increased risk of stillbirth, abruption and pre-eclampsia in women with thrombophilia, but also concluded that heparin was beneficial as a treatment and prevention (Kupferminc et al, 2011).

Clearly, large randomized trials are required to clarify the management of thrombophilia in pregnancy especially with a history of either adverse obstetric outcome (abruption, pre-eclampsia) or pregnancy loss. There are currently 2 ongoing randomized trials, which may proffer more guidance. The TIPPS: Thrombophilia in Pregnancy Prophylaxis trial is investigating antithrombotic therapy in women with congenital thrombophilia and previous pregnancy loss ([http://www.ClinicalTrials.gov; identifier: NCT00967382] and the other trial is the Effectiveness of Dalteparin Therapy as Intervention in Recurrent Pregnancy Loss [http://www.ClinicalTrials.gov; identifier: NCT00400387).

7. References

Altintas A, Pasa S, Akdeniz N *et al.* (2007) Factor V Leiden and G20210A prothrombin mutations in patients with recurrent pregnancy loss: data from the southeast of Turkey Ann Hematol. Oct; 86(10): 727-31.

Ajzner E, Balogh I, Szabo T, Marosi A, Haramura G, Muszbek L. (2002) Severe coagulation factor V deficiency caused by 2 novel frameshift mutations: 2952delT in exon 13 and 5493insG in exon 16 of factor 5 gene. *Blood*; 99:702-705.

Amer L, Kisiel W, Searles R et al (1990) Impairment of the protein C anticoagulation pathway in a patient with systemic lupus erythematosus anticardiolipin antibodies and thrombosis. *Thromb. Res*; 57:247-258.

Aparicio C and Dahlback B (1996) Molecular mechanisms of activated protein C resistance: properties of factor V isolated from an individual with homozygosity for the Arg506 to Gln mutation in the factor V gene. *Biochemical Journ*; 313:467-472.

Balasch J, Reverter JC, Fabregues F et al (1997) First trimester repeated abortion is not associated with activated protein C resistance. *Hum Reprod* 12:1094-1097.

Bates SM, Consultative Hematology: The Pregnant Patient (2010) *Hematology*: 166-72

Bates SM, Greer IA, Pabinger I et al. (2008) Venous thrombo-embolism, thrombophilia, antithrombotic therapy and pregnancy: American College of Chest Physicians Evidence Based Clinical Practice Guidelines (8th edition). *Chest*; 133:844-86

Bertina RM, Koelaman BP, Koster T et al (1994) Mutation in blood coagulation factor V associated with resistance to activated protein C. *Nature*; 369:64-67.

Bertina RM. Molecular risk factors for thrombosis. (1999) *Thromb Haemost*; 82:601-609.

Bokarewa MI, Blomback M, Egberg N, Rosen S. (1994) A new variant of interaction between phospholipid antibodies and the protein C system. *Blood Coagulation and Fibrinolysis*; 5:37-41

Brenner B, Hoffman R, Carp H *et al* for the LIVE–ENOX Investigators (2005) Efficacy and safety of two doses of enoxaparin in women with thrombophilia and recurrent pregnancy losses: the LIVE–ENOX study. *J Thromb Haemost*; 3: 227–9.

Brenner B, Mandel H, Lanir N et al (1997) Activated protein C resistance can be associated with recurrent fetal loss. *Brit J Haem* 97:551-554

Brenner B. Antithrombotic prophylaxis for women with thrombophilia and pregnancy complications. (2003) *Thromb Haemost*; 1:2070-2.

Brill-Edwards P, Ginsberg JS, Gent M et al (2000) Safety of withholding heparin in pregnant women with a history of venous thromboembolism. *N Eng J Med*; 343(20): 1439-44.

Carp H, Dolitzky M, Inbal A (2003)Thromboprophylaxis improves the live birth rate in women with consecutive recurrent miscarriages and hereditary thrombophilia. *J Thromb Haemost*; 1: 433–8.

Chan WP, Lee CK, Kwong YL, Lam CK, Liang R. (1998) A novel mutation of Arg 306 of factor V gene in Hong Kong Chinese.*Blood;* 91:1135-1139.

Clark P,Brennand J, Conkie J A, Mc Call F, Greer I A, Walker ID (1998) Activated protein C rsensitivity, protein C, protein S and coagulation in normal pregnancy. *Thromb Haemos* 79 (6); 1166-1170.

Clark R, Armitage J, Lewington S, Collins R. (2007) B-vitamin treatment trialists' collaboration of homocysteine-lowering trilas for prevention of vascular disease: protocol for a collaborative meta-analysis. *Clin Chem lab Med;* 45 (12): 1575-81

Coumans AB, Huijgens PC, Jakobs C, Sohorts R, de Visser JI, van Pampus MG, Dekker GA. (1999) Haemostatic and metabolic abnormalities in women with unexplained recurrent abortion. *Hum Reprod;* 14(1): 211-214.

Dahlback B. (1980) Human coagulation factor V purification and thrombin-catalyzed activation. *J Clin Invest;* 66:583-591

Dahlback B, Carlsson M, Svensson PJ. (1993) Familial thrombophilia due to a previously unrecognised mechanism characterised by poor anticoagulant response to activated protein C. Prediction of a cofactor to activated protein C. *Proceedings of the National Academy of Sciences of the United States of America;* 90:1004-1008.

Dahlback B. Factor V gene mutation causing inherited resistance to activated protein C as a basis for venous thrombo-embolism. (1995) .*J intern Med;* 237:221-227

Dawood F, Farquharson R, Quenby S, Toh C. H. (2003) Acquired activated protein C resistance maybe a risk factor for recurrent fetal loss. *Fertil Steril;* 80:649-650.

Dawood F, Mountford RG, Farquharson RG, Quenby S (2007) Genetic polymorphisms on the factor V gene in women with recurrent miscarriage and acquired APCR. *Human Reproduction;* Vol 22 (9): 2546-2453.

de Visser MC, Rosendaal F R & Bertina R M. (1999) A reduced sensitivity for activated protein C in the absence of factor V Leiden increases the risk of venous thrombosis. *Blood;* 93:1271-1276

Di Simone N, Caliandro D, Castellani R, Ferrazzani S, De Carolis S, Caruso A. (1999) Low-molecular weight heparin restores invitro trophoblast invasiveness and differentiation in presence of immunoglobulin G fractions obtained from patients with antiphospholipid syndrome. *Hum Rep;* 14(2): 489-495.

Dizon-Townson DS, Meline L, Nelson LM, et al. (1997) Fetal carriers of the factor V Leiden mutation are prone to miscarriage and placental infarction. *Am J Obstet Gynecol;* 177:402-405.

Egeberg O. Inherited antithrombin deficiency casuing thrombophilia. *Thromb Diath Haemorrh* 1965; 13:516-30.

Finan RR, Tamim H, Ameen G, Sharida HE, Rashid M, Almawi WY. (2002) Prevalence of factor V G1691A (Factor V-Leiden) and prothrombin G20210A gene mutations in a recurrent miscarriage population. *Am J Haem;* 71:300-305

Freyburger G, Javorschi S, Labrouche S and Bernard P. (1997) Proposal for objective evaluation of the performance of various functional APC-resistance tests in genotyped patients. *Thromb Haemost;* 78:1360-1365

Foka ZJ, Lambropoulos AF, Saravelos H et al. (2000) Factor V Leiden and prothrombin G20210A mutations, but not methyltetrahydrofolate reductase C677T, are associated with recurrent miscarriages. *Hum Reprod;* 15:458-462.

Folkeringa N, Leendert J, Brouwer P *et al.* Reduction of high fetal loss rate by anticoagulant treatment during pregnancy in antithrombin, protein C or protein S deficient women.2007 *Br J Haematol.*136, 656-661.

Freyburger G, Javorschi S, Labrouche S and Bernard P. (1997) Proposal for objective evaluation of the performance of various functional APC-resistance tests in genotyped patients. *Thromb Haemost;* 78:1360-1365

Gerhardt A, Scharf R. E, Beckmann M. W *et al.* (2000) Prothrombin and factor V mutations in women with a history of thrombosis during pregnancy and the puerperium. *N Engl J Med.;* 342:374-80.

Gewirtz AM, Shapiro C, Shen YM, Boyd R, Colman RW. (1992) Cellular and molecular regulation of factor V expression in human megakaryocytes. *J Cell Physiol;* 153:277-287

Gharavi AE, Pierangeli SS, Levy RA. et al. (2001) Mechanisms of pregnancy loss in antiphospholipid syndrome. *Clin Obstet Gynecol.;* 44:11-19.

Gonzales Ordonez AJ, Rodriguez JMM, Martin L, Alvarez V Coto E. (1999) The O blood group protects against venous thromboembolism in individuals with the factor V Leiden but not the prothrombin (factor IIG20210A) mutation. *Blood Coag Fibrin;* 10:303-307.

Grandone E, Margaglione M, Colaizzo D et al (1997) Factor V Leiden is associated with repeated and recurrent unexplained fetal losses. *Thromb Haemost* 77(5):822-824

Greengard JS, Sun X, Xu X, Fernandez JA, Griffin JH, Evatt B. (1994) Activated protein C resistance caused by Arg506Gln mutation in factor Va. *Lancet;* 343:1361-1362.

Gris JC, Quere I, Monpeyroux F et al. (1999) Case control study of the function of thrombophilic disorders in couples with late foetal losses and no thrombotic antecedent- the Nimes Obstetricians & Haematologists Study 5 (NOHA5). *Thromb. Haemost;* 81; 891-899.

Gris J. C, Mares P. (2005) The long and winding road towards LMWH for pregnancy loss. *J Thromb Haemost;* 3:224-6.

Griffin JH, Evatt B, Wideman C, Fernandez JA. (1993) Anticoagulant protein C pathway defective in a majority of thrombophilic patients. *Blood;* 82:1989-1993.

Jenny R, Pittman D, Toole J et al. (1987) Complete Cdna and derived amino acid sequence of human FV. *Proc Natl Acad Sci* USA; 84:4846-4850

Hatzis T, Cardamakis E, Drivalas E et al. (1999) Increased resistance to activated preotein C and factor V Leiden in recurrent abortions:review of other hypercoagulability factors. *Eur J Contracept Reprod Health Care;* 4:135-144.

Heeb MJ, Kojima Y, Greengard JS, Griffin JH. (1995) Activated protein C resistance: molecular mechanisms based on studies using purified Gln506-factor V. *Blood;* 85:3405-3411.

Henkens CMA, Bom VJ, Seinen AJ, van der Meer J. (1995) Sensitivity to activated protein C: influence of oral contraceptives and sex. *Thromb and Haemost;* 73:402-404

Holmes ZR, Regan L, Chilcott I, Cohen H. (1999) The C677T MTHFR gene mutation is not predictive of risk for recurrent fetal loss. *Br J Haematol.;* 105:98-101.

Hooper WC, Dilley A, Ribiero MJ et al (1996) A racial difference in the prevalence of the Arg506 Gln mutation. *Thromb Res;* 81:577-581.

Kaandorp S, Di Nisio M, Goddijn M, Middeldorp S. (2009) Aspirin or anticoagulants for treating recurrent miscarriage in women without antiphospholipid syndrome (Review). The Cochrane Library Issue 1.

Kiechl S, Muigg A,Santer P, Mitterer M, Egger G, Oberhollenzer M, Oberhollenzer F,Mayr A, Gasperi A, Poewe W, Willeit J. (1999) Poor response to activated protein C as a prominent risk predictor of advanced atherosclerosis and arterial disease. *Circulation*; 99:614-619

Kupferminc MJ, RimonE, Many A et al. (2011) Low molecular weight heparin treatment during subsequent pregnancies of women with inherited thrombophilia and previous severe pregnancy complications. *J Matern Fetal Neonatal Med.* 2011 Jan 13. [Epub ahead of print]

Koster T, Rosendaal FR, Briet E, van der Meer FJM, Colly, LP, Treinekens PH, Poort SR, Vandenbroucke JP, Bertina RM. (1993) Venous thrombosis due to a poor anticoagulant response to activated protein C. Leiden Thrombophilia study. *Lancet*; 342:1503-1506.

Kostka H, Sieger G, Schwarz T, Gehrisch S, Kuhlisch E, Schellong S and Jaross W. (2000) Frequency of polymorphisms in the B-domain of factor V gene in APC-resistant patients. *Thromb Res*; 99:539-547.

Kraaijenhagen RA, Anker PS, Koopman MMW, Reitsma PH, Prins MHH, van den Ende A, Buller HR. (2000) High plasma concentration of factor VIIIc is a major risk factor for venous thromboembolism. *Thrombosis Haemost*; 83:5-9.

Kujovic JL (2011) Prothrombin related thrombophilia. In: Gene Reviews, March 2011

Kujovic JL. (2004) Thrombophilia and pregnancy complications. *Am J Obst Gyne.*; 191:412-424.

Kumar KS, Govindaiah V, Naushad SE, Devi RR, Jyothy A. (2003) Plasma homocysteine levels correlated to interactions between folate status and methylene tetrathydrofolate reductase gene mutation in women with unexplained recurrent pregnancy loss. *J Obstet Gynaecol*; 23:55-58.

Kupferminc MJ, Eldor A, Steiman N, Many A, Bar-Am A, Jaffa A. (1999) Increased frequency of genetic thrombophilia in women with complications of pregnancy. *NEJM*; 340:9-13.

Lassere M, Empson M (2004) Treatment of antiphospholipid syndrome in pregnancy- a systematic review of randomized therapeutic trials. *Thromb Res* 114:419-26.

Lensen RP, Rosendaal FR, Koster T, Allaaart CF, de Ronde H, Vandenbroucke JP, Reitsma PH, Bertina RM. (1996) Apparent different thrombotic tendencies in patients with factor V Leiden and protein C deficiency due to selection of patients. *Blood*: 88:4205-4208.

Lindqvist P.G, Svensson P. J, Marsaal K *et al.* (1999) Activated protein C resistance (FV: Q506) and pregnancy. *Thromb Haemost*; 81:532-7.

Lindqvist P. G, Merlo J. (2006) The natural course of women with recurrent fetal loss. *J Thromb Haemost.*; 4(4):896-7.

Lissak A, Sharon A, Fruchter O, Kassel A, Sanderovitz J, Abramovica H. (1999) Polymorphism for mutation of cytosine to thymine at location 677 in the methylene reductase gene is associated with recurrent early fetal loss. *Am J Obst Gynec*; 181:126-130.

Lissalde-Lavigne G, Fabbro-Peray P, Cochery-Nouvellon E, et al. (2005) Factor V Leiden and prothrombin G20210A polymorphisms as risk factors for miscarriage during a first intended pregnancy: the matched case-control 'NOHA first' study. *J Thromb Haemost.* 3:2178–2184.

Lockwood CJ (2002) Inherited thrombophilias in pregnant patients: detection and treatment paradigm. *Obstet and Gynecol;* 99:333-341.

Lowe, GDO,Rumley A, Woodward M, Morrison CE, Philippou, H, Lane DA, Tunstall-Pedoe H (1997) Epidemiology of coagulation factors, inhibitors and activation markers: The third Glasgow MONICA survey1. Illustrative reference ranges by age, sex and hormone use. *British Journal Haem;* 97:775-784

Lu D, Kalfatis M, Mann KG, Long GL. (1996) Comparison of activated protein C/protein S-mediated inactivation of human factor VIII and factor V. *Blood;* 87:4708

Luddington R, Jackson A, Pannerselvam S, Brwon K, Baglin T. (2000) The factor V R2 allele: risk of venous thromboembolism, factor V levels and resistance to activated protein C. *Thrombo Haemost;* 83:204-208

Lunghi B,Iacovelli L, Gemmat D et al. (1996) Detection of New Polymorphic markers in the factor V gene: association with factor V levels in plasma. *Thrombosis and Hameostasis;* 75 (1): 45-48.

Lund M, Nielsen H. S, Hviid T. V. Hereditary thrombophilia and recurrent pregnancy loss: a retrospective cohort study of pregnancy outcome and complications. *Hum Reprod* 2010. Vol 25 No. 12 pp2978-2984.

Mak IY, Brosens JJ, Christian M et al (2002) Regulated expression of signal transducer and activator of transcription, Stat 5,and its enhancement of PRL expression in human endometrial stromal cells in vitro. *J Clin Endo Meta;* 87(6): 2581-8

Many A, Elad R, Yaron Y, Eldor A, Lessing JB, Kupferminc MJ. (2002); Third –trimester unexplained intrauterine fetal death is associated with inherited thrombophilia. *Obstet Gynecol.* 99:684-687.

Martinuzzo M, Forastiero, R, Adamczuk Y, Cerrato G, Carreras LO. (1996) Activated protein C resistance in patients with anti-beta2 glycoprotein-I antibodies. *Blood Coag & Fibrin.* 7:702-704

Mazzorana M, Cornillou B, Baffet G, Hubert N, Eloy R, Guguen-Guilluozo C. (1989) Biosynthesis of factor V by normal adult rat hepatocytes. *Thromb Res;* 54:655-675

Miletich JP, Sherman L, Broze GI. (1987) Absence of thrombosis in subjects with heterozygous protein C deficiency. *NEJM;* 317:991-996.

Mousa HA, Alfirevic Z (2000) Do placental lesions reflect thrombophilia state in women with adverse pregnancy outcome? *Hum Reprod.* 8:1830-3.

Nelen WL, Blom HJ, Steegers EA, den Heijer M, Thomas CM, Eskes TK. (2000) Homocysteine and folate levels as risk factors for recurrent early pregnancy loss. *Obstet Gynecol;* 95:519-524.

Nelen WL, Blom HJ, Steegers EA, den Heijer M, Eskers TK. (2000) Hyperhomocysteinaemia and recurrent early pregnancy loss: a meta-analysis. *Fertil Steril;* 74(6): 1196-9.

Nesheim ME, Taswell JB, Mann KG. (1979) The contribution of bovine factor V and factor Va to the activity of prothrombinase. *J Biol Chem;* 254:10952-10962

Nicolaes GAF, Thomassen MCLGD, van Oerle R, Hamulyak K, Hemker HC, Tans G, Rosing J (1996) A prothombinase-based assay for detection of resistance to activated protein C. *Thromb. Haem.*76: 404-410.

Oosting JD, Derksen RH, Bobbink IW, Hackeng, TM, Bouma, BN, de Groot, PG (1993) Antiphospholipid antibodies directed against a combination of phosphoplipids with prothrombin, protein C, or protein S: an explanation for their pathogenic mechanism. *Blood*;81:2618-2625

Ozawa T, Niiya K, Sakutagawa N. (1996) Absence of factor V Leiden in Japanese (letter). *Thromb Res.*; 81:595-596.

Perry DJ. Hyperhomocystenaemia. Baillieres Best Practice Res Clin Haematol 1999; 12:451-477.

Pihusch R, Buchholz T, Lohse P et al (2001) Thrombophilic gene mutations and recurrent spontaneous abortion: prothrombin mutation increases the risk in the first trimester. *Am J Reprod Immunol;* 46:124-131.

Poort SR, Rosendaal FR, Reitsma PH, Bertina RM. (1996) A common genetic variation in the 3′ untranslated region of the prothrombin gene is associated with elevated plasma prothrombin levels and an increase in venous thrombosis. *Blood;* 88:3698-3703.

Preston F E, Rosendaal F R, Walker A I D et al. (1996) Increased fetal loss in women with heritable thrombophilia. *Lancet;* 348: 913-916.

Pittman DD, Tomkinson KN, Kaufman RJ (1994) Post-translational requirements for functional factor V and factor VIII secretion in mammalian cells. *J Biol Chem;* 269:17329

Quenby S, Mountfield S, Cartwright JE et al (2004) Effects of low-molecular weight and unfractionated heparin on trophoblast function. *Obstet Gynecol;* 104 (2): 354-61

Quere I, Bellet H, Hoffet M, Janbon C, Mares P, Gris JC. (1998) A woman with five consecutive fetal deaths: case report and retrospective analysis of hyperhomocysteinaemia prevalence in 100 consecutive women with recurrent miscarrriages. *Fertil Steril;* 69:152-154.

Rai R, Backos M, Rushworth F, Regan L. (2000) Polycystic ovaries and recurrent miscarriage-a reappraisal. *Hum Reprod;* 15 (3): 612-615.

Rai R, Cohen H, Dave M and Regan L. (1997) Randomised controlled trial of aspirin plus heparin in pregnant women with recurring miscarriage associated with antiphospholipid antibodies. *BMJ;* 314: 253-257.

Rai R, Shlebak A, Cohen H et al (2001) Factor V Leiden and acquired activated protein C resistance among 1000 women with recurrent miscarriage. *Hum Reprod* 16:5 961-965

Rai R, Backos M, Elgaddal S *et al.* (2002) Factor V Leiden and recurrent miscarriage-prospective outcome of untreated pregnancies. Hum Reprod. Feb; 17(2): 442-5.

Raziel A, Kornberg Y, Friedler S, Schachter M, Sela BA, Ron-El R. (2001) Hypercoagulable thrombophilic defects and hyperhomocysteinemia in patients with recurrent pregnancy loss. *Am J Reprod Immunol* 45(2): 65-71

Rees DC,Cox M and Clegg JB. (1995) World distribution of factor V Leiden. *Lancet*;345:1133-1134.

Rey E, Kahn S. R, David M, Shrier I. Thrombophilic disorders and fetal loss: a meta analysis. *Lancet* 2003 361:901-8.

Reznikoff-Etievant MF, Cayol V, Carbonne B, Robert A, Coulet F, Milliez J (2001) Factor V Leiden and G20210 A prothrombin mutations are risk factors for very early recurrent miscarriage. *BJOG* 108:1251-1254

Ridker PM, Hennekens CH, Selhub J, Miletich JP, Manilow MR, Stampfer MJ. (1997) Interrelation of hyperhomocystenaemia, factor V Leiden, and risk of future venous thromboembolism. *Circulation*; 95:1777-1782.

Ridker PM, Miletich JP, Buring JE, Ariyo AA, Price DT (1998) Factor V Leiden mutation as a risk factor for recurrent pregnancy loss. *Ann Intern Med* 128:1000-1003

Rintelen C, Pabinger I, Knobl P, Lechner K, Mannhalter C. (1996) Probability of recurrence of thrombosis in patients with and without factor V Leiden. *Thrombosis and Haemostasis*;75:229

Robert A, Aillaud MF, Eschwege V, Randrianjohany A, Scarabin Y, Juhan-Vague I. (2000) ABO blood group and risk of venous thrombosis in heterozygous carriers of factor V Leiden. *Thromb Haem*; 83:630-631.

Robertson L, Wu O, Langhorne P *et al* (2006). The Thrombosis Risk and Economic Assessment of Thrombophilia Screening (TREATS) Study. Thrombophilia in Pregnancy; a systematic review. *Br J Haematol*; 132:171-196.

Rodger M A, Betancourt MT, Clark P, Pelle G, Lindqvist et al. (2010) The Association of Factor V Leiden and Prothrombin Gene Mutation and Placenta-Mediated Pregnancy Complications: A Systematic Review and Meta-analysis of Prospective Cohort Studies. *Plos Med*; 7 (6): e1000292.

Rosendaal, FR, Koster T, vandenbroucke JP, Reitsma PH. (1995) High risk of thrombosis in patients homozygous for FV Leiden (activated protein C resistance). *Blood*; 85:1504-1508.

Rosendaal FR. (1999) Risk factors for venous thrombotic disease. *Thromb Haemost*; 82:610-619.

Rosing J, Tans G, Nicolaes GA, Thomassen MC, van Oerle R, van der Ploeg PM, Heijnen P, Hamulyak K, Hemker HC. (1997) Oral contraceptives and venous thrombosis: different sensitivities to activated protein C in women using second and third generation oral contraceptives. *British Journ Haem*; 97:233-238

Rosing J, Tans G. (1997) Factor V. *Int J Biochem. Cell Biol*; 29:1123-1126

Rosing J, Tans G, Govers-Riemslag JWP, Zwaal RFA, Hemker HC. (1980) The role of phospholipids and factor Va in the prothrombinase complex. *J Biol Chem*; 255:274-283

Roque H, Paidas M. J, Funai E. F *et al (*2004) Maternal thrombophilias are not associated with early pregnancy loss. *Thromb Haemost*; 91:290-5.

Sabadell J, Castellas M, Alijotas-Reig J *et al.* (2010) Inherited antithrombin deficiency and pregnancy: Maternal and fetal outcomes. *Eur J Obstet Gynecol Reprod Biol.* 149 47-51.

Sanson BJ, Friederich PW, Simioni P, Zanardi S, Hilsman MV, Girolami A et al. The risk of abortion and stillbirth in antithrombin-, protein C-, and protein S -deficient women. *Thromb Haemost* 1996; 75:387-388.

Sarig G, Younis JS, Hoffman R, Lanir N, Blumenfeld Z, Brenner B (2002) Thrombophilia is common in women with idiopathic pregnancy loss and is associated with late pregnancy wastage. *Fertil Steril* 77(2): 342-347

Sebire NJ,Backos M,El Gaddal S et al (2003) Placental pathology,antiphospholipid antibodies,and pregnancy outcome in recurrent miscarriage patients. *Obstet Gynecol*;101(2):258-63

Selighsohn U and Zivelin A(1997) Thrombophilia as a multigenic disorder. *Thromb Haemost*:78(1):297-301

Serrano F, Lima M. L, Lopes C *et al.* (2010) Factor V Leiden and prothrombin G20210A in Portuguese women with recurrent miscarriage: is it worthwhile to investigate? Arch Gynecol Obstet

Sikkema JM, Franx A, Bruinse HW, van der Wijk NG, de Valk HW, Nikkels PG. (2002) Placental pathology in early onset pre-eclampsia and intra-uterine growth restriction in women with and without thrombophilia. *Placenta.* 4:337-42

Silver R. M, Zhao Y, Spong C. Y. *et al.* (2010) Prothrombin Gene G20210A Mutation and Obstetric Complications. *Obstet Gynaecol.* Vol. 115: 1

Simmons A. (1997) Hematology: a combined theoretical and clinical approach. 2nd ed:Butterworth-Heineman, Masachusetts.

Stirling Y, Woolf L, North WRS. et al. (1984) Haemostasis in normal pregnancy. *Thromb Haemost;* 52:176-182.

Soria JM, Almasy L, Souto JC, Buil A et al. (2003) Anew locus on chromosome 18 that influences normal variation in activated protein C resistance phenotype and factor VIII activity and its relation to thrombosis susceptibility. *Blood;* 101(1): 163-167

Svensson PJ and Dahlback B. (1994) Resistance to activated protein C as a basis for venous thrombosis. *NEJM;* 330:517-522.

Tait RC, Walker ID, Islam SIAM, Mc Call F, Conkie JA, Mitchell R, Davidson JF. (1993) Influences of demographic factors on antithrombin activity in a healthy population. *Brit. J. Haem;* 84:476-478.

Tal J, Schliamser LM, Leibovitz Z, Ohel G, Attias D (1999) A possible role for activated protein C resistance in patients with first and second trimester pregnancy failure. *Hum Rep* 14:1624-1627

Toole JJ, Knopf JL, Wozney JM et al. (1984) Molecular cloning of a cDNA encoding human antihaemophilic factor. *Nature;* 312:342-347.

Tracy PB, Eide LL, Bowie EJW, Mann KG. (1982) Radioimmunoassay of factor V in human plasma and platelets. *Blood;* 60:59-63

Urbanus R. T, Derksen R. H, de Groot P. G. (2008) Current insight into diagnostics and pathophysiology of the antiphospholipid syndrome. *Blood Rev;* 22(2): 93-105.

Van Boven HH, Reitsma PPH, Rosendaal FR, Bayston TA, Chowdury V, Bauer KA, Scharrer I, Conard J (1996) Factor V Leiden (FVR506Q) in families with inherited antithrombin deficiency. *Thromb Haemostasis.;* 75:417-421.

Vehar GA, Keyt B, Eaton D, Rodriguez H, O' Brien DP, Rotblat F et al. (1984) Structure of human factor VIII gene. *Nature;* 312: 337-342.

Villareal C, Garcia-Aguirre, Hernandez C, Vega O, Borbolla J R,Collados MT. (2002) Congenital thrombophilias associated to obstetric complications. *Journal of Thromb and Thrombolys;* 14(2): 163-169.

Voorberg J, Roelse J, Koopman R, Buller H, Berends F, ten Cate JW, Mertens K, van Mourik JA. (1994) Association of idiopathic venous thromboembolism with single point mutation at Arg506 of factor V. *Lancet;* 343:1535-1536.

Vossen C. Y, Preston F. E, Conard J *et al.* (2003) Hereditary thrombophilia and fetal loss: a prospective follow-up study. *Thromb Haemost,* 2:592-596.

Walker I D, Greaves M, Preston F E. (2001) British Society of Haematology Guideline. *Brit J Haem;* 114:512-528.

Walker I D. (1998) Inherited coagulation disorders and thrombophilia in pregnancy (In) Recent advances in Obstetrics and Gynaecology; 20:Chapter 3:35-64.

Williamson D, Brown K,Luddington R,Baglin C,Baglin I. (1998) FV Cambridge: a new mutation Wramsby ML, Sten-Linder M, Bremme K. (2000) Primary habitual abortions are associated with high frequency of factor V Leiden mutation. *Fertil Steril* 74(5): 987-991

Wilson DB, Salem HH, Mruk JS, Majerus PW. (1984) Biosynthesis of coagulation factor V by a human hepatocellular carcinoma cell line. *J Clin Invest*; 73:654-661

Younis JS, Brenner B, Ohel G, Tal J, Lanir N, Ben-Ami, M (2000) Activated protein C resistance and Factor V Leiden mutation can be associated with first- as well as second -trimester recurrent pregnancy loss. *Am J Rep Immunology* 43: 31-35

Zoller B and Dahlback B. (1994) Linkage between inherited resistance to activated protein C and factor V gene mutation in venous thrombosis. *Lancet*; 343:1536-1538.

Zoller B, Berntsdotter A, Garcia de Frutos P, Dahlback B. (1995) Resistance to activated protein C is an additional genetic risk factor in hereditary deficiency of protein S. *Blood*; 85:351

7

The Impact of Inherited Thrombophilia on Placental Haemostasis and Adverse Pregnancy Outcomes

Joanne M. Said
The Royal Women's Hospital
The University of Melbourne
Australia

1. Introduction

While the last century has seen substantial developments in our understanding of many human diseases, there are still vast gaps in our knowledge about many physiological and pathological processes. This is particularly so in obstetrics, where advances in care have resulted in significant declines in both maternal and perinatal mortality in developed countries. Yet, despite this, conditions such as pre-eclampsia, fetal growth restriction, stillbirth, miscarriage and placental abruption remain to a large extent idiopathic. Prediction and prevention of these complications remains limited, with timely delivery representing the only effective treatment strategy in cases of pre-eclampsia, fetal growth restriction and placental abruption. This will often result in the delivery of a premature infant who requires the investment of significant community and family resources - financial, physical, intellectual and emotional - to develop their full potential. The longer term sequelae of fetal growth restriction such as adult onset diabetes, hypertension and obesity, (Barker et al. 1993) and the effects of prematurity such as chronic lung disease (Askie et al. 2005) and neurodevelopmental impairment (Guellec et al. 2011) represent significant additional burdens. Any improvements that can be made in our understanding and treatment of these serious human pregnancy disorders, therefore has the potential to impact significantly not only on maternal well being, but also on the well-being of future generations.

A consistent finding among patients experiencing many of these complications is that of areas of thrombosis on histological examination of the placenta (Salafia et al. 1995a; Salafia et al. 1995b). This has prompted the suggestion that disturbances in coagulation may contribute to the aetiology of these conditions. The recognition of the association between inherited thrombophilias and venous thromboembolism has sparked significant interest in the possibility that inherited thrombophilias may also play a role in these pregnancy complications. In this review, the current state of understanding regarding inherited thrombophilia and adverse pregnancy outcome will be critically examined.

2. Inherited thrombophilias and adverse pregnancy outcomes: The limitations of case control studies

The association between inherited thrombophilias and adverse pregnancy outcomes has been intensely debated for the past 15 years. Early case-control studies suggested significant associations between maternal inherited thrombophilias and pregnancy complications such as pre-eclampsia (Dekker et al. 1995; van Pampus et al. 1999; Kupferminc et al. 2000), fetal growth restriction (Martinelli et al. 2001; Agorastos et al. 2002), placental abruption (Wiener-Megnagi et al. 1998; Kupferminc et al. 1999), stillbirth (Preston et al. 1996; Many et al. 2002) and recurrent miscarriage (Grandone et al. 1997; Younis et al. 2000). Despite the potential for confounding (de Vries et al. 2009) and bias (Sibai 2005) inherent in these early case control studies, their great strength is the fact that they examined the association between thrombophilias and severe, early onset complications. These complications are rare but extremely serious by virtue of the increased likelihood of long term maternal and perinatal sequelae. Follow up case control studies often included patients with milder forms of the condition, later onset of disease and delivery at more advanced gestations, and as a result, often failed to confirm the significant associations between thrombophilias and adverse pregnancy outcomes demonstrated in early case control studies. This is best exemplified by contrasting two studies investigating the association between fetal growth restriction and inherited thrombophilia (Infante-Rivard et al. 2002; Kupferminc et al. 2002). Kupferminc and colleagues restricted their analysis to the subgroup of women delivering severe early onset growth restricted babies with a birthweight below the 3rd centile and antenatal ultrasound evidence of oligohydramnios (Kupferminc et al. 2002) while Infante-Rivard used the more liberal definition of birthweight less than the 10th centile (Infante-Rivard et al. 2002). Kupferminc and colleagues calculated the highly significant odds ratio of 4.5 (2.3 - 9.0) for the association between any inherited thrombophilia and fetal growth restriction (FGR), whereas Infante-Rivard concluded that an association between fetal growth restriction and inherited thrombophilias did not exist. Such a difference is likely to be due to differences in the clinical definitions chosen. On the one hand Kupferminc's FGR population represents a small unique subgroup representing less than 0.2% of their entire obstetric population (Kupferminc et al. 2002). Meanwhile Infante-Rivard's FGR population represents a much broader group which is likely to include many women with healthy babies that are merely constitutionally small. This is further supported by the low rates of significant placental pathology in this group (Infante-Rivard et al. 2002). Most importantly, however, the majority of Infante-Rivard's cohort are likely to have excellent perinatal outcomes with low rates of prematurity and associated morbidity, a finding that contrasts starkly with the high perinatal mortality (approximately 60%), universal prematurity and associated morbidity described in Kupferminc's study (Kupferminc et al. 2002). While it is true that a statistically significant association is seen with the Kupferminc study, it must be emphasised that this is a highly specific, high risk population and these findings cannot necessarily be extrapolated to general obstetric populations.

The limitation to the study validity that is imposed by varying clinical definitions is evident not just with fetal growth restriction as described above, but also pre-eclampsia, fetal loss and placental abruption. Studies investigating the relationship between miscarriage and thrombophilias have variably defined recurrent miscarriage as two or more first trimester losses (Younis et al. 2000), three or more first trimester losses (Rai et al. 2001) or any number of second trimester losses (Raziel et al. 2001). Furthermore, miscarriage and stillbirth have not infrequently been combined making dissection of individual associations very difficult (Preston et al. 1996).

The potential for publication bias in case control studies with positive association studies being rapidly published while studies that do not confirm these associations have been delayed has also been suggested in several meta-analyses that examined the potential impact of publication bias (Howley et al. 2005; Facco et al. 2009). In addition, many of the early "positive" studies were published in high impact journals (Dekker et al. 1995; Preston et al. 1996; de Vries et al. 1997; Kupferminc et al. 1999; Rey et al. 2003) and were thus rapidly disseminated amongst the obstetric and haematology communities. Rapid translation of these preliminary research findings into clinical practice has also been a key issue. This has happened simply because thrombophilia tests were readily available to clinicians who were keen to take advantage of them. Furthermore, the publication of eminent guidelines (Bates et al. 2004) and influential articles (Kupferminc et al. 1999) advising of the merits of testing women who experience adverse pregnancy events (before the appearance of evidence to support treatment or prophylaxis for subsequent pregnancies) has resulted in the very high uptake of thrombophilia testing by obstetricians. This has confounded ongoing rigorous research examining the efficacy of testing and treatment in this field.

Another significant limitation of case-control studies is the variation in the ethnic distribution of inherited thrombophilias. A number of studies have now highlighted the significant ethnic variation in the prevalence of various thrombophilias (Rees et al. 1995; Herrmann et al. 1997; Said et al. 2006; Said et al. 2008) but it is important to note that even within predominantly Caucasian populations, significant ethnic variation in the prevalence of inherited thrombophilias exists by virtue of different migration patterns (Said et al. 2006). Failure to take into account the specific prevalence of inherited thrombophilias in the ethnic group being studied, and account for the potential interaction of other co-inherited thrombophilias, can result in studies that are underpowered and thus unable to answer questions regarding the association between inherited thrombophilias and adverse obstetric outcomes.

3. Meta-analysis of case control studies

A number of meta-analyses examining the association between inherited thrombophilias and adverse pregnancy outcomes on the basis of case control studies have been undertaken (McLintock et al. 2001; Alfirevic et al. 2002; Rey et al. 2003; Howley et al. 2005; Lin and August 2005; Robertson et al. 2006; Facco et al. 2009). Meta-analyses of case control studies are limited by the significant heterogeneity of the included studies but nevertheless attempt to provide a clinically relevant evidence base to support decision making regarding testing for inherited thrombophilias in these obstetric conditions. As stated previously however, meta-analyses have limited validity due to the effects of publication bias and clinical heterogeneity.

As with case control studies, meta-analyses examining the association between inherited thrombophilias and pre-eclampsia have invariably concluded that overall, the strength of association may be weak at best with the greatest association observed with severe early onset disease. Lin and August included a total of 31 published studies and 7522 patients in their meta-analysis and calculated a modest odds ratio of 1.81 (1.14 - 2.87) for the association between the factor V Leiden mutation and pre-eclampsia overall and an odds ratio of 2.24 (1.28 - 3.94) for severe pre-eclampsia (Lin and August 2005). In contrast a statistically significant association was not observed with either the prothrombin gene mutation or the MTHFR 677 polymorphism. Once again, however, funnel plot analysis for publication bias suggested the possibility of publication bias due to the absence of smaller, negative studies available for inclusion in the meta-analysis.

A comprehensive review of published studies investigating genetic risk factors for placental abruption revealed a positive association between the prothrombin gene mutation (OR 6.67,

3.21 - 13.88, 7 included studies) and the factor V Leiden mutation (OR 2.35, 1.62 – 3.41, 10 studies) (Zdoukopoulos and Zintzaras 2008). Interestingly the strength of these associations increased significantly when studies comprising non-Caucasian women were excluded since both these mutations are more frequently present in Caucasian compared to non-Caucasian populations.

Rey and colleagues took up the challenge of dissecting the associations between inherited thrombophilias and fetal loss in their meta-analysis published in The Lancet in 2003 (Rey et al. 2003). After categorising fetal loss as early recurrent loss and late non-recurrent loss (after 19 weeks), they concluded first trimester recurrent fetal loss was associated with factor V Leiden (OR 2.01, 1.13 - 3.58) and prothrombin gene mutation (OR 2.05, 1.18 - 3.54) while late non-recurrent loss was associated with factor V Leiden (OR 3.26, 1.82 – 5.83), prothrombin gene mutation (OR 2.30, 1.09 – 4.87) and protein S deficiency (OR 7.39, 1.28 – 42.83) (Rey et al. 2003).

The relationship between fetal growth restriction and inherited thrombophilias has been the subject of several meta-analyses of case control studies (Dudding and Attia 2004; Howley et al. 2005; Robertson et al. 2006; Facco et al. 2009) The most recent of these meta-analyses reported a very modest overall summary odds ratio for the association between factor V Leiden and fetal growth restriction of 1.23 (1.04 – 1.44), however, when cohort studies were removed from the analysis the OR was 1.91 (1.17 - 3.12) (Facco et al. 2009). Further exploration of the data confirmed the effects of publication bias by demonstrating a significant odds ratio when early (pre-2004) studies were analysed (OR 2.04, 1.05 – 3.96, 6 studies) whereas a non-significant odds ratio was calculated when publications from 2004 - 2008 were included (OR 1.19, 0.02 – 2.39, 8 studies) (Facco et al. 2009).

4. Prospective cohort studies

While case control studies and their meta-analyses provide important data about the association between inherited thrombophilias and adverse pregnancy outcomes, they have an important limitation in that they cannot examine the "natural history" of thrombophilias and hence cannot ascribe causality. Prospective cohort studies are necessary to address this question of the potential for causality. In contrast to case control studies, prospective cohort studies need to recruit participants prior to the onset of any disease state and hence often require large numbers, making them costly and time consuming. However, undertaking prospective cohort studies in the setting of pregnancy has several advantages. Firstly, in contrast to prospective cohort studies investigating risk factors for cardiovascular disease and cancer, the time period is quite short and can be restricted to the duration of the pregnancy (ie 9 months) rather than the many years it may take for cardiovascular disease or cancers to develop in asymptomatic people. Secondly, pregnant women (at least in developed countries) are far more likely to attend for medical care at an early (asymptomatic) phase allowing non-biased ascertainment. Finally, many of the endpoints are easily measurable, routinely collected and not subject to observer or recall bias (e.g. birthweight, gestation at delivery, mode of delivery etc).

A number of prospective cohort studies have now been undertaken in a variety of different ethnic populations. These prospective cohort studies have confirmed that inherited thrombophilias are indeed common with prevalence estimates for the factor V Leiden mutation ranging from 2.7% (Murphy et al. 2000; Dizon-Townson et al. 2005) to 10.9%

(Lindqvist et al. 1999). Likewise the prothrombin gene mutation is seen in 2.4% (Said et al. 2010a) to 6.2% (Salomon et al. 2004) of women.

Three prospective cohort studies have examined only the association between factor V Leiden and adverse pregnancy events, and all failed to detect a statistically significant difference in the rate of pregnancy complications such as pre-eclampsia, fetal growth restriction, placental abruption or stillbirth amongst carriers of this mutation (Lindqvist et al. 1999; Dizon-Townson et al. 2005; Clark et al. 2008) (although one did show an association between neonatal death and factor V Leiden (Clark et al. 2008)). Dudding et al examined both factor V Leiden and prothrombin gene mutation and concluded that neither mutation was associated with the development of either pre-eclampsia or fetal growth restriction (Dudding et al. 2008). Another study examined factor V Leiden and MTHFR 677 and found no significant increase in the risk of adverse pregnancy outcomes although the small sample size (n=584) and low prevalence of factor V Leiden (2.7%) meant that this cohort was underpowered to detect a significant difference (Murphy et al. 2000). Three studies investigated factor V Leiden, prothrombin gene mutation and also the MTHFR 677 polymorphism (Salomon et al. 2004; Karakantza et al. 2008; Said et al. 2010a). No significant correlation was seen between any of these thrombophilias and adverse pregnancy outcomes in the study from Israel (Salomon et al. 2004). The second study, in a relatively small Greek cohort of 392 women, reported significant associations between factor V Leiden and MTHFR 677 and placental abruption (Karakantza et al. 2008). Said et al also reported significant associations between factor V Leiden and stillbirth (OR 8.85, 1.60 – 48.92), prothrombin gene mutation and placental abruption (OR 12.15, 2.45 - 60.39) and a composite outcome comprising severe pre-eclampsia, small for gestational age (below the 5th centile), placental abruption and stillbirth (OR 3.58, 1.20 – 10.61) in a cohort of 1707 asymptomatic nulliparous women (Said et al. 2010a). In contrast, Silver et al reported no association between the prothrombin gene mutation and adverse pregnancy events in a larger cohort of 4167 women (Silver RM et al. 2010). However, most importantly, all prospective cohort studies have confirmed that carriers of these inherited thrombophilias can experience completely uncomplicated pregnancies (Rodger et al. 2010; Said et al. 2010a).

An interesting finding from the Australian prospective cohort study (Said et al. 2010a) was the observation that homozygous carriers of the MTHFR 1298 polymorphism appeared to be at reduced risk of adverse pregnancy outcomes, and in particular fetal growth restriction. While the MTHFR 1298 polymorphism is not generally regarded as a thrombophilia in its own right and does not appear to be associated with hyperhomocysteinaemia, heterozygous coinheritance of the MTHFR 677 and MTHFR 1298 polymorphisms does appear to be associated with hyperhomocysteinaemia. Said et al have attributed their curious finding to the fact that the two MTHFR polymorphisms were in linkage disequilibrium suggesting that the protective effect observed with MTHFR 1298 homozygosity may in fact be due to the fact that these patients were protected from the risk of hyperhomocysteinaemia associated with homozygosity of MTHFR 677 (Said et al. 2010a). This possibility further supports the notion that absence of association in many prospective cohort studies may be because of failure to test for the wider range of "known" thrombophilias as well as the cumulative effect of common, less thrombogenic thrombophilias or unknown thrombophilias. Few studies have examined the MTHFR 1298 polymorphism to date to confirm or refute these findings.

5. Meta-analysis of cohort studies

A meta-analysis of these prospective cohort studies was published in 2010 (Rodger et al. 2010). This meta-analysis included 10 studies with 21,833 women and found no statistically significant increase in the risk of pre-eclampsia amongst women carrying the factor V Leiden mutation (OR 1.23, 0.89 - 1.70) (Rodger et al. 2010) (Figure 1). Likewise, the prothrombin gene mutation did not appear to confer an increase in the risk of pre-eclampsia with a pooled odds ratio of 1.25 (0.79 - 1.99) when 6 studies including 14,254 women were included (Rodger et al. 2010) (Figure 2). Similar non-significant findings were observed for the association between both of these thrombophilic mutations and placental abruption and delivery of a small for gestational age baby. In fact the only statistically significant association observed in this detailed meta-analysis was the significant association between pregnancy loss and the factor V Leiden mutation (Figure 1). It is important to note, however, the significant heterogeneity in the definition of pregnancy loss in the included studies, which comprised spontaneous miscarriage or stillbirth variably (Rodger et al. 2010).

This meta-analysis was adequately powered to detect an absolute increase of 2% in the rate of pre-eclampsia in carriers of the factor V Leiden mutation (from 3.2% to 5.2%) and an absolute increase of 3% in carriers of the prothrombin gene mutation. However, despite the large numbers of patients included in this meta-analysis, the study had inadequate power to detect a two-fold increase in the risk of placental abruption amongst carriers of the prothrombin gene mutation.

However, even with such a large meta-analysis failing to confirm significant associations between individual inherited thrombophilias and adverse pregnancy outcomes, several interpretations remain. First, of course, it is quite plausible that thrombophilia is simply not causative of these pregnancy complications. However, an interaction between inherited thrombophilia in susceptible people remains possible. Such an interaction may well result in augmentation of the pathological processes leading to conditions such as pre-eclampsia, or fetal growth restriction in susceptible people, resulting in earlier onset and more severe disease in these people. Such an explanation would be supported by the apparent contradiction between case-control studies and prospective cohort studies. An alternative possibility is that additional, as yet unidentified thrombophilias may result in a cumulative effect that determines the disease phenotype once a critical threshold is reached. This hypothesis is supported by observations from case-control studies that demonstrate the presence of multiple inherited thrombophilias being more commonly found in women with more severe complications than in apparently asymptomatic women. This issue would be relevant in the many case-control and cohort studies that only examine a single thrombophilic polymorphism rather than a panel of common polymorphisms.

A key feature of the association between inherited thrombophilias and pregnancy complications that has been particularly borne out by the prospective cohort studies is the lack of specificity between individual thrombophilias and particular complications. For example both the factor V Leiden mutation and the prothrombin gene mutation have been variably associated with normal pregnancy outcomes, fetal growth restriction, pre-eclampsia, placental abruption, stillbirth and recurrent miscarriage. Conversely, the phenotype of these disorders appears identical regardless of which thrombophilic mutation (if any) is carried. In addition, in a patient who carries one of these mutations, it is unclear what additional modifying factors will determine the precise outcome.

Study or Subgroup	FVL (+)^ Events	Total	FVL (-)^ Events	Total	Weight	Odds Ratio M-H, Fixed, 95% CI
1.1.1 Pregnancy Loss						
Said 2010	2	93	4	1633	1.1%	8.95 [1.62, 49.51]
Clark 2008	1	142	71	3802	12.7%	0.37 [0.05, 2.70]
Karakantza 2008	4	13	47	379	5.4%	3.14 [0.93, 10.60]
Rodger 2007 (1)	3	133	28	2811	6.2%	2.29 [0.69, 7.64]
Lindqvist 2006	13	270	73	2210	37.9%	1.48 [0.81, 2.71]
Dizon-Townson 2005	8	134	264	4751	34.1%	1.08 [0.52, 2.23]
Murphy 2000	3	16	24	572	2.7%	5.27 [1.41, 19.73]
Subtotal (95% CI)		**801**		**16158**	**100.0%**	**1.52 [1.06, 2.19]**
Total events	34		511			
Heterogeneity: Chi² = 12.13, df = 6 (P = 0.06); I² = 51%						
Test for overall effect: Z = 2.26 (P = 0.02)						
1.1.2 Pre-eclampsia						
Said 2010	5	93	98	1633	16.5%	0.89 [0.35, 2.24]
Clark 2008	3	141	63	3731	7.4%	1.27 [0.39, 4.08]
Dudding 2008	17	243	204	4206	34.1%	1.48 [0.88, 2.46]
Karakantza 2008	0	13	8	379	1.0%	1.62 [0.09, 29.52]
Rodger 2007 (1)	4	128	76	2783	10.7%	1.15 [0.41, 3.19]
Lindqvist 2006	5	257	34	2137	11.8%	1.23 [0.48, 3.17]
Dizon-Townson 2005	5	134	141	4751	12.3%	1.27 [0.51, 3.14]
Salomon 2004	1	38	28	605	5.3%	0.56 [0.07, 4.21]
Murphy 2000	0	13	12	548	1.0%	1.59 [0.09, 28.26]
Subtotal (95% CI)		**1060**		**20773**	**100.0%**	**1.23 [0.89, 1.70]**
Total events	40		664			
Heterogeneity: Chi² = 1.64, df = 8 (P = 0.99); I² = 0%						
Test for overall effect: Z = 1.24 (P = 0.22)						
1.1.3 SGA						
Said 2010	10	93	179	1633	11.1%	0.98 [0.50, 1.92]
Dudding 2008	33	587	368	7282	33.5%	1.12 [0.78, 1.61]
Rodger 2007 (1)	9	128	188	2783	9.9%	1.04 [0.52, 2.09]
Lindqvist 2006	23	257	221	2137	27.9%	0.85 [0.54, 1.34]
Dizon-Townson 2005	10	124	403	4428	13.1%	0.88 [0.46, 1.69]
Salomon 2004	5	38	62	603	4.1%	1.32 [0.50, 3.51]
Murphy 2000	0	13	9	548	0.3%	2.10 [0.12, 38.02]
Subtotal (95% CI)		**1240**		**19414**	**100.0%**	**1.00 [0.80, 1.25]**
Total events	90		1430			
Heterogeneity: Chi² = 1.59, df = 6 (P = 0.95); I² = 0%						
Test for overall effect: Z = 0.01 (P = 0.99)						
1.1.4 Placental Abruption						
Said 2010	0	93	9	1633	11.3%	0.91 [0.05, 15.83]
Karakantza 2008	3	13	12	379	6.8%	9.18 [2.23, 37.68]
Rodger 2007 (1)	3	128	39	2783	36.9%	1.69 [0.51, 5.54]
Lindqvist 2006	2	257	11	2137	25.8%	1.52 [0.33, 6.88]
Dizon-Townson 2005	0	134	31	4751	19.1%	0.56 [0.03, 9.15]
Subtotal (95% CI)		**625**		**11683**	**100.0%**	**1.85 [0.92, 3.70]**
Total events	8		102			
Heterogeneity: Chi² = 5.98, df = 4 (P = 0.20); I² = 33% (0 - 75%)						
Test for overall effect: Z = 1.72 (P = 0.08)						

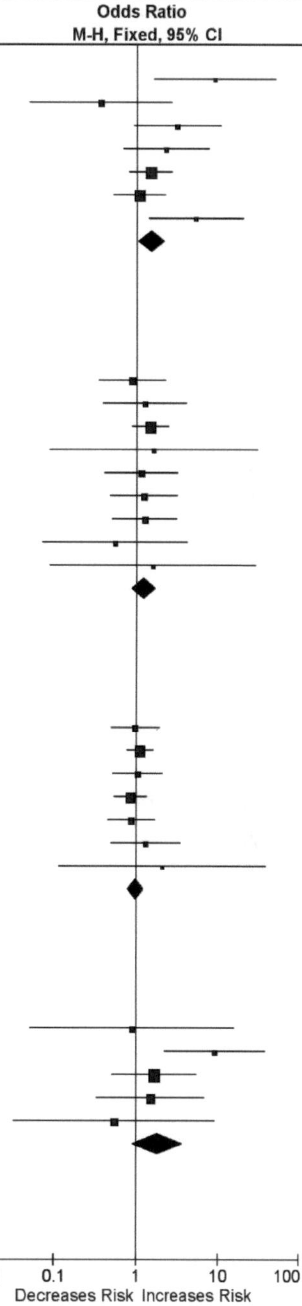

(1) Abstract
^ Homozygous or heterozygous

Fig. 1. Meta-analysis of pregnancy complications in women who are heterozygous or homozygous for factor V Leiden. (Rodger et al. 2010)

Study or Subgroup	PGM (+)^ Events	PGM (+)^ Total	PGM (-)^ Events	PGM (-)^ Total	Weight	Odds Ratio M-H, Fixed, 95% CI
2.1.1 Pregnancy Loss						
Silver 2010	9	157	238	4010	81.4%	0.96 [0.49, 1.91]
Said 2010	1	41	5	1685	1.1%	8.40 [0.96, 73.56]
Karakantza 2008	2	12	49	380	12.0%	1.35 [0.29, 6.35]
Rodger 2007 (1)	1	61	28	2879	5.5%	1.70 [0.23, 12.68]
Subtotal (95% CI)		**271**		**8954**	**100.0%**	**1.13 [0.64, 2.01]**
Total events	13		320			
Heterogeneity: Chi² = 3.69, df = 3 (P = 0.30); I² = 19%						
Test for overall effect: Z = 0.43 (P = 0.67)						
2.1.2 Pre-eclampsia						
Silver 2010	6	157	123	4010	30.9%	1.26 [0.54, 2.90]
Said 2010	3	41	100	1685	15.3%	1.25 [0.38, 4.12]
Dudding 2008	5	239	85	4176	31.2%	1.03 [0.41, 2.56]
Karakantza 2008	0	12	8	380	1.9%	1.75 [0.10, 32.09]
Rodger 2007 (1)	2	60	75	2851	10.4%	1.28 [0.31, 5.32]
Salomon 2004	3	40	26	603	10.4%	1.80 [0.52, 6.22]
Subtotal (95% CI)		**549**		**13705**	**100.0%**	**1.25 [0.79, 1.99]**
Total events	19		417			
Heterogeneity: Chi² = 0.56, df = 5 (P = 0.99); I² = 0%						
Test for overall effect: Z = 0.95 (P = 0.34)						
2.1.3 SGA						
Silver 2010	17	157	338	4010	33.4%	1.32 [0.79, 2.21]
Said 2010	5	41	184	1685	11.3%	1.13 [0.44, 2.92]
Dudding 2008	16	591	162	7251	35.0%	1.22 [0.72, 2.05]
Rodger 2007 (1)	5	60	190	2851	10.6%	1.27 [0.50, 3.22]
Salomon 2004	5	39	62	602	9.7%	1.28 [0.48, 3.40]
Subtotal (95% CI)		**888**		**16399**	**100.0%**	**1.25 [0.92, 1.70]**
Total events	48		936			
Heterogeneity: Chi² = 0.10, df = 4 (P = 1.00); I² = 0%						
Test for overall effect: Z = 1.46 (P = 0.15)						
2.1.4 Placental Abruption						
Silver 2010	2	157	24	4010	37.4%	2.14 [0.50, 9.15]
Said 2010	2	41	7	1685	6.6%	12.29 [2.47, 61.08]
Karakantza 2008	0	12	15	380	20.6%	0.94 [0.05, 16.67]
Rodger 2007 (1)	0	60	40	2851	35.3%	0.57 [0.03, 9.44]
Subtotal (95% CI)		**270**		**8926**	**100.0%**	**2.02 [0.81, 5.02]**
Total events	4		86			
Heterogeneity: Chi² = 5.94, df = 3 (P = 0.11); I² = 49% (0 - 83%)						
Test for overall effect: Z = 1.50 (P = 0.13)						

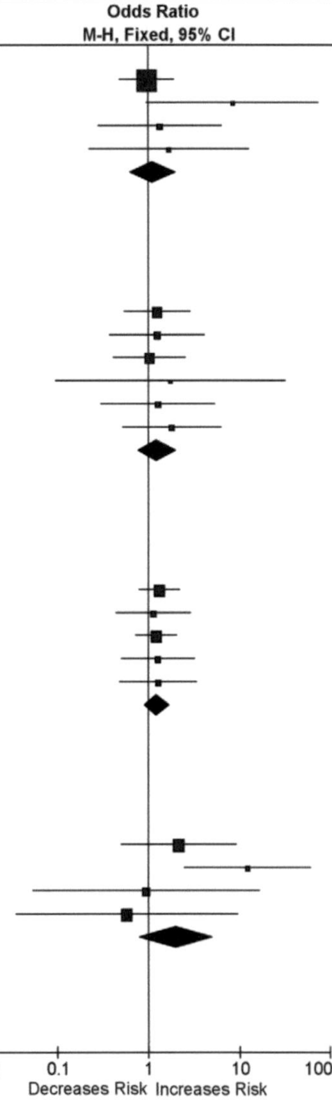

(1) Abstract
^ Homozygous or heterozygous

Fig. 2. Meta-analysis of pregnancy complications in women who are heterozygous or homozygous for prothrombin gene mutation. (Rodger et al. 2010)

Given the range of potential thrombophilias that could be investigated in an individual, the lack of specificity with disease states and the possibility of "unknown" or unidentified thrombophilias contributing to the phenotype, the appropriateness of investigating women for inherited thrombophilias to predict the risk for future pregnancy complications must be questioned. Thrombophilia testing is expensive. Furthermore there are conflicting data concerning the subsequent risks of recurrent adverse pregnancy outcomes such as pre-eclampsia (van Rijn et al. 2006; Facchinetti et al. 2009) in women who carry an inherited thrombophilia compared to those who don't, so the benefits of detecting these markers remain uncertain. This in turn makes the rationale of treating subsequent pregnancies with prophylactic heparins questionable. An alternative approach is to treat the disease phenotype rather than simply the test result!

6. Placental thrombotic lesions and inherited thrombophilias

Placental vasculopathy is a histopathological diagnosis which is increasingly being recognised in association with a variety of clinical pathologies including pre-eclampsia, fetal growth restriction, placental abruption and stillbirth. In addition, a number of reports regarding the association between these pathologic features and cerebral palsy have been published (Arias et al. 1998; Kraus and Acheen 1999). Redline and Pappin were amongst the first to report these specific placental lesions and their association with adverse neonatal outcomes. In addition they defined the pathologic criteria for diagnosis of this condition (Redline and Pappin 1995). While Kraus and Acheen (Kraus and Acheen 1999) have demonstrated that these lesions precede fetal death in cases of stillbirth, the precise pathophysiological mechanism resulting in the vascular thrombosis and fibrosis is unknown. Nevertheless it has been considered plausible that procoagulant states such as thrombophilias may contribute.

Many and colleagues (Many et al. 2001) investigated the contribution of maternal thrombophilias to the pathologic placental features in women with severe pregnancy complications and concluded that placental abnormalities such as infarcts and fibrinoid necrosis were more common in the placentae of women with pregnancy complications and thrombophilia compared to those with the same complications without thrombophilia. Of note, however, the women with thrombophilia and complications delivered at an earlier gestation and had lower birthweight babies compared to their non-thrombophilic counterparts. Thus whether these differences truly represent a difference in thrombophilia state or simply a difference in phenotypic state must be questioned. Likewise, Gogia and Machin (Gogia and Machin 2008) investigated the association between the specific placental lesions of maternal floor infarction (n=40), massive perivillous fibrin deposition (n=87) and fetal thrombotic vasculopathy (n=7) and identified a range of maternal thrombophilic markers in 40%, 23% and 71% respectively of the women with these placental histopathological diagnoses. The prevalence of thrombophilias in these women was significantly higher than the background prevalence of these same thrombophilias in the published literature.

In contrast, Mousa and Alfirevic (Mousa and Alfirevic 2000) were unable to detect a difference in placental histopathology amongst 43 thrombophilic women with adverse pregnancy outcome, who were compared to 36 non-thrombophilic women with the same adverse pregnancy outcomes. The validity of this study has however been questioned given that histopathological examination was performed as part of routine clinical investigation and management rather than being performed in a rigorous standardised manner, thereby leaving the final results and therefore conclusions potentially subject to bias (Khong et al. 2001). Likewise, Kahn et al examined the association between inherited thrombophilias and placental lesions reflecting underperfusion in a nested case-control study, and concluded that although the placental lesions were more common in cases of pre-eclampsia compared to controls, there was no correlation with maternal thrombophilia (Kahn et al. 2009).

In one of the largest studies to date, Rogers and colleagues prospectively collected and examined 105 placentae from women carrying the factor V Leiden mutation and 225 controls matched for maternal age, ethnicity and hospital (Rogers et al. 2010). They reported an increase in the frequency of syncytial knots (adjusted OR 3.6, 1.5 - 8.7 after controlling for hypertension, pre-eclampsia, small for gestational age fetus and preterm delivery before 35 weeks) and hypervascular villi (adjusted OR 3.4, 1.2 - 9.4 after controlling for mode of delivery) in placentae from women who were heterozygous for the factor V Leiden mutation. In contrast to the previous studies, this study did not demonstrate an increase in the frequency of placental infarcts, small for gestational age placentae or fetal thrombotic vasculopathy. An important limitation of this study, however, was that although testing for the prothrombin gene mutation and MTFR 677 polymorphism were performed, the numbers were too small to assess whether these polymorphisms also contributed to the placental pathological findings. Furthermore, subjects did not undergo testing for other known thrombophilias, raising the possibility that the pathologic lesions observed in control subjects may also be attributable to other thrombophilias

7. Fetal thrombophilias

It is of course plausible that it is the fetal thrombophilic status that is the strongest predictor of adverse pregnancy outcomes, fetal thrombotic vasculopathy and associated placental lesions. Given that inherited thrombophilias are generally inherited in an autosomal dominant fashion, the fetus would only have a 50% chance of inheriting maternal thrombophilias and this may explain why not all pregnancies appear to be affected. Placental tissue carries (in most cases) the same genotype as the fetus. A thrombophilic tendency in the placenta could therefore be conferred via the inheritance of paternally derived thrombophilias. The possibility that it is the fetal genotype, rather than the maternal, contributing to the development of fetal growth restriction was first suggested by a case report describing dizygotic twins with severe growth discordance. The patient had a past history of fetal growth restriction, placental abruption and pulmonary embolism and was found to be a compound heterozygote for the two MTHFR polymorphisms (677 and 1298) (Khong and Hague 2001). The twins demonstrated differential inheritance of the parental MTHFR genes, with the placenta of the smaller twin also demonstrating features of thrombotic vasculopathy. While dizygotic twins provide a unique opportunity for assessing the possible impact of fetal inheritance of thrombophilias, it is important to remember that a number of twins will have significant growth discordance which will partly relate to unequal utero-placental share, aside from any difference in thrombophilia state.

Ariel and colleagues investigated the association between fetal thrombophilia status and placental lesions but were unable to identify a statistically significant difference in the prevalence of placental thrombotic lesions between neonatal or maternal carriers of thrombophilia (Ariel et al. 2004). Rogers also investigated the potential contribution of fetal thrombophilias to the histopathologic appearance and found an increase in the frequency of avascular villi in placentae from 50 infants who carried the factor V Leiden mutation (Rogers et al. 2010). Forty of these infants inherited the mutation from the mother while 10 inherited it from the father. Of note, fetal inheritance of factor V Leiden was not associated with fetal thrombotic vasculopathy, placental infarction or small for gestational age placentae (Rogers et al. 2010).

An Australian study (Gibson et al. 2006) reported a significant association between fetal inheritance of the prothrombin gene mutation (heterozygous or homozygous) and fetal growth restriction (birthweight less than the 10th centile) in babies born prior to 28 weeks (odds ratio 5.71, 95% CI 1.49 - 21.93). Subgroup analysis for those babies with a birthweight less than the fifth centile also confirmed this finding.

Livingston also undertook a case control study investigating the relationship between maternal and fetal inherited thrombophilias and pre-eclampsia (Livingston et al. 2001). Although the large population of African American patients included in the study (and thus low prevalence of inherited thrombophilias) may have biased this study, Livingston concluded that neither maternal nor fetal inherited thrombophilias were associated with pre-eclampsia

Given these various reports, the association between inherited thrombophilias and placental thrombotic lesions appears to be weak at best and there are numerous confounding issues that must be considered such as the presence of additional maternal medical disorders, pregnancy complications and the complexities of the maternal-fetal genetic and immune interactions. Therefore recommendations for routine testing of entire families on the basis of placental findings (as suggested by Gogia (Gogia and Machin 2008)) are thus premature and raise concerns about the ethical implications of testing asymptomatic carriers.

8. The role of anticoagulants in preventing pregnancy complications in thrombophilic women

Despite the contradictory findings of studies investigating the association between inherited thrombophilias and adverse pregnancy outcomes, anticoagulant treatment for pregnant women who carry inherited thrombophilias has been embraced by many on the basis of small, non-randomised studies (Riyazi et al. 1998; Kupferminc et al. 2001; Ogueh et al. 2001; Grandone et al. 2002) and several larger randomised controlled trials with methodological limitations (Gris et al. 2004; Brenner et al. 2005). The rationale for anticoagulant treatment relies on the effect of anticoagulants in treating venous thromboembolism. A number of large scale randomised controlled trials investigating the role of low molecular weight heparins in preventing miscarriage in women who experience recurrent miscarriages have recently reported negative results (Clark et al. 2010; Kaandorp et al. 2010; Visser et al. 2011).

Meanwhile, the FRUIT study, (FRagmin®) in pregnant women with a history of Uteroplacental Insufficiency and Thrombophilia: a randomised trial (FRUIT) ISRCTN87325378), has recently been completed and demonstrated a small but statistically significant reduction in the risk of recurrent early onset pre-eclampsia or small for gestational age infant in thrombophilic women with a previous history of early onset pre-eclampsia or fetal growth restriction (de Vries et al. 2011). This multicentre trial randomised 139 thrombophilic women with prior adverse pregnancy outcomes (pre-eclampsia or small for gestational age infant with delivery prior to 34 weeks) to receive low molecular weight heparin (Fragmin®) (dosage adjusted for maternal weight) and aspirin 80mg or aspirin 80mg alone. Overall there was a statistically significant reduction in the primary outcome of pre-eclampsia or small for gestational age infant requiring delivery prior to 34 weeks, $p=0.012$ without any significant increase in the risk of adverse effects (de Vries et al. 2011).

While these data are encouraging, it must be emphasised that thrombophilic women with a history of prior adverse pregnancy outcomes such as those included in this study, represent only a very small proportion of the overall subgroup of women at risk of these serious pregnancy events and that many of these women do in fact achieve successful pregnancy outcomes with the far less expensive, less invasive and simple treatment regime of low dose aspirin which has been shown in an individual patient data meta-analysis to reduce the risk of recurrent pre-eclampsia and fetal growth restriction by up to 10% (Askie et al. 2007). The findings of the FRUIT study need to be confirmed in other, larger populations before this treatment should be recommended and certainly before this practice is extrapolated to other subgroups of thrombophilic patients (eg those with a prior stillbirth). The TIPPS study (Thrombophilia in Pregnancy Prophylaxis Study, ISRCTN87441504) is an ongoing multicentred randomised trial that will provide further data in this regard and may help to resolve some of these dilemmas.

However, as stated previously, the vast majority of women with these pregnancy complications do not have an identifiable thrombophilic marker, yet the mechanisms contributing to thrombotic lesions within the placenta remain uncertain. Moreover, the potential for anticoagulant prophylaxis to be of benefit in these women, as well as in women with identified thrombophilias, is limited by our lack of knowledge and understanding about the mechanisms involved in regulation of haemostasis in the placenta and potential actions of heparins in this organ.

9. Regulation of haemostasis in the placenta

Thrombotic lesions are observed commonly in placentae from women who experience pregnancy complications (Salafia et al. 1995a; Salafia et al. 1995b). Mechanisms regulating haemostasis within the placenta remain poorly understood (Sugimura et al. 2001; Lockwood et al. 2011; Said 2011). However, there is clear evidence of enhanced activation of the coagulation and fibrinolytic systems within both the uteroplacental and systemic circulations of women with pre-eclampsia compared to those with uncomplicated pregnancies (Higgins et al. 1998). As described previously, analysis of the published case-control studies reporting associations between inherited thrombophilias and adverse pregnancy events suggest that these associations are strongest with the more severe and earlier onset complications rather than with milder, later-onset conditions suggesting in fact that thrombophilias may exacerbate an underlying tendency toward the condition rather than causing it per se.

In vivo, coagulation and inflammatory pathways are intimately related (reviwed by Esmon (Esmon 2005)). The coagulation cascade is triggered with the exposure of tissue factor at the site of injury. Tissue factor is abundantly expressed in the decidua and first trimester trophoblast cells. Thus, invasion of the decidua during the first trimester by extravillous trophoblast cells is accompanied by profound local thrombin generation (which ultimately activates platelets and allows conversion of fibrinogen to fibrin) which protects against local haemorrhage. At the same time inflammatory processes are triggered which result in the production of inflammatory cytokines such as tumour necrosis factor-α (TNF-α), endotoxin and CD40 ligand, all of which induce tissue factor expression on the surface of white blood cells (especially monocytes), thereby augmenting the coagulation cascade (Esmon 2005). Furthermore, inflammatory mediators such as interleukin 6 (IL 6) increase both platelet numbers and platelet activation (Esmon 2005). These factors all contribute to the systemic procoagulant state observed in pregnancy. However, this system must be tightly regulated locally to prevent uncontrolled thrombosis. Thrombomodulin is also widely expressed on trophoblast cells (Isermann et al. 2003; Weiler 2004). The binding of thrombin to thrombomodulin results in activation of protein C. There is a modest but progressive increase in systemic protein C levels during the first half of pregnancy which may help to regulate haemostasis (Said et al. 2010b). Furthermore, it is now recognized that activated protein C plays an important role in the regulation of the inflammatory system through suppression of Tumour Necrosis Factor-α (TNFα) and inflammatory cytokine expression (Esmon 2001; Toltl LJ et al. 2008), which is mediated by protein C inhibition of Nuclear Factor-κB (NF-κB) translocation (Murakami et al. 1997).

Proteoglycans are macromolecules located within vessel walls and these are also abundantly expressed in human placentae. Being membrane bound, they act locally with exceptionally low levels detectable in maternal plasma (Giri and Tollefsen 2006). Proteoglycans were previously regarded as simply structural molecules responsible only for maintaining the "shape" and structural integrity of organs. It is now known that these molecules have important biological functions including anticoagulant properties, interactions with growth factors (particularly angiogenic growth factors such as VEGF and PlGF) (Santra et al. 2008) and anti-inflammatory properties, making them a potentially important group of candidate molecules in regulating placental haemostasis and potentially playing a role in the pathogenesis of pregnancy disorders (Schaefer and Iozzo 2008; Whitelock et al. 2008; Said 2011). Proteoglycans comprise a core protein to which sulphated glycosaminoglycans (GAG) chains are covalently linked. There are four types of GAG chains located in the blood vessel wall: Chondroitin Sulphate (CS), Dermatan Sulphate (DS), Heparan Sulphate (HS) and Hyaluronan (HA). (Iozzo 2005) Placentae contain two major types of proteoglycans; those containing heparan sulphate (syndecans, perlecan) (Jokimaa et al. 1998) and those containing dermatan sulphate (decorin and biglycan) (Murthi et al. 2010; Swan et al. 2010). HS chains bind Antithrombin (AT) – a potent inhibitor of thrombin - through a pentasaccharide sequence, and DS chains bind Heparin Cofactor II (HCII) through a highly charged sequence (Chen and Liu 2005). GAG bound AT and HCII undergo a conformational change, which in turn facilitates the inhibition of thrombin (Brinkmeyer et al. 2004). The cellular localization of proteoglycans to endothelium and cells in contact with circulating blood, suggest an important role for these molecules in localized anticoagulation. Previous studies have demonstrated significant reductions in mRNA expression of decorin (Swan et al. 2010) and biglycan (Murthi et al. 2010) in placentae from pregnancies affected by fetal growth restriction (FGR) compared to gestation matched control placentae using semi-quantitative RT-PCR (relative to the house keeping gene GAPDH). Warda et al also demonstrated a significant reduction in the expression of GAG synthesizing enzymes in preeclamptic placentae compared to controls (Warda et al. 2008). This reduction translated to a significant alteration in GAG structure raising the possibility that the altered GAG structure may have functional corollaries which may contribute to the development of pre-eclampsia.

Proteoglycans also play important roles in angiogenic pathways by acting as receptors for growth factors. Disordered angiogenesis has been implicated as a key pathogenic mechanism contributing to pregnancy disorders such as pre-eclampsia and fetal growth restriction (comprehensively reviewed by Young et al (Young et al. 2010)) Vascular endothelial growth factor (VEGF) plays an important role in stabilizing the endothelium in mature blood vessels (Maharaj et al. 2008). Placental growth factor (PlGF) has structural homology to VEGF and is thought to amplify VEGF signalling (Autiero et al. 2003). VEGF and PlGF are highly expressed by invasive cytotrophoblasts involved in spiral artery remodeling. However, in preeclamptic pregnancies, VEGF and PlGF levels are substantially lower than non-preeclamptic controls (Young et al. 2010). The soluble form of the VEGF receptor fms-like tyrosine kinase (sFlt1), an antagonist of VEGF, is significantly elevated in pre-eclamptic pregnancies (Young et al. 2010). Similarly transforming growth factor ß (TGF-ß) and endoglin (Eng) levels are higher in pre-eclamptic pregnancies compared to controls although whether this is a primary pathologic mechanism or a compensatory mechanism resulting from ongoing placental ischemia remains uncertain. sFlt1 and sEng, the soluble forms of FLt1 and Eng respectively are released into maternal plasma during pre-eclampsia and exert their antiangiogenic effects on maternal endothelium leading to a state of generalized endothelial dysfunction (Young et al. 2010).

The interaction between haemostatic pathways and angiogenic pathways is further illustrated by the finding that thrombin significantly augments first trimester (but not term) decidual expression of sFlt-1 (Lockwood et al. 2007). Thus, dysregulation of the complex haemostatic pathway by any one of a range of possible mechanisms during the first trimester, has the potential to lead to a cascade of events which may collectively lead to the pathophysiological processes observed in pregnancies complicated by adverse events such as pre-eclampsia.

The combination of endothelial dysfunction, altered blood flow dynamics secondary to abnormal vasculature and the hypercoagulable state of pregnancy provides a plausible background for the development of intravascular microthrombi, which in turn can result in a positive feedback loop leading to greater tissue ischaemia, ongoing oxidative stress and endothelial dysfunction thus perpetuating intravascular thrombosis and ultimately leading to the characteristic placental lesions we observe in pregnancy disorders such as pre-eclampsia, placental abruption, fetal growth restriction and stillbirth. It is plausible that dysregulation of these processes are far more important in leading to the pathogenesis of adverse pregnancy events than inherited thrombophilias.

10. The role of anticoagulants in "non-thrombophilic" patients

Recent randomised controlled trials (RCTs) investigating the role of low molecular weight heparins (LMWH) in preventing adverse pregnancy outcomes in non-thrombophilic women have suggested beneficial effects (Rey et al. 2009; Gris JC et al. 2010) raising the possibility that it is a primary placental haemostatic defect contributing to the pathogenesis of these conditions rather than a maternal thrombophilia. Data from these RCT's are supported by non-randomised observational studies in which non-thrombophilic women with previous obstetric complications and associated evidence of placental vasculopathy had improved obstetric outcomes when treated with LMWH in subsequent pregnancies (Kupferminc et al. 2011). These studies are indeed promising and suggest the more rational use of anticoagulants using an appropriate "phenotype" driven approach (ie on the basis of disease severity and corroborating placental histopathological findings) rather than just a genotype (presence of thrombophilia) driven approach. However a note of caution must be applied. Firstly, the precise mechanism by which low molecular weight heparins achieve beneficial obstetric outcomes remains obscure. Heparin is a synthetic glycosaminoglycan with augmented anticoagulant activity. Whether heparins produce their therapeutic effects in these pregnancy situations via their anticoagulant action or whether through non-anticoagulant (inflammatory or angiogenic mechanisms as discussed previously) has not yet been determined. Understanding these mechanisms may provide the basis for developing more efficacious and safe agents. Secondly, none of the randomised trials published to date have been adequately powered to assess uncommon but serious potential consequences of treatment. Although low molecular weight heparins are generally regarded as "safe"(Greer and Nelson-Piercy 2005), they have important implications for labour epidural use

(Horlocker et al. 2010) and risks of wound bleeding and haematoma (van Wijk et al. 2002) following operative delivery. These comparatively minor risks are particularly important given the third issue which is the fact that prophylaxis is given to prevent recurrence of placental mediated complications, but untreated women appear to only have a risk of at most 25-30% (van Rijn et al. 2006; Rey et al. 2009) for these recurrent complications, therefore potentially 70% or more of these women are exposed to this treatment without necessarily needing it. Strategies to better predict who will benefit from such therapy are urgently needed but what does appear clear is that prediction on the basis of presence or absence of a known inherited thrombophilia is not a useful or worthwhile strategy.

Kingdom et al attempted to better stratify women by incorporating a range of tests of placental function prior to including women in a pilot randomised trial of unfractionated heparin in women at risk of placental mediated obstetric complications (Kingdom et al. 2011). However, even despite this rigorous screening process, only 12% of women developed pre-eclampsia and 25% of the infants had intrauterine growth restriction in the standard care arm (Kingdom et al. 2011). The high prevalence of placental pathology, however was confirmed with only 5/31 normal placentae (4 in the unfractionated heparin group and one in the standard care group) identified. Although this study was underpowered to determine whether unfractionated heparin is beneficial in this setting, it does highlight the need for improved identification and stratification of patients who may benefit from this somewhat invasive therapy. Furthermore, the choice of unfractionated heparin in this study contrasts with that of previous studies which predominantly use low molecular weight heparins.

11. Conclusions

Inherited thrombophilias are common amongst women of reproductive age. However, we can be reassured by the prospective cohort studies and the meta-analysis of such studies that the majority of asymptomatic women who carry these inherited thrombophilias will not experience adverse pregnancy outcomes. What is less certain is the potential adjuvant role that thrombophilias may play in women at increased risk for other reasons of these complications or in women who are developing these complications. Also of concern is the large number of women who experience adverse pregnancy complications who do not carry a recognisable inherited or acquired thrombophilia. Understanding the precise mechanisms regulating coagulation within the placenta will be an important priority in order to establish the most efficacious therapeutic options for this majority of women experiencing these complications. Only then should the effects of and differences between the variety of available anticoagulants be investigated to ensure that these therapeutic agents are used in the most effective and rational manner to either treat or prevent serious adverse pregnancy events.

12. References

Agorastos, T., A. Karavida, et al. (2002). "Factor V Leiden and prothrombin G20210A mutations in pregnancies with adverse outcome." *Journal of Maternal-Fetal & Neonatal Medicine.* 12(4): 267-73.

Alfirevic, Z., D. Roberts, et al. (2002). "How strong is the association between maternal thrombophilia and adverse pregnancy outcome? A systematic review." *Eur J Obstet Gynecol Reprod Biol* 101(1): 6-14.

Arias, F., R. Romero, et al. (1998). "Thrombophilia: a mechanism of disease in women with adverse pregnancy outcome and thrombotic lesions in the placenta." *Journal of Maternal-Fetal Medicine.* 7(6): 277-86.

Ariel, I., E. Anteby, et al. (2004). "Placental pathology in fetal thrombophilia." *Human Pathology* 35(6): 729-733.

Askie, L. M., L. Duley, et al. (2007). "Antiplatelet agents for prevention of pre-eclampsia: a meta-analysis of individual patient data." *The Lancet* 369(9575): 1791-1798.

Askie, L. M., D. J. Henderson-Smart, et al. (2005). "Management of infants with chronic lung disease of prematurity in Australasia." *Early Human Development* 81(2): 135-142.

Autiero, M., A. Luttun, et al. (2003). "Placental growth factor and its receptor, vascular endothelial growth factor receptor-1: novel targets for stimulation of ischemic tissue revascularization and inhibition of angiogenic and inflammatory disorders." *Journal of Thrombosis & Haemostasis* 1(7): 1356-1370.

Barker, D., P. Gluckman, et al. (1993). "Fetal nutrition and cardiovascular disease in adult life." *The Lancet* 341: 938-941.

Bates, S., I. Greer, et al. (2004). "Use of Antithrombotic Agents During Pregnancy. The Seventh ACCP Conference on Antithrombotic and Thrombolytic Therapy." *Chest.* 126(3): 627S - 644S.

Brenner, B., R. Hoffman, et al. (2005). "Efficacy and safety of two doses of enoxaparin in women with thrombophilia and recurrent pregnancy loss: the LIVE-ENOX study." *J Thromb Haemost* 3(2): 227-229.

Brinkmeyer, S., R. Eckert, et al. (2004). "Reformable intramolecular cross-linking of the N-terminal domain of heparin cofactor II." *European Journal of Biochemistry* 271(21): 4275-4283.

Chen, J. and J. Liu (2005). "Characterization of the structure of antithrombin-binding heparan sulfate generated by heparan sulfate 3-O-sulfotransferase 5." *Biochimica et Biophysica Acta (BBA) - General Subjects* 1725(2): 190-200.

Clark, P., I. D. Walker, et al. (2008). "The GOAL study: a prospective examination of the impact of factor V Leiden and ABO(H) blood groups on haemorrhagic and thrombotic pregnancy outcomes." *British Journal of Haematology* 140(2): 236-240.

Clark, P., I. D. Walker, et al. (2010). "SPIN (Scottish Pregnancy Intervention) study: a multicenter, randomized controlled trial of low-molecular-weight heparin and low-dose aspirin in women with recurrent miscarriage." *Blood* 115(21): 4162-4167.

de Vries, J. I., W. J. Kist, et al. (2009). "Confounded thrombophilia studies in preeclampsia." *American Journal of Obstetrics and Gynecology* 201(5): e11-e12.

de Vries, J. I., M. G. Van Pampus, et al. (2011). "Fractionated heparin in pregnant women with a history of uteroplacental insufficiency and thrombophilia, a randomized trial (The FRUIT study)." *Reprod Sci* 18(3 (Supplement)): 352A: S199.

de Vries, J. I. P., G. A. Dekker, et al. (1997). "Hyperhomocysteinaemia and Protein S deficiency in complicated pregnancies." *British Journal of Obstetrics & Gynaecology* 104: 1248 - 1254.

Dekker, G. A., J. I. de Vries, et al. (1995). "Underlying disorders associated with severe early-onset preeclampsia." *Am J Obstet Gynecol* 173(4): 1042-8.

Dizon-Townson, D., C. Miller, et al. (2005). "The relationship of the factor V Leiden mutation and pregnancy outcomes for the mother and fetus." *Obstetrics & Gynecology* 106(3): 517-524.

Dudding, T., J. Heron, et al. (2008). "Factor V Leiden is associated with pre-eclampsia but not with fetal growth restriction: a genetic association study and meta-analysis." *Journal of Thrombosis and Haemostasis* 6(11): 1868-1875.

Dudding, T. E. and J. Attia (2004). "The association between adverse pregnancy outcomes and maternal factor V Leiden genotype: a meta-analysis." *Thromb Haemost* 91(4): 700-11.

Esmon, C. T. (2001). "Protein C anticoagulant pathway and its role in controlling microvascular thrombosis and inflammation." *Critical Care Medicine* 29(7 (Supplement)): S48-S52.

Esmon, C. T. (2005). "The interactions between inflammation and coagulation." *British Journal of Haematology* 131(4): 417-430.

Facchinetti, F., L. Marozio, et al. (2009). "Maternal thrombophilia and the risk of recurrence of preeclampsia." *American Journal of Obstetrics and Gynecology* 200(1): 46.e1-46.e5.

Facco, F., W. You, et al. (2009). "Genetic Thrombophilias and Intrauterine Growth Restriction: A Meta-analysis." *Obstet Gynecol* 113(6): 1206-1216.

Gibson, C. S., A. H. MacLennan, et al. (2006). "Associations between fetal inherited thrombophilia and adverse pregnancy outcomes." *American Journal of Obstetrics & Gynecology* 194: 947 -94.

Giri, T. K. and D. M. Tollefsen (2006). "Placental dermatan sulfate: isolation, anticoagulant activity, and association with heparin cofactor II." *Blood* 107(7): 2753-2758.

Gogia, N. and G. A. Machin (2008). "Maternal Thrombophilias Are Associated with Specific Placental Lesions." *Pediatric & Developmental Pathology* 11(6): 424-429.

Grandone, E., V. Brancaccio, et al. (2002). "Preventing adverse obstetric outcomes in women with genetic thrombophilia." *Fertility & Sterility.* 78(2): 371-5.

Grandone, E., M. Margaglione, et al. (1997). "Factor V Leiden is associated with repeated and recurrent unexplained fetal losses." *Thromb Haemost* 77(5): 822-824.

Greer, I. A. and C. Nelson-Piercy (2005). "Low-molecular-weight heparins for thromboprophylaxis and treatment of venous thromboembolism in pregnancy: a systematic review of safety and efficacy." *Blood* 106(2): 401-407.

Gris JC, Chauleur C, et al. (2010). "Enoxaparin for the secondary prevention of placental vascular complications in women with abruptio placentae. The pilot randomised controlled NOH-AP trial " *Thromb Haemost* 104(4): 771-779.

Gris, J. C., E. Mercier, et al. (2004). "Low-molecular-weight heparin versus low dose aspirin in women with one fetal loss and a constitutional thrombophilic disorder." *Blood* 103(10): 3695 - 3699.

Guellec, I., A. Lapillonne, et al. (2011). "Neurologic Outcomes at School Age in Very Preterm Infants Born With Severe or Mild Growth Restriction." *Pediatrics* 127(4): e883-e891.

Herrmann, F. H., M. Koesling, et al. (1997). "Prevalence of Factor V Leiden Mutation in various populations." *Genetic Epidemiology* 14: 403 - 411.

Higgins, J. R., J. J. Walshe, et al. (1998). "Hemostasis in the uteroplacental and peripheral circulations in normotensive and pre-eclamptic pregnancies." *American Journal of Obstetrics & Gynecology.* 179(2): 520-6.

Horlocker, T. T., D. J. Wedel, et al. (2010). "Regional anesthesia in the patient receiving antithrombotic or thrombolytic therapy: American society of regional anesthesia and pain medicine evidence-based guidelines (Third edition)." *Reg Anesth Pain Med* 35(1): 64-101.

Howley, H. E., M. Walker, et al. (2005). "A systematic review of the association between factor V Leiden or prothrombin gene variant and intrauterine growth restriction." *American Journal of Obstetrics & Gynecology* 192: 694-708.

Infante-Rivard, C., G.-E. Rivard, et al. (2002). "Absence of Association of Thrombophilia Polymorphisms with Intrauterine Growth Restriction." *New England Journal of Medicine* 347(1): 19-25.

Iozzo, R. V. (2005). "Basement membrane proteoglycans: from cellar to ceiling." *Nat Rev Mol Cell Biol* 6(8): 646-656.

Isermann, B., R. Sood, et al. (2003). "The thrombomodulin-protein C system is essential for the maintenance of pregnancy." *Nature Medicine* 9(3): 331-337.

Jokimaa, V., P. Inki, et al. (1998). "Expression of syndecan-1 in human placenta and decidua " *Placenta* 19(2-3): 157-163.

Kaandorp, S. P., M. t. Goddijn, et al. (2010). "Aspirin plus Heparin or Aspirin Alone in Women with Recurrent Miscarriage." *New England Journal of Medicine* 362(17): 1586-1596.

Kahn, S. R., R. Platt, et al. (2009). "Inherited thrombophilia and preeclampsia within a multicenter cohort: the Montreal Preeclampsia Study." *Am J Obstet Gynecol* 200(2): 151.e1-151.e9.

Karakantza, M., G. Androutsopoulos, et al. (2008). "Inheritance and perinatal consequences of inherited thrombophilia in Greece." *Int J Gynecol Obstet* 100(2): 124-9.

Khong, T. Y. and W. M. Hague (2001). "Biparental contribution to fetal thrombophilia in discordant twin intrauterine growth restriction." *American Journal of Obstetrics & Gynecology.* 185(1): 244-5.

Khong, T. Y., L. Moore, et al. (2001). "Thrombophilias and adverse pregnancy outcome." *Human Reproduction.* 16(2): 395-7.

Kingdom, J., M. Walker, et al. (2011). "Unfractionated heparin for second trimester placental insufficiency: a pilot randomized trial." *J Thromb Haemost* epub 20 June 2011.

Kraus, F. and V. Acheen (1999). "Fetal thrombotic vasculopathy in the placenta: cerebral thrombi and infarcts, coagulopathies, and cerebral palsy." *Human Pathology* 30(7): 759-769.

Kupferminc, M., E. Rimon, et al. (2011). "Low molecular weight heparin versus no treatment in women with previous severe pregnancy complications and placental findings without thrombophilia." *Blood Coagul Fibrinolysis* 22(2): 123-126.

Kupferminc, M. J., A. Eldor, et al. (1999). "Increased frequency of genetic thrombophilia in women with complications of pregnancy." *N Engl J Med* 340(1): 9-13.

Kupferminc, M. J., G. Fait, et al. (2000). "Severe preeclampsia and high frequency of genetic thrombophilic mutations." *Obstet Gynecol* 96(1): 45-9.

Kupferminc, M. J., G. Fait, et al. (2001). "Low-molecular-weight heparin for the prevention of obstetric complications in women with thrombophilias." *Hypertens Pregnancy.* 20(1): 35-44.

Kupferminc, M. J., A. Many, et al. (2002). "Mid-trimester severe intrauterine growth restriction is associated with a high prevalence of thrombophilia." *BJOG* 109(12): 1373-6.

Lin, J. and P. August (2005). "Genetic thrombophilias and preeclampsia: a meta-analysis." *Obstet Gynecol* 105(1): 182-192.

Lindqvist, P. G., P. J. Svensson, et al. (1999). "Activated protein C resistance (FV:Q506) and pregnancy." *Thromb Haemost* 81(4): 532-7.

Livingston, J. C., J. R. Barton, et al. (2001). "Maternal and fetal inherited thrombophilias are not related to the development of severe preeclampsia." *Am J Obstet Gynecol* 185(1): 153-7.

Lockwood, C. J., S. J. Huang, et al. (2011). "Decidual Hemostasis, inflammation, and angiogenesis in pre-eclampsia." *Semin Thromb Hemost* 37(2): 158-164.

Lockwood, C. J., P. Toti, et al. (2007). "Thrombin Regulates Soluble fms-Like Tyrosine Kinase-1 (sFlt-1) Expression in First Trimester Decidua: Implications for Preeclampsia." *The American Journal of Pathology* 170(4): 1398-1405.

Maharaj, A. S. R., T. E. Walshe, et al. (2008). "VEGF and TGF-Î² are required for the maintenance of the choroid plexus and ependyma." *The Journal of Experimental Medicine* 205(2): 491-501.

Many, A., R. Elad, et al. (2002). "Third-trimester unexplained intrauterine fetal death is associated with inherited thrombophilia." *Obstetrics & Gynecology.* 99(5 Pt 1): 684-7.

Many, A., L. Schreiber, et al. (2001). "Pathologic features of the placenta in women with severe pregnancy complications and thrombophilia." *Obstetrics & Gynecology.* 98(6): 1041-4.

Martinelli, P., E. Grandone, et al. (2001). "Familial thrombophilia and the occurrence of fetal growth restriction." *Haematologica.* 86(4): 428-31.

McLintock, C., R. North, et al. (2001). "Inherited thrombophilias: implications for pregnancy associated venous thromboembolism and obstetric complications." *Current Problems in Obstetrics, Gynaecology and Fertility* 24: 115-149.

Mousa, H. A. and Z. Alfirevic (2000). "Do placental lesions reflect thrombophilia state in women with adverse pregnancy outcome?" *Human Reproduction.* 15(8): 1830-1833.

Murakami, K., K. Okajima, et al. (1997). "Activated protein C prevents LPS-induced pulmonary vascular injury by inhibiting cytokine production." *American Journal of Physiology. Lung Cellular and Molecular Physiology* 272(2): L197-202.

Murphy, R. P., C. Donoghue, et al. (2000). "Prospective evaluation of the risk conferred by factor V Leiden and thermolabile methylenetetrahydrofolate reductase polymorphisms in pregnancy." *Arteriosclerosis, Thrombosis and Vascular Biology* 20: 266-270.

Murthi, P., F. A. Faisal, et al. (2010). "Placental Biglycan Expression is Decreased in Human Idiopathic Fetal Growth Restriction." *Placenta* 31(8): 712-717.

Ogueh, O., M. F. Chen, et al. (2001). "Outcome of pregnancy in women with hereditary thrombophilia." *Int J Gynaecol Obstet* 74(3): 247-53.

Preston, F. E., F. R. Rosendaal, et al. (1996). "Increased fetal loss in women with heritable thrombophilia." *The Lancet.* 348(9032): 913-6.

Rai, R., A. Shlebak, et al. (2001). "Factor V Leiden and acquired activated protein C resistance among 1000 women with recurrent miscarriage." *Hum Reprod* 16(5): 961-965.

Raziel, A., Y. Kornberg, et al. (2001). "Hypercoagulable thrombophilic defects and hyperhomocysteinemia in patients with recurrent pregnancy loss." *Am J Reprod Immunol* 45(2): 65-71.

Redline, R. W. and A. Pappin (1995). "Fetal thrombotic vasculopathy: The clinical significance of extensive avascular villi." *Human Pathology* 26(1): 80-85.

Rees, D. C., M. Cox, et al. (1995). "World distribution of factor V Leiden." *Lancet* 346: 1133 - 1134.

Rey, E., P. Garneau, et al. (2009). "Dalteparin for the prevention of recurrence of placental-mediated complications of pregnancy in women without thrombophilia: a pilot randomized controlled trial." *J Thromb Haemost* 7(1): 58-64.

Rey, E., S. R. Kahn, et al. (2003). "Thrombophilic disorders and fetal loss: a meta-analysis." *Lancet.* 361(9361): 901-8.

Riyazi, N., M. Leeda, et al. (1998). "Low-molecular-weight heparin combined with aspirin in pregnant women with thrombophilia and a history of preeclampsia or fetal growth restriction: a preliminary study." *Eur J Obstet Gynecol Reprod Biol* 80(1): 49-54.

Robertson, L., O. Wu, et al. (2006). "Thrombophilia in pregnancy: a systematic review." *Br J Haematol* 132(2): 171-196.

Rodger, M. A., M. T. Betancourt, et al. (2010). "The Association of Factor V Leiden and Prothrombin Gene Mutation and Placenta-Mediated Pregnancy Complications: A Systematic Review and Meta-analysis of Prospective Cohort Studies." *PLoS Med* 7(6): e1000292.

Rogers, B. B., V. Momirova, et al. (2010). "Avascular Villi, Increased Syncytial Knots, and Hypervascular Villi Are Associated with Pregnancies Complicated by Factor V Leiden Mutation." *Pediatric and Developmental Pathology* 13(5): 341-347.

Said, J. M. (2011). "The role of proteoglycans in contributing to placental thrombosis and fetal growth restriction." *Journal of Pregnancy*: Article ID 928381.

Said, J. M., S. P. Brennecke, et al. (2006). "Ethnic differences in the prevalence of inherited thrombophilic polymorphisms in an asymptomatic Australian prenatal population." *Hum Biol* 78(4): 403-12.

Said, J. M., S. P. Brennecke, et al. (2008). "The prevalence of inherited thrombophilic polymorphisms in an asymptomatic Australian antenatal population." *Australian & New Zealand Journal of Obstetrics & Gynaecology* 48(6): 536-41.

Said, J. M., J. R. Higgins, et al. (2010a). "Inherited Thrombophilia Polymorphisms and Pregnancy Outcomes in Nulliparous Women." *Obstetrics & Gynecology* 115(1): 5-13.

Said, J. M., V. Ignjatovic, et al. (2010b). "Altered reference ranges for protein C and protein S during early pregnancy: Implications for the diagnosis of protein C and protein S deficiency during pregnancy." *Thromb Haemost* 103(5): 875-1108.

Salafia, C. M., V. K. Minior, et al. (1995a). "Intrauterine growth restriction in infants of less than thirty-two weeks' gestation: Associated placental pathologic features." *American Journal of Obstetrics & Gynecology* 173(4): 1049 - 1057.

Salafia, C. M., J. C. Pezzullo, et al. (1995b). "Placental pathologic features of preterm preeclampsia." *American Journal of Obstetrics & Gynecology* 173(4): 1097 - 1105.

Salomon, O., U. Seligsohn, et al. (2004). "The common prothrombotic factors in nulliparous women do not compromise blood flow in the feto-maternal circulation and are not associated with preeclampsia or intrauterine growth restriction." *American Journal of Obstetrics & Gynecology* 191(6): 2002-9.

Santra, M., S. Santra, et al. (2008). "Ectopic decorin expression up-regulates VEGF expression in mouse cerebral endothelial cells via activation of the transcription factors Sp1, HIF1α, and Stat3." *Journal of Neurochemistry* 105(2): 324-337.

Schaefer, L. and R. V. Iozzo (2008). "Biological Functions of the Small Leucine-rich Proteoglycans: From Genetics to Signal Transduction." *Journal of Biological Chemistry* 283(31): 21305-21309.

Sibai, B. (2005). "Thrombophilia and Severe Preeclampsia. Time to screen and treat in future pregnancies?" *Hypertension* 46: 1252-1253.

Silver RM, Zhao Y, et al. (2010). "Prothrombin gene G20210A mutation and obstetric complications." *Obstetrics & Gynecology* 115(1): 14-20.

Sugimura, M., R. Ohashi, et al. (2001). "Intraplacental coagulation in intrauterine growth restriction: cause or result?" *Semin Thromb Hemost* 27(2): 107-13.

Swan, B., P. Murthi, et al. (2010). "Decorin expression is decreased in human idiopathic fetal growth restriction." *Reproduction, Fertility and Development* 22(6): 949-955.

Toltl LJ, Swystun LL, et al. (2008). "Protective effects of activated protein C in sepsis." *Thrombosis & Haemostasis* 100(4): 582 - 592

van Pampus, M. G., G. A. Dekker, et al. (1999). "High prevalence of hemostatic abnormalities in women with a history of severe preeclampsia." *American Journal of Obstetrics & Gynecology.* 180(5): 1146-50.

van Rijn, B. B., L. B. Hoeks, et al. (2006). "Outcomes of subsequent pregnancy after first pregnancy with early-onset preeclampsia." *American Journal of Obstetrics and Gynecology* 195(3): 723-728.

van Wijk, F. H., H. Wolf, et al. (2002). "Administration of low molecular weight heparin within two hours before caesarean section increases the risk of wound haematoma." *BJOG: an International Journal of Obstetrics & Gynaecology* 109(8): 955-957.

Visser, J., V.-M. Ulander, et al. (2011). "Thromboprophylaxis for recurrent miscarriage in women with or without thrombophilia HABENOX*: A randomised multicentre trial." *Thromb Haemost* 105(2): 295-301.

Warda, M., F. Zhang, et al. (2008). "Is human placenta proteoglycan remodeling involved in pre-eclampsia?" *Glycoconjugate Journal* 25(5): 441-450.

Weiler, H. (2004). "Mouse models of thrombosis: thrombomodulin." *Thrombosis & Haemostasis* 92(3): 467-77.

Whitelock, J. M., J. Melrose, et al. (2008). "Diverse Cell Signaling Events Modulated by Perlecan " *Biochemistry* 47(43): 11174-11183.

Wiener-Megnagi, Z., I. Ben-Shlomo, et al. (1998). "Resistance to activated protein C and the Leiden mutation: High prevalence in patients with abruptio placentae." *American Journal of Obstetrics and Gynecology* 179(6): 1565-1567.

Young, B. C., R. J. Levine, et al. (2010). "Pathogenesis of Preeclampsia." *Annual Review of Pathology: Mechanisms of Disease* 5(1): 173-192.

Younis, J. S., B. Brenner, et al. (2000). "Activated protein C resistance and factor V Leiden mutation can be associated with first as well as second-trimester recurrent pregnancy loss." *Am J Reprod Immunol* 43(1): 31-35.

Zdoukopoulos, N. and E. Zintzaras (2008). "Genetic risk factors for placental abruption. A HuGE review and meta-analysis." *Epidemiology* 19(2): 309-323.

8

Infertility and Inherited Thrombophilia

Ricardo Barini, Adriana Goes Soligo,
Joyce Annichino-Bizzachi and Egle Couto
State University of Campinas, UNICAMP
Brazil

1. Introduction

Infertility is a condition that affects between one-fifth and one-sixth of couples of reproductive age. It is defined as a reduction in or a lack of ability to reproduce and its cause may lie either in the male or female partner (Stedman, 2006). According to the American Society for Reproductive Medicine, infertility should be considered when pregnancy fails to occur after one year of regular sexual activity without the use of any contraceptive method.

In view of its high incidence, infertility currently constitutes a significant health issue. The social structure prevalent today in which women are conditioned to consider motherhood at a later age results in an increase in the number of couples seeking medical assistance to fulfill their dream of having children (Neuspiller, 2003). Nevertheless, the forms of treatment available today within the realm of assisted reproduction result in a pregnancy rate of approximately 40%, an unsatisfactory percentage, since it means that the majority of couples are still denied the opportunity to conceive (Qublan, 2006; Vaquero et al., 2006). In 30% of the couples currently undergoing treatment for infertility, the factors preventing them from becoming pregnant have yet to be identified (Grandone, 2005).

The majority of the studies conducted to evaluate failure to conceive in assisted reproduction have focused on the problems that occur following laboratory fertilization, i.e. implantation of the embryo in the woman's uterus (Vaquero et al., 2006). Various studies have concentrated on improving factors associated with the embryo, such as the quality and quantity of embryos, and on female factors. Some that need to be taken into consideration include improving endometrial receptivity and identifying intervening factors associated with immunological response and the genetic characteristics of the woman, including her potential for coagulation during pregnancy and implantation of the embryo (Glueck, 2000).

Because of the success rate of 34%, the assisted reproduction clinics try to improve the pregnancy rate by transferring more than one embryo. This procedure has as a consequence, another problem of great significance and social impact, which is the multiple pregnancy (Haggarty, 2006).

Recently, a hypothesis has been raised that the same factors associated with the occurrence of recurrent pregnancy loss may also affect the early phase of the embryo implantation process (Vaquero et al., 2006). The possible causes for a failure in embryo implantation have been widely investigated; however, there is no consensus in the literature on this subject.

The qualities of the embryo and endometrial receptivity are believed to represent significant factors in the failure of in vitro fertilization (IVF) (Simur et al, 2009). The hematological changes that lead to hypercoagulability, with a consequent increase in the occurrence of thrombosis, have been cited as factors that hamper the process of embryo implantation (Grandone, 2001; Sarto, 2001; Vaquero et al., 2006). Hence, thrombophilia should be considered an adverse factor in cases of embryo implantation failure.

Thrombophilia may be congenital or acquired and is related to changes in hemostatic mechanisms, characterized by an increased tendency for the blood to clot and a consequent risk of thromboembolism (Machac at el., 2006). Congenital factors suspected of being responsible for this propensity for thrombosis are: protein C deficiency, protein S deficiency, antithrombin III deficiency, the presence of factor V Leiden, a mutation in the 20210^A allele of the prothrombin gene and a mutation in the methylenetetrahydrofolate reductase (MTHFR) enzyme gene (D'Amico, 2006).

The hereditary causes of thrombophilia have been investigated since 1956, when Jordan and Nandorff introduced the term thrombophilia. In 1965, it had been identified the antithrombin deficiency as a cause of genetic thrombophilia.These studies have become wider in 80 years, when the deficiencies of proteins C and S were described and, later, in 1994, description of factor V Leiden. (Reitsma, 2007). About 40% of thrombosis cases with arterial or venous occlusion are hereditary. Venous thromboembolism often occurs as a result of mixed factors. In general, thrombophilia should be considered a multifactorial disorder and not as an expression of a single genetic abnormality (Buchholz, 2003).

The relationship between thrombophilic factors and infertility should be taken into consideration because of the possibility of alterations in hemostasis of a thrombophilic nature at the implantation site. This vascular change affects trophoblast invasion and placental vasculature, hampering implantation of the embryo (Sarto, 2001).

We performed a review of the pertinent literature to evaluate whether any relationship exists between thrombophilia and the presence of infertility.

A literature review was performed for the 1996-2010 period using the Medline and Lilacs databases on the following websites: www.bireme.br and www.pubmed.com. The key words used to search for relevant papers were: thrombophilia, infertility, blood coagulation, embryo implantation failure and hyperstimulation syndrome.

2. Thrombophilia and infertility

Compared to fertile women, a finding of a higher incidence of thrombophilia in women submitted to repeat cycles of in vitro fertilization (IVF) and implantation failure has become increasingly common. Azem et al. conducted a case-control study including 45 women with implantation failure, 44 fertile women and 15 infertile women who had, however, become pregnant at their first IVF attempt. The women evaluated were submitted to tests to investigate the following thrombophilic factors: prothrombin gene mutation, MTHFR gene mutation, the presence of factor V Leiden, and antithrombin, protein C and protein S deficiency. A high frequency of thrombophilia was found in the subgroup of women with implantation failure (17.8%) compared to the group of fertile women and the group of women who became pregnant at the first IVF attempt (a frequency of 8.9% in both groups). This fact reinforces the association of this pathology with vascular impairment and a consequent difficulty in embryo implantation (Azem, 2004).

Grandone et al. also reported similar results in a case-control study involving a smaller sample of women (18 women with implantation failure and 216 fertile controls) (Grandone, 2001). The results of the two abovementioned studies, although indicative of a possible association between thrombophilia and failed implantation, do not positively confirm this association.

On the other hand, Martinelli et al. conducted a case-control study with the largest sample size evaluated up to the present time and found no evidence of a higher frequency of thrombophilia in infertile women. A total of 234 infertile women were compared with 234 fertile women. The women with implantation failure were not, however, evaluated as a separate group. Antiphospholipid antibodies (lupus anticoagulant and anticardiolipin antibody), factor V Leiden mutation, prothrombin mutation and MTHFR mutation were evaluated. No evidence was found of any association between the thrombophilic factors and infertility (Martinelli, 2003).

Vaquero et al. evaluated 59 women with implantation failure and 20 fertile women in a case-control study and failed to find a higher occurrence of congenital thrombophilia in the infertile population. Nevertheless, a higher rate of acquired thrombophilia and thyroid antibodies was found in the infertile population (Vaquero et al., 2006).

In a prospective study conducted by Bellver et al., 119 women were evaluated. Thirty-two Caucasian women included in the control group were egg donors with no endocrine or autoimmune disorders, with normal karyotype and no history of obstetric pathology. A second group consisted of 31 women with infertility of no apparent cause, while a third group was composed of 26 women with implantation failure and a fourth group consisted of 30 women who had a history of recurrent pregnancy loss. The group of women with implantation failure and the recurrent pregnancy loss group had been diagnosed as normal prior to implantation. The following factors were investigated in these four groups: protein C, protein S, antithrombin III, lupus anticoagulant, activated protein C resistance, IgG and IgM anticardiolipin antibodies, homocysteine, factor V Leiden, prothrombin mutation, MTHFR mutation, thyroid-stimulating hormone (TSH), free thyroxine, antithyroid peroxidase antibody and antithyroglobulin antibody. In the group of women with implantation failure, a higher prevalence was found of activated protein C resistance and lupus anticoagulant, as well as the presence of more than one thrombophilic factor. Thyroid autoimmunity was more common in the group of women with implantation failure and in the group with infertility of no apparent cause (Bellver et al., 2008). The authors suggest an association between thrombophilia and implantation failure, but do not recommend screening for all infertile women. Moreover, they raise the hypothesis of an association between thyroid autoimmunity and infertility of no apparent cause and embryo implantation failure (Bellver et al., 2008).

In 2009, a Turkish group published the findings of a study in which the relationship between thrombophilia and implantation failure was evaluated. This was a case-control study comparing a group of 51 women with implantation failure and a group of 50 fertile women. Three hereditary thrombophilic factors were evaluated: the presence of factor V Leiden, MTHFR mutation and prothrombin mutation. No statistically significant difference was found in the frequency of thrombophilic factors between the groups evaluated. Nevertheless, a finding of at least one thrombophilic factor (62.7%) was more common in the group of women with implantation failure compared to the control group (53.9%). Although this difference was not statistically significant, the authors suggest that the difference may become significant if the sample population were larger (Simur et al., 2009).

In 2010, Casadei et al. published a case-control study that included a total of 300 women, 100 with infertility of no apparent cause and 200 fertile women. The following hereditary factors were investigated: factor V Leiden (G1691A), prothrombin gene mutation (G20210A) and MTHFR enzyme mutation (C677T). This study found no difference in the frequencies of thrombophilic factors between the two populations evaluated (Casadei, 2010).
Also in 2010, Sharif et al. conducted a prospective cohort study and analyzed 273 cases of implantation failure (two or more transfer of good quality embryos without the occurrence of pregnancy). In this group, serial ultrasound examinations, hysteroscopy and research of hereditary and acquired thrombophilias were performed. One hundred and twelve patients had abnormal tests and 84 out of these women had tested positive for thrombophilia (63 hereditary thrombophilia and 21 acquired thrombophilias). This study confirms the importance of microthrombosis deployment in the implantation site as a factor that prevents the trophoblastic invasion and subsequent embryo implantation (Sharif, 2010).
A study was recently published on the prevalence of thrombophilia in a fertile and infertile female population in Brazil. This study found a high frequency of thrombophilia among infertile women. Although this was a prevalence study, i.e. no comparison was made between the two groups, thrombophilia was more common in the group of infertile women. Women with implantation failure were not evaluated as a separate group (Soligo, 2007).
The association between thrombophilia and infertility remains controversial; however, studies have tended to associate this coagulation disorder with implantation failure. In 2008, Qublan conducted a case-control study to evaluate the use of low-molecular-weight heparin for the treatment of embryo implantation failure in view of the association between thrombophilia and implantation failure. Although the exact mechanism behind implantation failure and infertility remains to be fully clarified, this study suggests that maternal blood vascularization with adequate syncytiotrophoblast invasion may be affected by microthrombosis at the implantation site. Furthermore, thrombophilia may also affect the various trophoblast functions including invasion, differentiation, proliferation and hormone function with consequent implantation failure (Qublan, 2008).
The table below shows a summary of the results of the studies evaluated:

Author/ year	Fertile women (n)	Infertile women (n)	Implantation failure (n)
Grandone, 2001	(-) 216		(+) 18
Martinelli, 2003	(-) 234	(-) 234	
Azem, 2004	(-) 44	(-) 15	(+) 45
Vaquero et al., 2006	(-) 20		(+) 59
Bellver, 2008	(-) 32	(-) 31	(+) 26
Simur, 2009	(-) 50		(+) 51
Casadei, 2010	(-) 200	(-) 100	

Legend:(+) A higher frequency of thrombophilia was found.
(-) A higher frequency of thrombophilia was not found.

Table 1. Thrombophilia in Fertile and Infertile Women

Combining the published data in the afore mentioned studies, there was no increased risk of thrombophilia between the groups of fertile women, infertile and implantation failure. The studies did not show statistical difference between the groups studied and highlight the limit of the sample for statistical evidence in cases of thrombophilia. There is also evidence that the normal MTHFR genotype is related to the ability to produce good quality embryos. This is a result of a prospective study to evaluate vitamin B12, folate and MTHFR gene mutation and their influence on the success of IVF programs (Haggarty, 2006).

The ovarian hyperstimulation syndrome (OHS) is a complication of ovulation induction in assisted reproduction treatment. It is estimated that 0.5% of women undergoing ovulation induction have OHS (Saul, 2009). This iatrogenic condition is characterized by an extensive clinical and laboratory manifestation, including an increase of ovarian volume, fluid into the extravascular space, intravascular volume depletion, rapid weight gain, hemoconcentration, leukocytosis, oliguria and electrolyte disturbance (Rongolino, 2003). It may also occur ovarian torsion, ascites, hydrothorax, liver dysfunction, thromboembolism, and renal failure. Despite technological advances there is still no effective strategy to eliminate this complication in cases of medical treatment of assisted reproduction. It is estimated, at present, different strategies of ovarian stimulation protocols for patients considered at risk. These patients considered at risk include young women suffering from polycystic ovaries, with or without hormonal abnormalities associated with the sonographic findings, previous history of high ovarian response to hormonal induction (Engmanan, 2008)

The exact origin of OHSS is unknown, but is related to arteriolar vasodilation and increased capillary permeability triggered by vasoactive substances. Factors belonging to the renin-angiotensin system, including cytokines, interleukins (IL-8 and IL-9), tumor necrosis factor-α, endothelin 1, vascular endothelial growth factor (VEGF) leading to increased vascular permeability. Currently, it is believed that increased platelet activation is related with the elevation of VEGF (Varnagy, 2008). Because the presence of hypercoagulable changes observed in the OHS has attracted the interest of evaluating a possible association of thrombophilic factors to the occurrence of OHSS (Dulitzky, 2002).

In 2002, Dulitzky et al. performed a prospective study to evaluate the presence of thrombophilic factors in women hospitalized due to severe OHS. It was conducted a case-control study, where twenty women hospitalized due to OHS were selected and forty-one women who underwent ovulation induction and did not develop OHS. The following thrombophilic factors were evaluated: antithrombin, protein C, protein S, antiphospholipid antibodies, mutation of Factor V and MTHFR gene mutation. Among the women studied, 85% of the women with OHS and 26.8% of non-OHS women had one or more associated thrombophilic factor. This study demonstrates the positive association between thrombophilia and OHS, as well as suggests a screening for thrombophilia in patients at risk for OHS (Dulitzky, 2002). However, Machaca et al., despite a higher prevalence of FVL mutation in the infertile population, did not find a higher incidence of OHSS in this group of women (Machac et al., 2006).

Fabregues et al, in 2004, conducted a case-control study to assess the frequency of thrombophilic factors in women with OHS and to assess the cost benefit of performing a screening for Factor V Leiden and prothrombin mutation in women who were undergoing IVF treatment. They studied three groups of women. In the first group twenty women with OHS were included. In group 2, with forty women, were included women undergoing IVF, but who did not develop OHS. In group 3, one hundred healthy women were included. All women were investigated for the following thrombophilic factors: Factor V Leiden, prothrombin gene mutation, antithrombin, protein C and S, lupus anticoagulant and anticardiolipin antibody. In this study, was not evidenced a higher frequency of thrombophilic factors in women with OHS, even were no differences between groups of fertile and infertile women. (Fabregues et al., 2004).

However, as the thrombophylic factors are of rare occurrence, the evaluation of such a small sample of patients, as in the above studies, may not be sufficient to establish the association between the proposed data.

3. Conclusion

Thrombophilia is rare, hence difficult to evaluate in the population. Consequently, to establish a precise correlation between this event and infertility, a study with a very large sample size would have to be conducted, rendering such an endeavor costly and difficult.

The studies available in the literature were conducted in small samples, a fact that may compromise the validity of the results obtained.

This literature review and the consequent analysis of the above mentioned studies tend to suggest that thrombophilia is indeed more common in infertile women, particularly in the subgroup with embryo implantation failure. Nevertheless, data in the literature up to the present moment remain controversial.

The importance of angiogenesis in embryo implantation must be taken into consideration, since thrombophilia may lead to the occurrence of microthrombosis at the implantation site. Therefore, screening for thrombophilia in infertile women, particularly in those with implantation failure, is pertinent.

Infertile women, who have tested positive for thrombophilia and who achieve their objective of becoming pregnant, merit particular attention during prenatal care. Obstetric care must be rigorous, since thrombophilia is known to be associated with an increased risk of complications during pregnancy such as preeclampsia, intrauterine growth restriction, placental abruption, premature delivery, recurrent pregnancy loss and chronic fetal distress in addition to ischemic events during pregnancy (Kuperfenic, 2000; Brenner, 2003; Couto, 2005; Ren, 2006).

4. References

Azem F, Many A, Yovel I, Amit A, Lessing JB, KupfermincMJ . Increased rates of trombophilia in women with repeated FIV failures. Human Reproduction 2004; 19 (2): 368-70.

Bellver J, Soares RS, Alvarez C, Munoz E, Ramírez A, Rubio C et al.The role of trombophilia and thyroid autoimmunity in unexplained infertility, implantation failure and recurrent spotaneous abortion. Human Reproduction 2008; 23 (2): 278-284.

Brenner B, KupfermincMJ. Inherited thrombophilia and poor pregnancy outcome. Best Pract Res Clin Obstet Gynaecol. 2003; 17(3):427-39.

Buchholz T, Thaler CJ. Inherited thrombophilia: impact on human reproduction. Am J Reprod Immunol 2003; 50 (1): 20-32.

Casadei L, Puca F, Privitera L, Zamaro V, Emidi E. Inherited thrombophilia in infertile women: implication in unexplain infertility. Fertil Steril 2010; 94(2): 755-7.

Couto E, Nomura ML, Barini R, Silva JL. Pregnancy-associated venous thromboembolism in combined heterozygous factor V Leiden and prothrombin G20210A mutations. São Paulo Med J. 2005; 123(6): 286-88.

D'Amico EA. Trombofilia. In: Lorenzi TF. Manual de Hematologia Propedêutica e Clínica. Rio de Janeiro: Guanabara koogan; 2006.p. 657-71.

Dulitzky M, Cohen SB, Inbal A, Seidman DS, Soriano D, Lidor A, Mashiach S, Rabinovici J. Increased prevalence of thrombofilia among women with severe ovarian hiperstimulation syndrome. Fertility and Sterility 2002; 77(3): 463-7.

Engman L, DiLuigi A, Schmidt D, Nulsen J, Maier D, Benadiva C. The use of gonadotropin-releasing hormone (GnRH) agonist to induce oocyte maturation after cotreatment with GnRH antagonist in high- risk patients undergoing in vitro fertilization prevents the risk of ovarian hyperstimulation syndrome: a prospective randomized controlled study. Fertil Steril 2008; 89(1):84-91.

Fábregues F, Tássies D, ReverterJC, Carmona F, Ordinas A, Balasch J. Prevalence of thrombophilia in women with severe ovarian hyperstimulation syndrome and cost-effectiveness os screening. Fertli Steril 2004; 81 (4): 989-95.

Glueck CJ, AwadallaSG, Philips H, Cameron D, Wang P, Fontaine RN. Polycistic ovary síndrome, infertility, familial trombophilia, recurrent loss of in vitro fertilized embryos, and miscarriage. Fertility and Sterility 2000; 74(2): 394-7.

Grandone E, Colaizzo D, Lo Bue A, Checola MG, Cittadini E, Margaglione M. Inherited thrombophilia and in vitro fertilization implantation failure. Fertility and Sterility 2001; 76 (1): 201-02.

Grandone E. Infertility and trombophilia.Thromb Res. 2005; 115(1):24-7.

Haggarty P, McCallum H, McBain H, Andrews K, Duthie S, Mc Neil G et al. Effect of B vitamins and genetics on success of in vitro fertilisation: prospective cohort study. Lancet 2006; 367: 1513-19.

Kupferminc Mj, Yair D, Bornstein NM, Lessing JB, Eldor A. Transient focal neurological deficits during pregnancy in carriers of inherited thrombophilia. Stroke 2000; 31(4):892-5.

Machac S, Lubusky M, Prochazka M, Streda R. Prevalece of inherited thrombophilia in patients with severe ovarian hyperstimulation syndrome. Biomed Pap Med Fac Univ Palacky Olomouc Czech Repub. 2006; 150 (2): 289-92.

Martinelli I, Taioli E, Ragni G, Levi-Setti P, Passamonti SM, Battagliolo T, Lodigiani C, Mannucci PM. Embryo implantation after assisted reproductive procedures and maternal thrombophilia. Haematologica 2003; 88(7):789-93.

Neuspiller F, Ardiles G. Conceitos e Epidemiologia em Medicina Reprodutiva. In: Scheffer BB, Remohí J, Garcia-Velasco J, Pellicer A, Simon C, editores. Reprodução Humana Assistida. 1ª. Edição São Paulo: Atheneu; 2003.p.1-12.

Qublan HS, Eid SS, Ababneh HÁ, AmarinZO, Smadi AZ, Al- Khafaji FF, KhaderYS. Acquired and inherited thrombophilia: implication in recurrent IVF and embryo tranfer failure. Hum Reprod. 2006; 21(10): 2694-8.

Qublan H, Amarin Z, Dabbas M, Farraj A-E, Beni-Merei Z, Al-Kash H, bdoor A-N, Nawasreh M, Malkawi S, Diab F, Al-Ahamad N, Balawneh M, Salim -Abu A. Low-molecular-weight heparin in the treatment of recurrent IVF-ET failure and thrombophilia: a prospective randomized placebo-controlled trial. Hum Fertility 2008; 11(4): 246-253.

Reistma PH, Rosendaal FR. Past and future of genetic research in thrombosis. J Thromb Haemost 2007; 5(1): 264-9.

Ren A, Wang J. Methylenetetrahydrofolate reductase C677T polymorphism and the risk of unexplained recurrent pregnancy loss: a meta-analysis. Fertility and Sterility 2006; 86(6): 1716-22.

Rongolino A, Coccia ME, Fedi S, Gori AM, Cellia AP, ScarselliGF ,Prisco D, Abbate R,. Hypercoagulability, high tissue factor and low tissue factor pathway inhibitor levels in severe hyperstimulation syndrome: possible association with clinical outcome. Blood Coagul Fibrinolysis 2003; 14(3): 277-82.

Sarto A, Rocha M, Geller M, Capmany C, Martinez M, Quintans, Donaldson M, Pasqualini RS. Tratamiento con enoxaparina adaptado a los programas de fertilidad en mujeres con aborto recurrente y trombofilia. Medicina (Buenos Aires) 2001; 61: 406-12.

Sharif KE, Ghunaim S. Management of 273 cases os recurrent implantation failure results of a combined evidence-based protocol. Reprod Biomed online 2010; 21: 373-380.

Saul T, Sosnson JM. Ovarian hyperstimulation syndrome.Am J EmergMéd 2009; 27(2): 253-4.

Simur A, Ozdemir S, Acar H, Colakoglu MC, Gorkemli H, Balci O, Nergis S. Repeated in vitro fertilization failure and its realation with thrmbophilia. Gynecol Obstet Invest. 2009; 67(2): 109-12.

Soligo AGS, Barini R, Carvalho ECC, Annichino-BizzacchiJ. Prevalência dos Fatores Trombofílicos em mulheres com infertilidade. Rev Bras Ginecol Obstet. 2007; 29(5): 235-240.

Stedman TL. Stedman's Medical Dictionary. 28ª edição. Baltimore, Maryland USA; 2006.p.970.

Vaquero E, Lazzarin N, Caserta D, Valensise H, Baldi M, Moscarini M, Arduii D. Diagnostic evaluation of women experiencing repeated in vitro fertilization failure. Eur J Gynecol Reprod Biol 2006; 125(1):79-84.

Varnagy A; Koppan M; Manfai Z; Busznyak C; Bodis J. Low- dose aspirin for prophylaxis of ovarian hyperstimulation syndrome. Fertil Steril 2008; 89(4): 1035-6.

9

Thrombophilia and Recurrent Pregnancy Loss

Gokalp Oner
Erciyes University / Department of Obstetric and Gynecology
Turkey

1. Introduction

Recurrent pregnancy loss (RPL) is usually defined as the loss of three or more consecutive pregnancies before 20 weeks of gestation. Within this definition is a large and heterogeneous group of patients with many different causes of miscarriage. RPL is a common clinical problem that occurs in approximately 1 % of reproductive-aged women. However, this frequency increases up to 5% when clinicians define RPL as two or more losses of pregnancy. In addition, epidemiological investigations have demonstrated that the frequency of subsequent pregnancy loss is 24% after two pregnancy losses, 30% after three and 40% after four successive pregnancy losses. In many cases, the etiology is unknown, but several hypotheses have been proposed, including chromosomal and uterine anatomic abnormalities, endometrial infections, endocrine abnormalities, antiphospholipid syndrome, inherited thrombophilias, alloimmune causes, genetic factors, exposure to environmental factors and unexplained causes. Recently, it has become clear that prothrombotic changes are associated with a substantial proportion of these fetal losses. Therefore, the role of thrombophilias in RPL has generated a great deal of interest. This heterogeneous group of disorders results in increased venous and arterial thrombosis. Although some thrombophilic states in RPL may be acquired such as antiphospholipid antibody syndrome (APAS), most are heritable such as hyperhomocyteinemia, activated protein C resistance, deficiencies in proteins C and S, mutations in prothrombin, and mutations in antithrombin III.

Data suggest that women with thrombophilia have an increased risk of pregnancy loss and other serious obstetric complications, including placental abruption, pre-eclampsia, intrauterine growth restriction and intrauterine fetal death. Recent attention has focused on thrombophilic factors that might be associated with pregnancy complications, including early pregnancy loss. Additionally pregnancy complications including idiopathic fetal loss are thought to result from placental under perfusion due to occlusive events, including thrombosis of placental vessels. Thrombosis of placental vessels is multicausal in nature and may involve both acquired and inherited risk factors, leading to RPL. It has been reported that genetic tendencies to thrombosis may also be associated with recurrent pregnancy loss. The three most common genetic markers for thrombophilia which are known to predispose to venous thrombosis are; factor V Leiden (FVL), methylenetetrahydrofolate reductase mutation (MTHFR, C677T) and prothrombin gene mutation (FII, G20210). In this chapter, we discuss the association of thrombophilia and RPL; these include important roles in management and treatment that appear to be required for normal pregnancy.

2. Recurrent pregnancy loss

Recurrent pregnancy loss (RPL) is usually defined as the loss of three or more consecutive pregnancies before 20 weeks of gestation or with fetal weights less than 500 grams. Within this definition is a large and heterogeneous group of patients with many different causes of miscarriage. RPL affects approximately 1 % of couples (1). However, this frequency increases up to 5% when clinicians define RPL as two or more losses of pregnancy (2) In addition, epidemiological investigations have demonstrated that the frequency of subsequent pregnancy loss is 24% after two pregnancy losses, 30% after three and 40% after four successive pregnancy losses (3). Additionally, recurrent risk for RPL may increase up to 50 percent even after six losses (4). Remarkably, the maternal and paternal age may approach the risk of pregnancy loss (Table 1) (5). Maternal age at conception and previous reproductive history are strong and independent risk factors for RPL. The chance of successful pregnancy in a woman aged 40 years or more and a man aged 40 years or more is poor. In many cases, the etiology is unknown, but several hypotheses have been proposed, including chromosomal and uterine anatomic abnormalities, endometrial infections, endocrine abnormalities, antiphospholipid syndrome, inherited thrombophilias, alloimmune causes, genetic factors, exposure to environmental factors and unexplained causes (Table 2) (6). The normal coagulation pathway is pivotal for the pregnancy outcomes (Table 3). Also any kind of disorder in coagulation pathway may cause thrombophilia that may be the reason of plasental insufficiency and PL (7). Recently, it has become clear that prothrombotic changes are associated with a substantial proportion of these fetal losses. Therefore, the role of thrombophilias in RPL has generated a great deal of interest. This heterogeneous group of disorders results in increased venous and arterial thrombosis. Although some thrombophilic states in RPL may be acquired such as antiphospholipid antibody syndrome (APAS), most are heritable such as hyperhomocyteinemia, activated protein C resistance, deficiencies in proteins C and S, mutations in prothrombin, and mutations in antithrombin III.

Maternal Age	Rate of PL (%)	Paternal Age	Rate of RPL (%)
< 20	12.2	< 20	12
20-24	14.3	20-24	11.8
25-29	13.7	25-29	15.7
30-34	15.5	30-34	13.1
35-39	18.7	35-39	15.8
40-44	25.5	40-44	19.5

Table 1. The relationship between the spontaneous pregnancy loss and the maternal and paternal age.

Etiology	Proposed Incidence (%)
Genetic Factors	**3.5-5**
Chromosomal, Single gene defects, Multifactorial	
Anatomic Factors	**12-16**
Congenital -Incomplete mullerian fusion or septum resorption -Diethylstilbestrol exposure -Uterine artey anomalies -Cervical incompetence Acquired -Cervical incompetence -Synechiae -Leiyomyomas -Adenomyomas	
Endocrine Factors	**17-20**
Luteal phase insufficiency, Polycystic ovarian syndrome, Diabetes mellitus, Thyroid disorders, Prolactin disorders	
Infectious Factors	**0.5-5**
Bacteria, Viruses, Parasites, Zoonotic, Fungal	
Immunologic and Trombotic Factors	**20-50**
Cellular mechanisms, Humoral mechanisms , Antiphospholipid Antibody Syndrome, Inherited Thrombophilias such as activated protein C resistance associated with mutations in factor V Leiden, deficiencies in protein C and S, mutations in the gene encoding methylene tetrahydrofolate reductase, mutations in the promoter region of the prothrombin, hyperhomocyteinemia,	

Table 2. Proposed Etiologies for Recurrent Spontaneous Abortion.

2.1 Antiphospholipid antibody syndrome

Pregnancy-specific antigens can elicit humoral responses, and patients with RPL can display altered humoral responses to endometrial and trophoblast antigens (8, 9). Nevertheless, most literature surrounding humoral immune responses and RPL focus on organ-nonspecific autoantibodies associated with APAS. Historically, these IgG and IgM antibodies were thought to be directed against negatively charged phospholipids. Those phospholipids most often implicated in RPL are cardiolipin and phosphatidylserine. Most recently, however, it has been shown that antiphospholipid antibodies often are directed against a protein cofactor, called β2 glycoprotein 1, that assists antibody association with the phospholipid (10). The association of these antiphospholipid antibodies with thrombotic complications has been termed the antiphospholipid syndrome, and although many of these

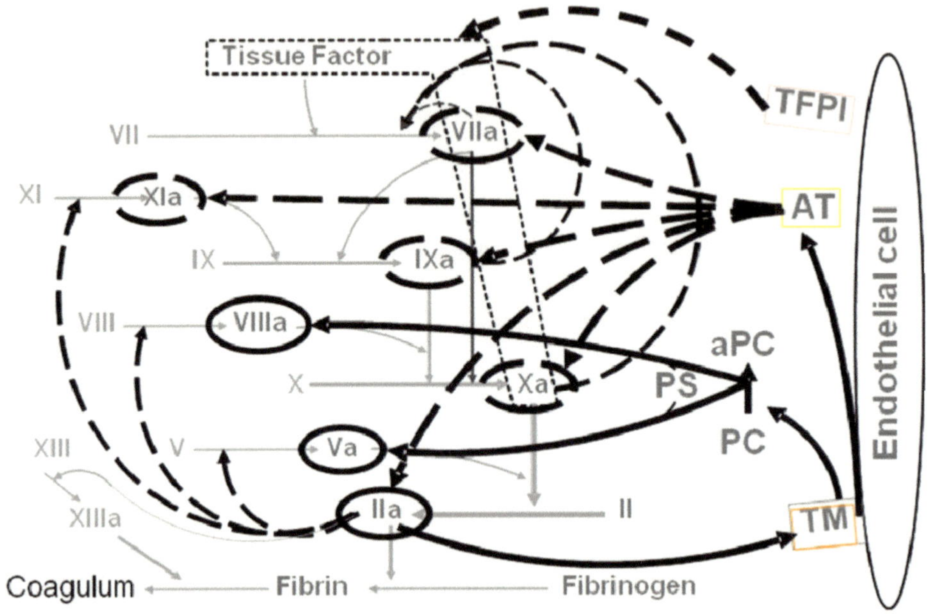

aPC: activated protein C
AT: Antithrombin
PC: Protein C
PS: Protein S
TAFI: Trombin activated fibrinolyse inhibitor
TM: Thrombomodulin

Table 3. Coagulation pathway and factors

complications are systemic, some are pregnancy specific—spontaneous abortion, stillbirth, intrauterine growth retardation, and preeclampsia (11).

Diagnosis of this syndrome requires at least one of each clinical and laboratory criterion (12). These are listed below.

Clinical

- One or more confirmed episode of vascular thrombosis of any type
- Venous
- Arterial
- Small vessel
- Pregnancy complications
- Three or more consecutive spontaneous pregnancy losses at less than 10 weeks of gestation
- One or more fetal deaths at greater than 10 weeks of gestation
- One or more preterm births at less than 34 weeks of gestation secondary to severe preeclampsia or placental insufficiency

Laboratory

(Testing must be positive on two or more occasions, 6 weeks or more apart.)

- Positive plasma levels of anticardiolipin antibodies of the IgG or IgM isotype at medium to high levels

- Positive plasma levels of lupus anticoagulant

The presence of antiphospholipid antibodies (anticardiolipin or lupus anticoagulant) during pregnancy is a major risk factor for an adverse pregnancy outcome (13). In large series of couples with recurrent abortion, the incidence of the APAS was between 3% and 5% (14). The presence of anticardiolipin antibodies among patients with known systemic lupus erythematosus portends less favorable pregnancy outcome (15).

A number of mechanisms whereby antiphospholipid antibodies might mediate pregnancy loss have been proposed. Antibodies against phospholipids have been proposed to cause fetal loss because these antibodies inhibit release of prostacyclin, a potent vasodilator and inhibitor of platelet aggregation. In contrast, platelets produce thromboxane A2 which is a vasoconstrictor that also promotes platelet aggregation. These autoantibodies have also been shown to inhibit protein C activation, which results in coagulation and fibrin C formation. Clinically, these events might lead to hypercoagulability and recurrent thrombosis within the placenta. Women with both a history of early fetal loss and high levels of these antibodies may have a 70 percent miscarriage recurrence (16). In a prospective study of 860 women screened for anticardiolipin antibody in the first trimester reported that 7 percent tested positive (17). Miscarriage developed in 25 percent of the antibody-positive group, compared with only 10 percent of the negative group. In another study, there was no association between early pregnancy loss and the presence of either anticardiolipin antibody or lupus anticoagulant (18).

2.2 Inherited thrombophilias

Thrombophilic disorders have generated considerable interest in the field of RPL. Thrombophilia is an important predisposition to thrombosis due to a procoagulant state. Several blood clotting disorders are grouped under the term of thrombophilia. In table 4, thrombophilic mutations were described. Amongst these, are activated protein C resistance (APCR), protein S deficiency, protein C deficiency, prothrombin mutation, antithrombin III deficiency and hyperhomocysteinaemia (methylenetetrahydrofolate reductase mutation, C677 T MTHFR). Clinical studies suggest that the underlying pathophysiological mechanism is mediated via hypercoagulation, leading to uteroplacental insufficiency with resultant pregnancy loss. The basis for the association between adverse fetal outcomes and heritable thrombophilias has focused on the mechanisms of impaired placental development and function secondary to venous or arterial thrombosis at the maternal-fetal interface. Activation of protein S synergizes with activated protein C, thereby inhibiting the actions of clotting factors V and VIII. Thus, proteins S and C have an anticoagulant effect. Decreased action of these proteins has been postulated to increase the risk for pregnancy loss. Mutation in the gene encoding factor V results in a protein that is resistant to the effects of activated protein C (aPC). The most common of a variety of mutations is at position 506 with a glutamine substitution for arginine, this FV:R506Q mutation is called the factor V Leiden mutation (19, 20, 21). The mutation results in a protein resistant to the effects of aPC. The net result is increased the cleavage of prothrombin to thrombin, which causes excessive coagulability. Inherited decreased or absent antithrombin III activity will lead to increased thrombin formation and clotting. Prothrombin gene mutation is signalled by a defect in clotting factor II at position G20210A. The relative risk for thrombosis in patients with this mutation is two-fold in heterozygotes. Individuals with hyperhomocysteinaemia exhibit a deficiency of folate due to the presence of the methylene tetrahydrofolate reductase mutation (MTHFR C677 T). The thrombotic risk is increased two-fold in homozygosity; and in the heterozygous state for Antithrombin III deficiency, the risk is 20- to 50-fold. APCR has emerged as the commonest genetic cause of thrombo-embolism. APCR is caused by a point mutation (Factor V Leiden, FVL) in 95% of cases. The risk of thrombosis is increased 5- to 10-fold in heterozygous carriers of FVL, and 100-fold in homozygosity (22, 23) Consistent with general thrombotic risk, carriage of combinations of two or more inherited thrombophilic defects has particularly strong association with adverse pregnancy outcomes (24, 25, 26). Considerable attention has been directed recently toward a possible relationship between thrombophilias and certain pregnancy complications other than venous thrombosis (27). Table 5 summarizes the findings of 79 studies systematically reviewed by Robertson and associates (28).

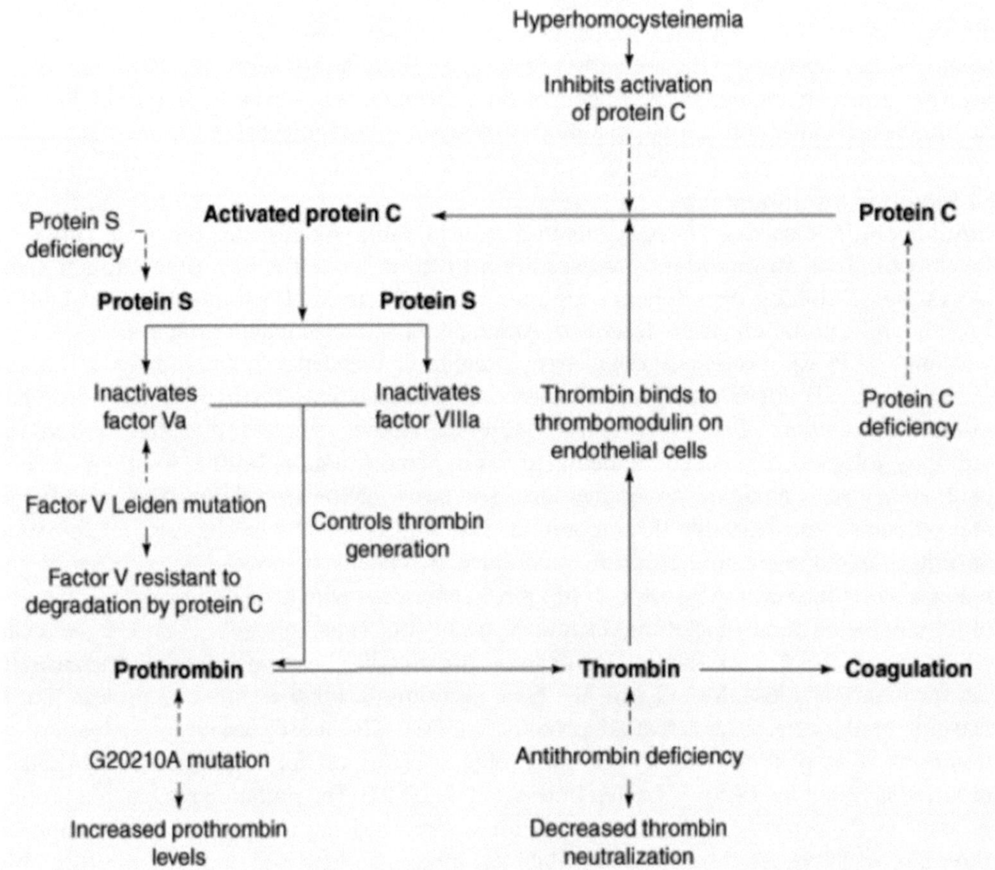

Table 4. Effects of inherited thrombophilia on the coagulation pathway.

Thrombophilia	Early Pregnancy Loss	Stillbirth	Preeclampsia	Placental Abruption	Fetal-Growth Restriction
FVL—homozygous	2.7 (1.3-5.6)	2.0 (0.4-9.7)	1.9 (0.4-7.9)	8.4 (0.4-171.2)	4.6 (0.2-115.7)
FVL—heterozygous	1.7 (1.1-2.6)	2.1 (1.1-3.9)	2.2 (1.5-3.3)	4.7 (1.1-19.6)	2.7 (0.6-12.1)
Prothrombin—heterozygous	2.5 (1.2-5.0)	2.7 (1.3-5.5)	2.5 (1.5-4.2)	7.7 (3.0-19.8)	2.9 (0.6-13.7)
MTHFR—homozygous	1.4 (0.8-2.6)	1.3 (0.9-1.1)	**1.4 (1.1-1.8)**	1.5 (0.4-5.4)	1.2 (0.8-1.8)
Hyperhomocysteinemia	**6.3 (1.4-28.4)**	1.0 (0.2-5.6)	**3.5 (1.2-10.1)**	2.4 (0.4-15.9)	N/A
Antithrombin deficiency	0.9 (0.2-4.5)	7.6 (0.3-196.4)	3.9 (0.2-97.2)	1.1 (0.1-18.1)	N/A
Protein C deficiency	2.3 (0.2-26.4)	3.1 (0.2-38.5)	5.2(0.3-102.2)	5.9 (0.2-151.6)	N/A
Protein S deficiency	3.6 (0.4-35.7)	**20.1 (3.7-109.2)**	2.8 (0.8-10.6)	2.1 (0.5-9.3)	N/A
Acquired activated protein C resistance	**4.0 (1.7-9.8)**	0.9 (0.2-3.9)	1.8 (0.7-4.6)	1.3 (0.4-4.4)	N/A
Anticardiolipin antibody	**3.4 (1.3-8.7)**	**3.3 (1.6-6.7)**	**2.7 (1.7-4.5)**	1.4 (0.4-4.8)	**6.9 (2.7-17.7)**
Lupus anticoagulant	**3.0 (1.0-8.6)**	2.4 (0.8-7.0)	1.5 (0.8-2.8)	N/A	N/A

Data presented as odds ratios (95-percent confidence intervals). Bolded numbers are statistically significant.
FVL = factor V Leiden, MTHFR = methylenetetrahydrofolate reductase, N/A = data not available.

Table 5. Obstetrical Complications Associated with Some Inherited and Acquired Thrombophilias

2.3 Treatment

The treatment of couples with recurrent miscarriage has traditionally been based on anecdotal evidence, personal bias, and the results of small uncontrolled studies. There are some treatment regimens for APAS that increase live birth rates. The American College of Obstetricians and Gynecologists (12) recommends low-dose aspirin—81 mg orally per day, along with unfractionated heparin—5000 units subcutaneously, twice daily. This therapy, begun when pregnancy is diagnosed, is continued until delivery. Although this treatment may improve overall pregnancy success, these women remain at high risk for preterm labor, prematurely ruptured membranes, fetal-growth restriction, preeclampsia, and placental abruption (4). The Cochrane review of immune therapy for RPL also addressed IVIg therapy and reported that its use did not alter pregnancy outcomes in patients with otherwise unexplained RPL (29). Although both vaginal and intramuscular progesterone therapy are associated with few minor side effects, their efficacy in the treatment of either unexplained RPL or RPL associated with TH cell dysregulation has never been investigated appropriately. The efficacy and side effects of prednisone plus low-dose aspirin was examined in a recent, large, randomized, placebo-controlled trial treating patients with autoantibodies and RPLs. Pregnancy outcomes for treated and control patients were similar; however, the incidence of maternal diabetes and hypertension and the risk of premature delivery were all increased among those treated with prednisone and aspirin(30). Treatment for thrombophilias remains contraversial, but may include heparin and aspirin. Recently, Cochrane Database review concluded that women with recurrent miscarriage and thrombophilia do not benefit from aspirin or heparin therapy (31) . Vitamins B6, B12, and folate are important in homocysteine metabolism and hyperhomocysteinemia is linked to RPL. Women with RPL and isolated fasting hyperhomocysteinemia should be offered supplemental folic acid (0.4–1.0 mg/day), vitamin B6 (6 mg/day), and possibly vitamin B12 (0.025 mg/day) (32).

3. References

[1] Stirrat GM. Recurrent miscarriage. Lancet 1990; 336: 673-675.
[2] Hogge, WA. et al. The clinical use of karyotyping spontaneous abortions. Am. J. Obstet. Gynecol. 2003; 189, 397–400.
[3] Regan, L. et al. Influence of past reproductive performance on risk of spontaneous abortion. BMJ 1989; 299, 541–545.
[4] Poland B, et al. Reproductive counseling in patients who have had a spontaneous abortion. Am J Obstet Gynecol 1977; 127: 685.
[5] Knudsen UB, et al. Prognosis of a new pregnancy following previous spontaneous abortions. Eur J Obstet Gynecol Reprod Biol. 1991; 39: 31-36.
[6] Rai, R. and Regan, L. Recurrent miscarriage. Lancet 2006; 368, 601–611.
[7] Reznikoff-Etievan MF, et al. Factor V Leiden and G20210A prothrombin mutations are risk factors for very early recurrent miscarriage. BJOG, 2001; 108(12):1251-1254.
[8] Hill JA, et al. T helper 1-type immunity to trophoblast antigens in women with recurrent spontaneous abortion. JAMA 1995;273:1933–1936.
[9] Eblen AC, et al. Alterations in humoral immune responses associated with recurrent pregnancy loss. Fertil Steril 2000;73:305–313.
[10] McNeil HP, et al. Anti-phospholipid antibodies are directed against a complex antigen that includes a lipid-binding inhibitor of coagulation: beta 2-glycoprotein I (apolipoprotein H). Proc Natl Acad Sci U S A 1990;87:4120–4124.
[11] Harris EN. Syndrome of the black swan. Br J Rheumatol 1986;26:324–326.
[12] American College of Obstetricians and Gynecologists: Antiphospholipid syndrome. Practice Bulletin No. 68, November, 2005.

[13] Out HJ, et al. A prospective, controlled multicenter study of the obstetric risks of pregnant women with antiphospholipid antibodies. Br J Obstet Gynaecol 1992;167:26-32.
[14] Hill JA. Sporadic and recurrent spontaneous abortion. Curr Probl Obstet Gynecol Fertil 1994;17:114-162.
[15] Kutteh WH, Lyda EC, Abraham SM, Wacholtz MC. Association of anticardiolipin antibodies and pregnancy loss in women with systemic lupus erythematosus. Fertil Steril 1993;60:449-455.
[16] Dudley DJ, et al. Antiphospholipid syndrome: A model for autoimmune pregnancy loss. Infert Reprod Med Clin North Am 1991; 2:149.
[17] Yasuda M, et al: Prospective studies of the association between anticardiolipin antibody and outcome of pregnancy. Obstet Gynecol 1995; 86: 555.
[18] Simpson JL, et al: Lack of association between antiphospholipid antibodies and first-trimester spontaneous abortion: prospective study of pregnancies detected within 21 days of conception. Fertil Steril 1998; 69:814.
[19] Cotter AM, et al. Elevated plasma homocysteine in early pregnancy: A risk factor for the development of severe preeclampsia. Am J Obstet Gynecol, 2001; 185:781-5.
[20] Aubard Y, et al. Hyperhomocysteinema and pregnancy review of our present understanding and therapeutic implications. Eur J Obstet Gynecol, 2000; 93: 157-65.
[21] Jeanine F. et al. Prenatal Screening for Thrombophilias: Indications and Controversies Clin Lab Med 2010; 30: 747-760.
[22] Kovalevsky G, et al. Evaluation of the association between hereditary thrombophilias and recurrent pregnancy loss: a meta-analysis. Arch Intern Med 2004; 164: 558 - 63.
[23] Rey E, et al. Thrombophilic disorders and fetal loss: a meta-analysis. Lancet 2003; 361: 901 - 08.
[24] Lockwood CJ. Inherited thrombophilias in pregnant patients: detection and treatment paradigm. Obstet Gynecol 2002;99:333-341.
[25] Lockwood CJ. Inherited thrombophilias in pregnant patients. Prenat Neonat Med 2001;6:3-14.
[26] Preston FE, et al. Increased fetal loss in women with heritable thrombophilia. Lancet 1996;348:913-916.
[27] De Santis M, et al: Inherited and acquired thrombophilia: Pregnancy outcome and treatment. Reprod Toxicol 2006; 22: 227.
[28] Robertson L, et al: Thrombophilia in pregnancy: A systematic review. Br J Haematol 2005; 132:171.
[29] Scott JR. Immunotherapy for recurrent miscarriage. Cochrane Database Syst Rev 2003; (1):CD000112.
[30] Laskin CA, et al. Prednisone and aspirin in women with autoantibodies unexplained recurrent fetal loss. N Engl J Med 1997;337:148-153.
[31] Kaandorp S, et al: Aspiring or anticoagulants for treating recurrent miscarriage in women without antiphospholipid syndrome. Cochrane Database Syst Rev (1):CD004734, 2009.

[32] de la Calle M, et al. Homocysteine, folic acid and B group vitamins in obstetrics and gynaecology. Eur J Obstet Gynecol Reprod Biol 2003;107:125–134.

10

Pathogenic Mechanisms of Thrombosis in Antiphospholipid Syndrome (APS)

Marina P. Sikara, Eleftheria P. Grika and Panayiotis G. Vlachoyiannopoulos
Department of Pathophysiology, School of Medicine, National University of Athens Greece

1. Introduction

The term "antiphospholipid syndrome" (APS) was coined in the early '80s to describe a unique form of acquired autoimmune thrombophilia, with clinical features of recurrent thrombosis and pregnancy morbidity, combined with the presence of antiphospholipid antibodies (aPL). aPL consist a heterogeneous group of autoantibodies, which recognize phospholipid-protein complexes or rather proteins with high affinity for phospholipids, such as β2-glycoprotein I (β2GPI) and prothrombin. This heterogeneity reflects the nature of the antigen recognized by each antibody and it is expressed with different pathogenic mechanisms. Although a broad spectrum of aPL exists, the universally accepted diagnostic aPL tests are lupus anticoagulant (LA); anticardiolipin (anti-CL); and anti–β2-glycoprotein I antibodies (anti-β2GPI) (Table 1). These autoantibodies interfere with physiological mechanisms of coagulation and fibrinolysis, leading the hemostatic balance towards coagulation. Moreover, it seems to affect the physiological function of various cells such as platelets, monocytes and endothelial cells (EC). However, not all aPL are pathogenic; transient increase in aPL during several infections has been observed. Although aPL can cause clinical manifestations of almost every organ in the body (e.g. blood vessels, brain, kidneys, lungs, gastrointestinal tract, placenta), the common hallmark of the syndrome is thrombosis, either arterial, venous or in the microcirculation.

2. Epidemiology

2.1 aPL in healthy population and other conditions

In healthy population, the incidence of aPL ranges from 1 to 5%. It has been shown to increase with age and especially with coexistence of chronic diseases [1]. Among various studies, there is great variation in the incidence of anti-CL antibodies in apparently healthy elderly subjects, ranging from 12 to 64% [2]. The prevalence of anti-β2GPI antibodies is calculated at 31.8%. These variations may be attributed to both methodological differences and choice of sample population. In general population, aPL are detected in about one out of five patients who suffered from cerebrovascular events (strokes) at the age under 50 years. The clinical suspicion is clearly enhanced in young patients with additional features of the syndrome. Moreover, aPL can be detected in various conditions such as infections, malignancies, vaccination and use of certain drugs. In these cases, aPL are usually transient, low-titre and normally independent of the presence of β2GPI. The prevalence of aPL in healthy obstetric population is difficult to be determined since aPL have been implicated in pregnancy morbidity. However, in two studies with large number of healthy pregnant women, aPL were identified in 0.7 and 5.3% respectively [3]. It has been reported that aPL are detected in 11-29% of women with preeclampsia [4].

Symbol/acronym	Description/explanation	Definition based on the detection assay
Anti-CL	Anti-cardiolipin	Antibodies detected against cardiolipin-a negatively charged phospholipid, which is used as antigen in an enzyme linked immunosorbent assay (ELISA). These antibodies recognize β2GPI which exists in abundance in bovine serum; this serum is used as a blocking agent (blocks the non-specific binding sites) in ELISA plates. β2GPI binds to cardiolipin.
Anti-β2 GPI	Antibodies recognizing β2 GPI independently of cardiolipin	Anti-β2GPI antibodies are detected by ELISA, but the polystyrene ELISA plates have been γ-irradiated and negative charges are generated on their surface. β2GPI binds to negatively charged irradiated plates in the absence of cardiolipin and is recognized by the anti-β2GPI antibodies
LA	Lupus Anticoagulant	Antibodies which interfere *in vitro* with the generation of thrombin from prothrombin, thus increasing the activated partial thromboplastin time (aPTT). The prolonged aPTT is not corrected by adding normal plasma in the detection system. These antibodies disrupt *in vitro* the prothrombinase complex (constituted by the activated coagulation factors V and X, prothrombin and phospholipids). Kaolin clotting time (KCT) and Dilute Russel Viper Venom Test (DRVVT) are two other ways to measure LA. Antibodies of the LA type usually recognize β2GPI or Prothrombin.
BFP-STS & VDRL test	Biological false positive serological tests for syphilis & Venereal Disease Research Laboratory test	Antibodies against phospholipids/cholesterol complexes

Table 1. Classification of antiphospholipid antibodies defined according to detection assay.

2.2 aPL in other systemic autoimmune diseases

APS can occur in association with other systemic autoimmune diseases, particularly Systemic Lupus Erythematosus (SLE). About 40% of patients with SLE have aPL, but less than 40%of them will eventually have thrombotic events [5]. Particularly, 37% of patients in the "Euro-Phospholipid" study was suffering from SLE, while 4% was associated with SLE-like disease [6]. It is well documented that thrombotic complications appear more frequently in patients with SLE and aPL, as compared to aPL positive patients without other systemic autoimmune disease[7,8]. The diagnosis of secondary APS clearly leads to a threefold increase of miscarriages, especially after the 20th week of gestation [9]. aPL have also been detected in other autoimmune diseases, such as rheumatoid arthritis (RA), with a frequency up to 28%.

3. Classification Criteria for APS

An international consensus statement on the APS classification was published in 1999, after the 8th International Symposium on the aPL in Sapporo [10]. The diagnosis of the syndrome requires the presence of at least one clinical event and one positive laboratory test for aPL, including lupus anticoagulant (LA) or anti-CL antibodies, or both, in medium-high titers, detected at least twice within 6 weeks . The classification criteria were revised in 2006, in Sidney, Australia [11]. Essentially, the clinical criteria remained unchanged while the laboratory criteria were modified in two significant points: (a) the time between two positive determinations was extended to 12 weeks and (b) anti-β2GPI antibodies (IgG and IgM) were included in the laboratory tests (Table 2).

After 30 years of intensive clinical and basic research, it is now well documented that LA is the strongest predictor of thrombosis [12-14]. Moreover, anti-β2GPI antibodies appear to be mainly responsible for the clinical manifestations that characterize the syndrome [15,16]. More specifically, a subpopulation of anti-β2GPI antibodies, raised against a cryptic epitope in domain I β2GPI (Arg39-Arg43), is highly correlated with clinical events and prognosis of the syndrome [17]. Several research groups suggest that patients positive for all three classes of antibodies (LA, anti-CL and anti-β2GI) are at the higher risk for venous/arterial thrombosis and pregnancy morbidity [18,19].

4. Clinical manifestations of APS

Clinical presentation of APS includes manifestations of various organs and systems, such as blood vessels, central nervous system (CNS), skin, kidney, gastrointestinal tract, heart, and placenta. The hallmark of the syndrome is thrombosis, either arterial or venous. Unlike the strict vaso-specific localization of thrombosis due to congenital thrombophilias (e.g. correlation between deficiency of protein C only with venous thromboembolic events), thrombosis in APS may occur in any vascular bed [20,21]. This "diffuse" thrombotic predisposition clearly indicates a multifactorial influence of autoantibodies in the haemostatic system. It is worth noting that thrombotic recurrences tend to occur in the same vascular distribution as the original event (i.e., arterial are followed by arterial and venous by venous thrombotic events)[22]. Venous thromboembolic events are the most common clinical manifestations of APS. The clinical expression of the syndrome can vary from mild (mild thrombocytopenia, livedo reticularis, leg ulcers, migraine) to severe (ischemic infarctions, recurrent miscarriages, valvular insufficiency) or destructive [multiple organ failure, catastrophic APS (CAPS)]. The clinical spectrum associated with the presence of aPL is extensive. The events included in the classification criteria of APS are described in (Table 3). Some clinical manifestations, such as valvular disease, livedo reticularis, thrombocytopenia and neurological manifestations, although not included in the diagnostic criteria of the syndrome, are frequently observed in patients with APS [11]. The thrombotic etiology for these events does not seem very likely, as they usually do not subside with antithrombotic therapy. The simultaneous presence of thrombotic and non thrombotic events in patients with APS leads to the logical conclusion that most of the aPL (and especially anti-β2GPI antibodies) interfere with many different biological mechanisms. Moreover, there is a subset of asymptomatic patients with permanently high titers aPL.

Antiphospholipid antibody syndrome (APS) is present if at least one of the clinical criteria and one of the laboratory criteria that follow are met

Clinical criteria

1. Vascular thrombosis

One or more clinical episodes of arterial, venous, or small vessel thrombosis§, in any tissue or organ. Thrombosis must be confirmed by objective validated criteria (i.e. unequivocal findings of appropriate imaging studies or histopathology). For histopathologic confirmation, thrombosis shouldbe present without significant evidence of inflammation in the vessel wall.

2. Pregnancy morbidity

a. One or more unexplained deaths of a morphologically normal fetus at or beyond the 10th week of gestation, with normal fetal morphology documented by ultrasound or by direct examination of the fetus, or
b. One or more premature births of a morphologically normal neonate before the 34th week of gestation because of: (i) eclampsia or severe preeclampsia defined according to standard definitions [11], or (ii) recognized features of placental insufficiency, or
c. Three or more unexplained consecutive spontaneous abortions before the 10th week of gestation, with maternal anatomic or hormonal abnormalities and paternal and maternal chromosomal causes excluded.

Laboratory criteria

1. Lupus anticoagulant (LA) present in plasma, on two or more occasions at least 12 weeks apart, detected according to the guidelines of the International Society on Thrombosis and Haemostasis (Scientific Subcommittee on LAs/phospholipid-dependent antibodies)
2. Anticardiolipin (aCL) antibody of IgG and/or IgM isotype in serum or plasma, present in medium or high titer (i.e. >40 GPL or MPL, or >the 99th percentile), on two or more occasions, at least 12 weeks apart, measured by a standardized ELISA
3. Anti-b2 glycoprotein-I antibody of IgG and/or IgM isotype in serum or plasma (in titer >the 99th percentile), present on two or more occasions, at least 12 weeks apart, measured by a standardized ELISA, according to recommended procedures

Modified from ref 11

Table 2. Classification criteria for antiphospholipid syndrome

The literature on the clinical manifestations of APS, although extensive, mostly includes a large number of case reports. Fortunately, since the beginning of the 21st century, significant multicenter studies on large series of patients provide reliable information as to the relative frequency of different clinical manifestations of the syndrome [21,23,24]. In a multicenter study of 1000 patients with APS, 53.1% of patients had primary APS while 36.2% had secondary APS (in association with SLE). The most common manifestations were deep venous thrombosis (38.9%), thrombocytopenia (29.6%), livedo reticularis (24.1%), stroke (19.8%) and pulmonary embolism (14.1%). Less frequent events included superficial thrombophlebitis (11.7%), transient ischemic attacks (11.1%), hemolytic anemia (9.7%) and epilepsy (7%). The fetal abortion was the primary event in 14% of female patients.

4.1 Venous thrombosis

As mentioned above, deep venous thrombosis is the most frequent clinical manifestation of APS. Other vascular sites which may be affected are the larger veins, such as the subclavian, the iliofemoral, the upper abdomen, portal vein, the axillary etc. Venous thrombosis has been described, with much less frequency, in almost every organ of the body, causing related clinical manifestations. Superficial thrombophlebitis, superior vena cava syndrome, renal vein thrombosis, adrenal infarction, Addison's syndrome, Budd Chiari syndrome, pulmonary hypertension, due to recurrent pulmonary embolism and diffuse pulmonary hemorrhage, due to micro-thromboses are some of the unusual venous thrombotic manifestations of the syndrome. Recent meta-analysis regarding the relationship (odds ratio, OR) of LA and IgG/IgM anti-CL antibodies with venous thrombosis, concludes that all studies report a significant correlation between LA and VTE, with an OR up to 16.2. The correlation of anti-CL with VTE is not confirmed [25]. Titers of anti-β2GPI antibodies seem to increase the OR for venous thrombosis up to 5 times [26].

4.2 Arterial thrombosis

Arterial thrombosis consists a main clinical feature of APS, but appears less frequently than venous [27]. The most common site of arterial thrombosis is the cerebral circulation, usually in the form of stroke or transient ischemic attack [21]. Thrombosis of coronary, renal artery or the mesentery has also been observed. A multicenter population-based study, which examined the risk of arterial thrombosis in patients who were treated with oral contraceptives (RATIO study, Risk of Arterial Thrombosis In relation to Oral contraceptives), showed that the presence of LA is a major risk factor for arterial thrombosis in women under 50 years, while anti-CL and anti-prothrombin antibodies did not increase the risk for ischemic stroke or myocardial infarction [28].

4.3 CNS involvement

The CNS involvement is co-responsible for high morbidity and mortality of the syndrome, with strokes and transient ischemic attack being the most common manifestations [29,30]. The neurological manifestations cover a fairly broad clinical spectrum and may include, apart from stroke and transient ischemic attack, also Sneddon's Syndrome, epilepsy, dementia, cognitive dysfunction, headaches/migraine, chorea, transverse and spotty myelitis, ocular symptoms, Guillain-Barré, psychosis and depression [31]. More specifically, the presence of anti-CL antibodies in SLE patients has been associated with cognitive disorders. Similarly, mild cognitive impairment has been recorded in more than 40% of patients with APS and focal white matter lesions [32].

4.4 Renal involvement

APS nephropathy is now recognized as a distinct entity from lupus nephritis [33]. The most common manifestations of renal involvement are thrombosis or stenosis of renal artery, kidney infarction, thrombosis of the renal vein and end-stage renal disease/renal failure [34]. Clinically, the so-called APS nephropathy is characterized by positive aPL in conjunction with vascular nephropathy, which presents with hypertension, low-grade proteinuria, and acute and/or chronic renal failure. The clinical suspicion of this clinical entity should always be placed in young patients with renal artery stenosis, high blood pressure and unexplained deterioration of renal function. The main histopathological findings are: a) thrombotic microangiopathy, as an expression of acute thrombosis, and b) fibrous intimal hyperplasia, arteriosclerosis, focal cortical atrophy, arterial and fibrous infarcts, as for chronic vascular lesions [34]. The biopsy proven renal damage is significantly correlated with LA, but not with anti-CL antibodies. A study from our department showed that patients with APS and kidney involvement develop hypertension, elevated serum creatinine levels, characteristic findings in renal biopsy as mentioned previously, and factors associated with poor renal prognosis [35]. Moreover, a large series of patients demonstrated that APS nephropathy is presented in 39.5% of patients with SLE and positive aPL, while only in 4.3% of SLE patients without aPL [36]. The APS nephropathy is strongly correlated with LA, anti-CL antibodies and livedo reticularis. The prognosis of nephritis in patients with SLE is rather poor in the presence of coexisting APS nephropathy.

4.5 Cardiovascular manifestations

Cardiac manifestations in APS include valvular disease, acute myocardial infarction (AMI), intracardial thrombi, myocardial microthrombosis and valvular lesions similar to Libman-Sacks endocarditis of SLE [37]. The latter represent the commonest manifestation in APS with prevalence up to 38% [38]. The valves of the left ventricle are most frequently involved, with mitral impairment observed in the majority of cases. It is well known that patients with valvular disease are at higher risk of arterial thromboembolic events [39]. In a multicenter prospective study, AMI was the presenting manifestation in 2.8% and reached up to 5.5% during the follow-up period [40]. A large prospective study found that high titers of anti-CL antibodies are an independent risk factor for AMI or sudden cardiac death [41]. Although some studies do not show a correlation between anti-CL and AMI, there should be a thorough check for aPL in patients aged under 45 with coronary artery disease or AMI without other risk factors.

4.6 Skin manifestations

Skin events in APS vary both in form and severity, with livedo reticularis and leg ulcers being the commonest [42]. Livedo reticularis is caused by stagnation of blood in dilated superficial capillary venules and its prevalence in APS is calculated at 24%, according to the study of Cervera et al [43,44]. This lesion represents the first manifestation of the syndrome in 17-40% of patients. The clinical features of such lesions, although nonspecific, can lead to the diagnosis of APS. Typically, the histopathological findings of skin biopsies do not reveal evidence of thrombosis (except in the case of CAPS). Livedo reticularis has been characterized as a major risk factor for arterial thrombosis and it is correlated with high titers of anti-CL antibodies [45]. Other cutaneous manifestations of the syndrome are leg ulcers, superficial thrombophlebitis, necrotizing vasculitis and gangrene.

4.7 Hematological manifestations

Several hematological manifestations such as thrombocytopenia, autoimmune hemolytic anemia, Evan's syndrome, bone marrow necrosis and thrombotic microangiopathy have been described in APS [46]. Thrombocytopenia, defined by platelet count less than 100-150x10^9/L, is found in approximately 20% of patients with primary APS and more than 40% of patients with secondary APS in SLE [21,47]. It is usually moderate and does not require any medical intervention. The mechanisms that may lead to thrombocytopenia in patients with APS are not clear. However, the characteristic combination of thrombocytopenia and thrombosis in APS patients suggests that aPL interact with platelets resulting in platelet aggregation and thrombosis. The prevalence of autoimmune hemolytic anemia in APS patients was calculated at 6.6% to 9.7% [23]. On the other hand, studies confirm the presence of aPL in patients with autoimmune hemolytic anemia at a rate ranging from 55 to 72% [48]. The pathogenesis of autoimmune hemolytic anemia is unclear. It has been assumed that anti-CL antibodies bind directly to the surface of red blood cells of patients with APS and hemolytic anemia, although the antigen recognized by aPL has not been identified.

5. Pathogenic mechanisms of thrombosis

Significant in vitro and in vivo studies confirm that aPL are pathogenic [49-51]. The exact mechanism by which these antibodies participate in the prothrombotic tendency of APS, remain to be clearly defined. However, it has been illustrated that the heterogeneity of antibodies is associated with multiple mechanisms of action [52]. These include briefly: the activation of cellular components (endothelial cells, platelets and monocytes), activation of the coagulation cascade, inhibition of the fibrinolytic system, inhibition of natural anticoagulant pathways and activation of the complement system.

5.1 Activation of cellular components

5.1.1 Activation of endothelial cells

The interaction of aPL with endothelial cells has until now been in frequent disputes and misunderstandings. Regarding the study of endothelium in the pathogenesis of APS, major questions have arisen: a) Under what conditions the aPL bind to the surface of endothelial cells in vitro and in vivo; b) What molecular structures on the surface of endothelial cells are responsible for the binding d) What signaling pathways are activated; **Table 4** summarizes the effects of aPL on endothelial cells.

In vitro studies have shown that β2GPI binds to immobilized endothelial cells, and allows the anti-β2GPI antibodies to bind to cells and induce a proinflammatory and procoagulant phenotype [53]. A clinical demonstration of endothelial dysfunction in APS patients is the increased level of circulating endothelial microparticles and endothelial cells in peripheral blood [54,55]. In vitro studies have shown that incubation of endothelial cells with aPL and β2GPI, induces the expression of significantly higher levels of adhesion molecules ICAM-1, VCAM-1 and E-selectin. In addition, production of IL-6 and altered metabolism of arachidonic acid, have been demonstrated [56-58]. Animal models suggest that human

Clinical and laboratory characteristics	Presence at the disease onset n (%)	Cumulative prevalence n (%)
Thrombophlebitis	28 (20.72)	57 (42.18)
Peripheral Arterial Thrombotic Event	6 (4.44)	12 (8.88)
Pericarditis	5 (3.7)	11 (8.14)
Myocarditis	1 (0.74)	1 (0.74)
Stroke (arterial)	10 (7.4)	32 (23.68)
Brain Microinfarcts/TIA	1 (0.74)	14 (10.36)
Brain Venous Thrombosis	1 (0.74)	1 (0.74)
Epilepsy/Seizures	2 (1.48)	19 (14.06)
Diplopia/Ocular disorders	1 (0.74)	23 (17.02)
Peripheral Neuritis	1 (0.74)	30 (22.2)
Lower Back Pain	1 (0.74)	15 (11.1)
Headache/Migraine	6 (4.44)	34 (25.16)
Pleurisy	3 (2.22)	12 (8.88)
Pulmonary Emboli	7 (5.18)	16 (11.84)
Pulmonary Arterial Hypertension	1 (0.74)	9 (6.66)
Nephritis	2 (1.48)	17 (12.58)
APS associated Nephropathy	1 (0.74)	6 (4.44)
Budd-Chiari Syndrome	1 (0.74)	1 (0.74)
Ascites	1 (0.74)	1 (0.74)
Myalgia	2 (1.48)	9 (6.66)
Arthralgia	25 (18.5)	67 (49.58)
Arthritis	9 (6.66)	21 (15.54)
Livedo Reticularis	2 (1.48)	48 (35.52)
Ischemic Leg Ulcers	2 (1.48)	5 (3.7)
Digital Gangrene	1 (0.74)	1 (0.74)
Maculopapular Rash	3 (2.22)	13 (9.62)
Malar Rash (Butterfly)	8 (5.92)	21 (15.54)
Mucosal Ulcers	6 (4.44)	15 (11.1)
Vasculitis Rash	1 (0.74)	5 (3.7)
Raynaud	10 (7.4)	34 (25.16)
Photosensitivity	8 (5.92)	20 (14.8)
Alopecia	4 (2.96)	22 (16.28)
Foetal Loss	23 (23) *	40 (40) *
Chronic Disease Anemia	1 (0.74)	23 (17.02)
Hemolytic Anemia	2 (1.48)	22 (16.28)
Thrombocytopenia	5 (3.7)	20 (14.8)
Leucopenia	1 (0.74)	40 (29.6)

*percentage (%) out of the total of female patients (N= 100)
Grika E. –Vlachoyiannopoulos P. submitted

Table 3. Prevalence of clinical and laboratory characteristics present on the onset of the disease as well as during the follow-up of 135 APS patients (89 PAPS, 46 SAPS). The mean (SD) disease duration was 8.8 years (5.3) and the mean (SD) duration of follow up 7.55 (4.89) years.

1	β 2GPI-dependent increased expression of adhesion molecules (ICAM-1, VCAM-1, E-selectin)
2	Increase of synthesis and secretion of pro-inflammatory cytokines (IL-1, IL-6)
3	Increased tissue factor expression/upregulation of tissue factor mRNA
4	Increase of endothelin-1 levels
5	Induction of apoptosis

Table 4. The effects of aPL antibodies on endothelial cells

polyclonal and monoclonal aPL activate endothelium and enhance clot formation in vivo [50,59]. Studying the effect of aPL in mice with genetic deletion of ICAM-1, E-selectin and P-selectin, it was demonstrated that aPL-mediated endothelial activation depends on a considerable extent by these molecules [60-62]. Some studies suggest the presence of elevated levels of soluble adhesion molecules and soluble cytokines in patients with aPL and history of thrombosis [63]. Pierangeli et al. examined the pathogenic properties of human anti-CL antibodies in vivo and in vitro. The researchers used an in vivo model of thrombosis in mouse femoral vein. It turned out that antibodies caused leukocyte adhesion to endothelial cells of the microvasculature and increased the expression of adhesion molecules (e.g. VCAM-1). Among the proposed mechanisms, which explain the prothrombotic and proinflammatory properties of aPL, an increased expression of tissue factor (TF) is included. Data on the increase in TF expression in patients with APS is supported by several researchers. Typically, Zhou et al. demonstrated that IgG from patients with APS increases the expression and function of TF in monocytes [64]. Moreover, they described increased levels of soluble TF (sTF) in the peripheral blood of patients with a history of thrombosis and aPL.

The study of the endothelium clearly indicates the potentially beneficial effect of statins in the therapeutic approach of patients. Meroni et al. demonstrated that fluvastatin inhibits the expression of adhesion molecules and IL-6 by endothelial cells [65]. Very recently, proteomic study of monocytes and endothelial cells in patients with APS who received fluvastatin for one month, confirmed a significant reduction in the expression of TF, PAR-1, 2 and VEGF, which is associated with inhibition of the p38MAPK and NF-kB pathway [66]. Furthermore, Shoenfeld et al, based on the immunoregulatory and possibly antithrombotic effect of vitamin D, studied the serum levels of vitamin in patients with APS and its in vitro effects in HUVEC. It was shown that ~ 50% of patients had vitamin D deficiency (<15ng/ml) which correlates with thrombotic complications and other clinical manifestations of the syndrome (neurological, ocular, livedo reticularis and skin ulcers). In vitro, vitamin D seems to suspend the anti-β2GPI-induced expression of TF [67].

The role of anti-endothelial antibodies, especially of anti-HSP60, in the mechanism of thrombosis was studied in LA positive patients with secondary APS [68]. These antibodies induce endothelial apoptosis and seem to be associated with increased incidence of thrombosis. The researchers suggest that anti-HSP60 bind to the surface of EC and induce expression of anionic phosphatidylserine, thus providing a target for aPL binding and promotion of a thrombotic phenotype.

The exact nature of aPL- receptors on the surface of endothelial cells remains obscure and is a key subject of current research. Initially, several studies have suggested the simple recognition of β2GPI, bound to the surface of endothelial cells (by the domain V), by anti-β2GPI antibodies. This observation emerged from the crystallographic study of β2GPI. This glycoprotein is a single-chain polypeptide chain composed of five domains (I-V), comprising patterns of the complement control protein family (sushi domains). All domains resemble each other, except for domain V that contains an additional carboxy- loop with positively charged amino acids lysine. From the crystal structure of human β2GPI, it was showed that the positively charged region interacts electrostatically with negatively charged phospholipids. Furthermore, a partially hydrophobic loop of the molecule has the ability to enter the phospholipid bilayer and is involved in cell binding of β2GPI [69]. Later, Zhang et al. demonstrated that β2GPI binding to endothelial annexin A2 promotes the activation of endothelium by anti-β2GPI antibodies, possibly through a mechanism of multiple connections (cross linking), thus inducing a procoagulant phenotype [70]. To note that annexin A2 lacks intracellular region and possibly a second adaptor protein participates in intracellular signal transduction. There is evidence that specific antibodies against annexin A2, regardless of aPL, have been detected in plasma from APS patients and seem to correlate with thrombotic events. These antibodies are able to activate EC in a manner similar to anti-β2GPI antibodies [71]. Besides annexin A2, various members of Toll-like receptors (TLRs) family have been proposed as potential receptors of β2GPI/anti-β2GPI complexes on the surface of endothelial cells. Several data suggest the involvement of TLR-4 in aPL-mediated activation of endothelial cells. An important study shows the activation of the molecular pathway of MyD88 (Myeloid Differentiation factor 88), which is associated with TLR-4 - a receptor of bacterial endotoxin or lipopolysacharide (LPS), by anti-β2GPI antibodies [72]. Binding of LPS with TLR-4 triggers the nuclear translocation of NF-kB, the p38MAPK phosphorylation and other intracellular events that lead to the expression of pro-inflammatory cytokines, adhesion molecules and TF [73]. Fischetti et al. showed that the in vivo formation of complexes β2GPI/anti-β2GPI on the endothelial surface induces the development of thrombus, only under the influence of LPS [74]. In similar results, concerning the requirement of a priming factor, conclude several in vivo animal models of thrombosis, which require either photochemical or mechanical injury of the vessel so that the aPL can exert their thrombotic properties. It is not clear why the formation of anti-β2GPI/β2GPI complexes on the endothelial surface cannot induce thrombosis without a priming factor [75]. It is generally accepted that other molecules (not specified so far) could act as protein receptors for β2GPI, since the glycoprotein lacks a recognized specific cell receptor. It is assumed that β2GPI binds to endothelial surface via a "multi-receptor" and the molecular signaling is initiated immediately upon binding of specific antibodies.

The study of signal transduction in aPL-mediated endothelial activation continues to be an important area of research. As it was originally shown, there is an increased expression of adhesion molecules by endothelium in vitro. Nowadays, several studies confirm the involvement of NF-kB nuclear translocation and phosphorylation of p38MAPK in, aPL-mediated, induction of transcription, expression and function of TF in endothelial cells and the production of proinflammatory cytokines (IL-6 and IL-8).

5.1.2 Activation of platelets

The thrombophilic tendency in combination with the observation that thrombocytopenia is a frequent manifestation in APS, led early on the assumption that platelet activation is an important factor in the pathogenesis of the disease [52]. It should be noted that the study of platelet as "experimental model" has some peculiarities: platelets as anucleated cell fragments cannot be cultivated in vitro, or studied by techniques of recombinant DNA and on the other hand, unlike endothelial cells, platelet samples can be purified in the absence heparin, leaving unaffected the β2GPI interaction with platelet membranes [76]. Several studies demonstrate platelet activation and aggregation by aPL, both in vitro and in vivo [77,78]. **Figure 1** summarizes the main pathogenic effects of aPL in platelets. It has been

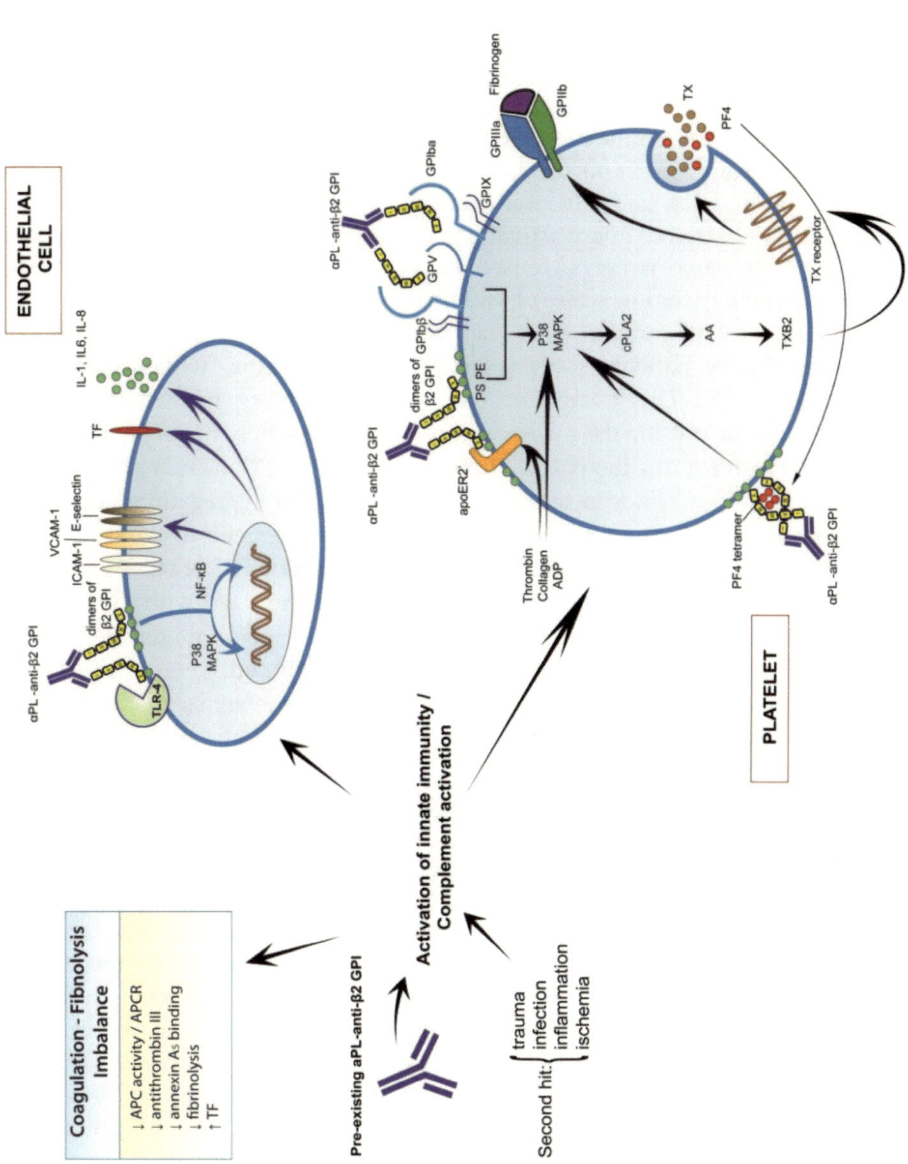

Fig. 1. A synopsis of the major and well characterized thrombogenic mechanisms of antiphospholipid (anti-β2GPI) antibodies: Pre-existing anti-β2GPI, probably under a second hit, activate components of innate immunity such as complement, endothelial cells, monocytes (not depicted) and platelets, as well as the coagulation system. More specifically, as shown by *in vitro* experiments, dimmers of β2GPI anchored to negatively charged phospholipids and TLR-4 are recognized by anti-β2GPI antibodies; then, P38-MAPK mediated endothelial cell activation takes place as depicted by ICAM-1, VCAM-1, E-selectin IL-1,-6,-8 and TF expression which change the phenotype of endothelial cells to a pro-coagulant form. On the other hand, dimmers of β2GPI induced, either, through β2GPI interaction with apo-ER2', or with GPIba, or with PF4 tetramers, activate platelets towards aggregation and release of PF4 and thromboxan B2. Coagulation-fibrinolysis imbalance is induced by the mechanisms depicted in the upper left panel.

demonstrated that aPL cannot bind to the surface of "intact" platelets, while they have the ability to bind to platelets with exposed negatively charged phospholipids in their membranes. Subactivating priming by known agonists, leading to phosphatidylserine exposure on the outer membrane seems to be a prerequisite for aPL to exert their pathogenic effects. One significant indication of platelet activation was the observation that patients with aPL and positive LA had increased urinary excretion of Thromboxane B2 (TXB2), a platelet metabolite secreted upon activation. Furthermore, purified F (ab ') 2 antibody fragments from the same patients, caused increased platelet aggregation and release of serotonin in the presence of low doses of thrombin.

A second indication of impaired platelet function in APS, is the observation that approximately 40% of patients show prolonged bleeding time, without accompanying bleeding tendency [79]. This assay depends only on primary hemostasis and thus is considered the classic test for the assessment of platelet function. Strong evidence of aPL-induced platelet activation is the enhanced expression of platelet membrane glycoproteins, particularly GPIIb-IIIa (fibrinogen receptor, critical in platelet aggregation) and GPIIIa [80]. More recently, Pierangeli et al. showed that in mice with genetic deletion of GPIIb-IIIa, passive immunization with aPL did not increase clot formation [81]. It has been also shown that blood clots are reduced in vivo, in mice that had been injected with monoclonal anti-GPIIb-IIIa antibodies. The possibility to include this type of inhibitors for the treatment of thrombotic events in patients with APS has not yet been confirmed.

A recent suggestion regarding platelet activation derived from the observation that patients with SLE and anti-β2GPI antibodies showed increased plasma levels of active von Willebrand factor (vWF), leading to platelet aggregation. It is assumed that under normal circumstances, β2GPI binds vWF, inhibiting its ability to promote adhesion and platelet aggregation, whereas in the presence of anti-β2GPI antibodies this anticoagulant effect is inhibited [82].

The activation of platelets by aPL, in vivo, has been supported by several groups. Joseph et al. studied in vivo the extent of platelet activation from patients with primary or secondary APS and SLE, using flow cytometry (FACS) and ELISA. They showed evidence of platelet activation as a significant increase in CD63 (a lysosomal membrane protein, which moves to the cell membrane after activation), increased binding of PAC-1 (a monoclonal IgM antibody against GPIIa-IIIb), the formation of platelet-leukocytes complexes and increased soluble p-selectin in patients' plasma [83]. Jankowski et al., studying a photochemically-induced thrombosis rat model, demonstrated that anti-β2GPI monoclonal antibodies with LA activity induced the formation of stable thrombi and large aggregates [51].

So far, two receptors have been proposed as mediators of platelet activation by aPL: a) the receptor of apolipoprotein E2' (apoER2') and b) glycoprotein GPIba (subunit of the platelet receptor GPIb/V/IX), which binds multiple ligands, including vWF. Involvement of apoER2' emerged from the research group of De Groot. They constructed chimeric dimers of β2GPI, which mimic the properties of anti-β2GPI/β2GPI complexes and showed an increase in the degree of platelet aggregation and adhesion to collagen [84]. The dimerization of the protein is of major importance, as monomeric β2GPI does not induce the same result. The researchers demonstrated by co-immunoprecipitation that dimeric β2GPI interacts with apoER2', which mediates the activation of platelets and the production of thromboxane. The specific inhibition of apoER2' by a specific monoclonal antibody resulted in reduced adhesion of platelets to collagen [85]. The role of apoER2' was recently investigated in an animal model of thrombosis. Passive immunization of apoER2'-/- mice with aPL purified from patients or monoclonal anti-β2GPI or β2GPI chimeric dimers, caused significantly reduced clots and reduced TF expression of vascular cells and macrophages, compared with immunization of control mice [86]. The role of GPIba as a β2GPI-receptor and potential mediator of platelet activation has been studied by in vitro binding assays and selective inhibition using specific antibodies [87]. It appeared that GPIba was able to bind directly β2GPI, suggesting a new mediator in platelet activation and thromboxane production by anti-β2GPI antibodies. It is well established that the intracellular signaling triggered by β2GPI/antiβ2GPI complexes in platelets involve the phosphorylation of p38MAPK which leads to activation of cytoplasmic phospholipase A2 (cPLA2), and ultimately the production of TXB2. However, these events are quite downstream in the intracellular cascade and several efforts have been undertaken to reveal more detailed information regarding the molecular intracellular events [88].

5.1.3 Activation of monocytes

Activation of monocytes by aPL has been extensively studied. The main findings include an increase of TF expression [89] and activity as well as the increased production of proinflammatory cytokines. The proposed β2GPI-receptors mediating monocyte activation are the members of toll-like receptors, TLR-2 and TLR-4, ApoER2' and annexin A2 [90-92]. Although annexin A2 lacks intracellular domain, its involvement is strongly supported by genetic modification experiments (knockdown). Therefore, it has been suggested that an additional adaptor protein should participate in the interaction.

5.2 Disruption of coagulation–fibrinolysis balance

5.2.1 Enhanced coagulation

It is assumed that although aPL cause delayed clotting times *in vitro*, these antibodies exert procoagulant effects *in vivo*, with accelerated thrombin formation. The exact pathogenic involvement of aPL in the coagulation cascade remains obscure. Apart from the aPL-mediated increase of tissue factor (TF) expression and activity by endothelial cells and monocytes, which has been proven by in vivo models, the direct role of aPL on coagulation events is controversial. Autoantibodies against thrombin have been detected in a subgroup (up to 43%) of patients with APS [93]. However, after the description by Krilis et al. of the possible interaction between β2GPI and thrombin, the results which support the presence of distinct antibodies against thrombin must be critically re-evaluated [94]. As mentioned above, the effects of LA are caused by either anti-β2GPI/β2GPI complexes, by competitively inhibiting the formation of prothrombinase complex *in vitro*, or by anti-prothrombin (PT) /prothrombin complexes [15]. It has been supported by several studies that although anti-PT antibodies are involved in the activity of LA, these antibodies by themselves are not associated with thrombosis. A recent multicenter study, completed in 2010, which included patients with APS and LA, concludes that 26% of patients were positive for anti-PT antibodies without any apparent correlation with clinical features of the syndrome [95].

Although initially coagulation factor XII was seen as a component of intrinsic coagulation pathway, it is now accepted that this factor has a more significant role in intrinsic fibrinolysis. Low plasma levels of factor XII in conjunction with presence of aPL has been described. Under current circumstances, the deficiency of factor XII does not cause bleeding but only prolonged aPTT, which can be taken as an expression of LA. This deficiency can participate in thrombotic events due to its role in fibrinolysis. It has been shown that anti-β2GPI antibodies inhibit the activation of factor XII, but at high concentrations of antibody the opposite effect was observed. On the other hand, when the plasma is enriched with β2GPI and excess of negatively charged phospholipids, there is again a reduction in the rate of production of activated XIIa [96]. Presence of autoantibodies to factor XII is associated with LA and appears to be distinct from anti-PT antibodies [97,98]. The presence of these antibodies leads to acquired deficiency of factor XII and presents a statistically significant association with recurrent fetal abortions in APS.

5.2.2 Impaired fibrinolysis

Research data suggest that impaired fibrinolysis may contribute to the thrombophilic tendency in APS [97,99-103]. Independent studies have shown an increased activity of plasminogen activator inhibitor-1 (PAI-1) and reduced tissue plasminogen activator (tPA) following venous obstruction in patients with APS. Another possible mechanism suggested that elevated levels of lipoprotein (a) in plasma of patients, which shares structural homology with plasminogen, could compete for binding to fibrin and interfere with plasmin-mediated degradation of fibrin [104]. Recent studies revealed plasmin as a potential antigen in APS and observed that one out of four patients had antibodies to plasmin, which potentially interfere with fibrinolysis. Furthermore, binding of tPA by some aPL with subsequent inhibition of plasminogen activation has been reported [105-107].

β2GPI has also been suggested to have a direct role in fibrinolysis, through direct interaction with components of plasminogen activation. It has been shown that β2GPI blocks the PAI-1-mediated inhibition of tPA in a dose dependent manner and that aPL prevent this inhibitory effect of β2GPI. In addition, monoclonal anti-β2GPI antibodies in the presence of β2GPI cause reduced endogenous fibrinolytic activity, even in the presence of excess clotting factor XIIa. Overall, these data indicate that aPL inhibit both endogenous and exogenous fibrinolysis. It has been supported that nicked β2GPI by plasmin, in the lysine-rich amino acid chain of domain V, has the ability to bind plasminogen and inhibit the formation of plasmin [108,109]. Recent data also give a role to β2GPI and regulation of the fibrinolytic system, showing that β2GPI interacts with tPA and causes tPA-dependent activation of plasminogen and that this process is inhibited by the presence of anti-β2GPI antibodies [110].

The role of annexin A2 in the mechanism of fibrinolysis is also interesting. Apart from this role as endothelial receptor of β2GPI/anti-β2GPI complexes, it is known that annexin A2 induces fibrinolysis by binding tPA and plasminogen. Autoantibodies against annexin A2 have been reported in patients with APS and appear to correlate with a history of thrombosis. These antibodies inhibit the ability of annexin A2 to induce tPA-mediated plasminogen activation and to inhibit fibrinolysis on the surfaces of the EC.

5.2.3 Resistance to natural anticoagulants

The protein C pathway is the most important natural anticoagulant pathway, activated in the presence of low concentrations of thrombin. The activated protein C (activated protein C, APC) exerts its anticoagulant effect through proteolytic inactivation of coagulation factors V and VIII. Apart from the mutation FV Leiden, the resistance in activated protein C activity (APC resistance, APCR) is associated with the occurrence of thrombosis in patients with APS and LA. The percentage of patients with aPL and APCR ranges between 17-75%. In a recent study, APCR was found in 44% of anti-CL/anti-β2GPI positive patients and in 55% of anti-PS/anti-PT positive patients [111-114]. Indeed, both anti-PT and anti-β2GPI antibodies assert to cause APCR [115]. These antibodies reduce the APC activity through competition with the latter for binding to phospholipid surfaces. Another possible mechanism through which aPL could cause APCR is the direct interaction between β2GPI and APC [116]. It has been shown that β2GPI interact directly with the APC, especially in the presence of anti-β2GPI antibodies, and therefore inhibits its activity. Furthermore, aPL with an affinity for proteins C and S have been described in APS patients with protein C or/and S deficiency. Cross-reactivity between β2GPI and APC, indicating that several anti-β2GPI antibodies recognized APC and vice versa, has also been proposed [117]. Protein C and/or S is associated with about five times increased risk of thrombosis, depending on severity of deficiency.

Annexin A5 is a plasma protein with high affinity to anionic phospholipids, thereby creating an anticoagulant "shield" in vascular cells and platelets. Rand et al. suggested that aPL could induce thrombosis and pregnancy morbidity, by competing with annexin A5 for binding to cell surfaces, thereby reducing its anticoagulant properties. However, it must be clarified whether this annexin A5 "shield" exists in vivo, as annexin A5 -/- mice showed no specific phenotype [118,119].

5.3 Activation of innate immunity/ complement activation

Complement activation appears to have a key role in the thrombophilic diathesis of APS. The involvement of complement was first suggested by the observation of increased activated complement components in plasma of patients with APS and history of thrombosis [120]. As mentioned above, aPL induce a proinflammatory and procoagulant phenotype in endothelial cells, monocytes and platelets. It is also well documented that activated complement components are able to bind and activate inflammatory cells and endothelial cells, either directly through C5b-9 membrane attack complex complex (MAC), or through effects mediated by C5a receptor. Furthermore, endothelial cells release TF upon activation by anaphylatoxin C5a. In an in vivo model of surgically induced thrombosis in mice prior to aPL injections, Pierangeli et al. demonstrated that complement activation plays an important role in the induction and stabilization of thrombosis and adhesion of leukocytes to endothelial cells. Mice with genetic deletion of the complement components C3, C5, or C5a receptor were resistant to aPL-induced thrombophilia [75,121,122]. Another in vivo study, with rats pretreated by intraperitoneal injection of bacterial LPS and later(after a few hours) injected with polyclonal IgG antibodies from patients with APS, concludes that thrombotic manifestations were mainly depended on the activation of factors C5 and C6 [74]. Therefore, it turns out that complement activation significantly participates in the pathophysiology of thrombosis in APS.

It remains unclear why only some people with aPL develop clinical manifestations of disease. It has been argued by several researchers that the activation of innate immunity plays a critical role in two separate stages: a) the "immune" phase, critical for aPL production and b) the "pathological "phase, in which autoantibodies become involved in the induction of thrombosis [123]. According to this model, aPL alone is insufficient to cause thrombosis and thus requires the concomitant triggering of innate immunity (e.g., a ligand for TLRs). During those two phases, the innate immunity can be triggered by various stimuli such as trauma, infection, inflammation or ischemia.

5.4 Controversial issues in the thrombogenic properties of aPL- A novel mechanism for platelet activation involving β2GPI/PF4 complexes

Despite the clinical diversity (several manifestations with thrombotic or non-thrombotic etiology) and laboratory heterogeneity (autoantibodies recognizing many different proteins) of APS, it is accepted that only anti-β2GPI antibodies are responsible for the clinical presentation of the syndrome [16]. More specifically, a subpopulation of anti-β2GPI antibody against a cryptic epitope (Arg39-Arg43) in domain I of β2GPI, which is highly correlated with clinical symptoms and prognosis of the syndrome, has been identified [17]. Undoubtedly, β2GPI has an important role in the pathophysiology of APS, yet not entirely clear even after 30 years of intensive research [124]. So far, the best explanation for the role of β2GPI is that anti-β2GPI in APS induce new functions to the glycoprotein.

The newest trend in the study of β2GPI, oriented to reveal conformational changes and / or post-translational modifications of the molecule, which are induced by specific conditions and appear to be associated with the pathogenesis of APS. Therefore, while monomeric β2GPI (due to lack of specific cellular receptor) binds with low affinity to cell membranes, in the presence of anti-β2GPI autoantibodies and upon induction of conformational changes, becomes a "sticky" protein that can easily bind to different cellular receptors. So far, two responsible factors for such tertiary variations have been suggested: the anionic phospholipids and anti-β2GPI antibodies. Very recently, it has been demonstrated that β2GPI can exist in two different conformations, a circular and a stretched one. In circulation, the glycoprotein lies with the circular conformation and adopts a stretched structure after interaction with autoantibodies [125]. The researchers propose that this change could lead to the exposure of a "recognition pattern", which explains why the protein interacts with many different protein receptors. On post-translational modifications of β2GPI, a large multicenter retrospective study was recently published, which concludes that in plasma of APS patients the proportion of oxidized form of β2GPI predominates [126]. It becomes clear that β2GPI is an enigmatic protein with significant "reserve" of new structures and functions that are induced after specific stimuli.

An important indication about the biology of β2GPI and the mechanisms of action of anti-β2GPI is the observation that the dimerization of the molecule on the surface of cell membranes is a critical step to initiate cellular activation. It was shown that the chimeric dimers of β2GPI have the ability to bind and activate platelets, even in the absence of anti-β2GPI antibodies [84]. Of course, the dimerization of ligands occurs in many known interactions with cellular transmembrane receptors. In most cases however, the dimerization of the ligand is induced by the transmembrane receptor, which has not been proven in the case of β2GPI.

In vivo models of passive or active immunization with purified antibodies or β2GPI from APS patients have demonstrated a clear direct relationship between aPL and the increased risk of thrombosis and fetal abortion [51,127,128]. Although the exact pathogenetic mechanisms have not been clarified, the involvement of cellular activation (EC, platelets and monocytes) is now well-documented. One of the most critical questions in the literature is to identify the main cellular receptors through which anti-β2GPI/β2GPI complexes exert their pathogenic effects. As presented in this review, several possible receptors have been proposed and nowadays, the research is evolving towards the identification of important ones and their exact role.

Our research towards this objective was based to a null hypothesis: platelet membrane proteins, which selectively bind to a β2GPI-affinity column, will be those that potentially interact with β2GPI in vivo[35]. Attempt was made to minimize nonspecific interactions: on the one hand, by the effect of neuraminidase on platelets, to remove large sialic groups from surface glycoproteins and on the other hand, by the purification of platelet membranes and subsequent extraction of membrane proteins. The study highlighted platelet factor 4 (PF4) as the dominant β2GPI-binding protein, after protein identification by mass spectroscopy. The interaction was studied by analytical methodology and confirmed by size exclusion chromatography, which illustrates the composition and stoichiometry of complexes. The important point of interaction is that PF4 contributes to the natural dimerization of β2GPI, enhancing the recognition of low-affinity anti-β2GPI antibodies, which in turn further stabilize the entire complex. With *in silico* approach, molecular dynamics interface suggested that the interaction consists of electrostatic interactions between the positively charged surface of the PF4 tetramers and negative amino acids in domains III-V of β2GPI, enhanced by the formation of hydrogen bonds. It is worth noting that in the proposed structure of the complex, the critical epitopes in subunit I of β2GPI are arranged in such a geometric conformation that fits perfectly with the geometry of two F(ab') fragments of an antibody.

The functional significance of the formed β2GPI/PF4 complexes studied both at the level of recognition by anti-β2GPI antibodies, and in the induction of platelet activation. The study of the antigenicity of β2GPI indicates that the sera of patients with APS recognize β2GPI/PF4 complexes more powerful than β2GPI alone. Moreover, the results of this study support the phosphorylation of platelet p38MAPK and production of thromboxane B2 (TXB2) by anti-β2GPI/β2GPI/PF4 complexes, after pretreatment of platelets with suboptimal doses of thrombin. The coexistence of anti-β2GPI and β2GPI seemed to be a prerequisite for p38MAPK phosphorylation, while the anti-β2GPI/β2GPI/PF4 complexes significantly enhance this effect.

These experimental data combined with literature information, on the importance of conformational changes of β2GPI and on the necessity of β2GPI dimerization, leads to the following logical model: the binding of β2GPI by PF4 tetramers result to the natural dimerization of β2GPI, which is crucial for interaction with phospholipid surfaces and could also contribute to the induction of conformational changes, thereby revealing cryptic epitopes of domain I. The latter is consistent with the finding of the stronger recognition of complexes from patients' antibodies.

An interesting observation that arose while guided the study was the known involvement of PF4 in the pathogenesis of heparin-induced thrombocytopenia and thrombosis syndrome (HITT) [129,130]. Given the clinical similarities of two immunologically-mediated thrombophilic conditions, APS and HITT, we recommend PF4 as a "common denominator" of their pathogenesis. One distinguishing point that emerged from this work is that while in HITT, platelet activation induced by heparin/PF4/HITT-antibodies complexes is mediated primarily by Fc fragments of antibodies and stimulation of FcgRIIa receptor, unlike in APS the effects of β2GPI/PF4/anti-β2GPI complexes on platelet activation is independent of the Fc fragments of the antibodies [35].

In summary, our study describes for the first time a new interaction between β2GPI and PF4. The main significance of this interaction is the stabilization of dimeric structures of β2GPI upon interaction with PF4, which facilitates the recognition by specific antibodies. The formation of anti-β2GPI/β2GPI/PF4 complexes induces platelet activation, mainly through the F (ab ') 2 fragments of specific antibodies.

5.5 Conclusions

APS is an autoantibody mediated thrombophilia induced by antibodies recognizing phospholipid binding proteins, mainly β2GPI and prothrombin. The mechanisms by which these antibodies induce thrombosis are now beginning to be understood and involve imbalance of coagulation-fibrinolysis, as well as platelet, endothelial cell and monocyte activation towards coagulation. The cellular activation requires dimerization of β2GPI as well as intracellular domains possessing adaptor proteins on the cell surface. The most well characterized ones are the apoER2′ and the GPIba (subunit of the platelet receptor GPIb/V/IX), while Annexin A2 and the receptors TLR-2 and -4 have also been implicated in the procoagulant process by some researchers. PF4 is a CXC-chemokine produced by platelets and monocytes; PF4 spontaneously forms tetramers in solution and these tetramers possess sites available for binding of 2 molecules of β2GPI in a way that PF4 favors a natural dimerization of β2GPI, which is then rather accessible for binding by the anti-β2GPI antibodies. The anti-β2GPI/β2GPI/PF4 complexes are immunogenic and thrombogenic, at least by activating platelets.

6. References

[1] Petri M. Epidemiology of the antiphospholipid antibody syndrome. J Autoimmun. 2000;15:145-151.

[2] Richaud-Patin Y, Cabiedes J, Jakez-Ocampo J, Vidaller A, Llorente L. High prevalence of protein-dependent and protein-independent antiphospholipid and other autoantibodies in healthy elders. Thromb Res. 2000;99:129-133.

[3] Katano K, Aoki A, Sasa H, Ogasawara M, Matsuura E, Yagami Y. beta 2-Glycoprotein I-dependent anticardiolipin antibodies as a predictor of adverse pregnancy outcomes in healthy pregnant women. Hum Reprod. 1996;11:509-512.

[4] Clark EA, Silver RM, Branch DW. Do antiphospholipid antibodies cause preeclampsia and HELLP syndrome? Curr Rheumatol Rep. 2007;9:219-225.

[5] Biggioggero M, Meroni PL. The geoepidemiology of the antiphospholipid antibody syndrome. Autoimmun Rev;9:A299-304.

[6] Cervera R, Boffa MC, Khamashta MA, Hughes GR. The Euro-Phospholipid project: epidemiology of the antiphospholipid syndrome in Europe. Lupus. 2009;18:889-893.

[7] Opatrny L, David M, Kahn SR, Shrier I, Rey E. Association between antiphospholipid antibodies and recurrent fetal loss in women without autoimmune disease: a metaanalysis. J Rheumatol. 2006;33:2214-2221.

[8] Danowski A, de Azevedo MN, de Souza Papi JA, Petri M. Determinants of risk for venous and arterial thrombosis in primary antiphospholipid syndrome and in antiphospholipid syndrome with systemic lupus erythematosus. J Rheumatol. 2009;36:1195-1199.

[9] Clowse ME, Magder LS, Witter F, Petri M. Early risk factors for pregnancy loss in lupus. Obstet Gynecol. 2006;107:293-299.

[10] Wilson WA, Gharavi AE, Koike T, et al. International consensus statement on preliminary classification criteria for definite antiphospholipid syndrome: report of an international workshop. Arthritis Rheum. 1999;42:1309-1311.

[11] Miyakis S, Lockshin MD, Atsumi T, et al. International consensus statement on an update of the classification criteria for definite antiphospholipid syndrome (APS). J Thromb Haemost. 2006;4:295-306.
[12] Galli M, Luciani D, Bertolini G, Barbui T. Lupus anticoagulants are stronger risk factors for thrombosis than anticardiolipin antibodies in the antiphospholipid syndrome: a systematic review of the literature. Blood. 2003;101:1827-1832.
[13] Tektonidou MG, Laskari K, Panagiotakos DB, Moutsopoulos HM. Risk factors for thrombosis and primary thrombosis prevention in patients with systemic lupus erythematosus with or without antiphospholipid antibodies. Arthritis Rheum. 2009;61:29-36.
[14] Martinez-Berriotxoa A, Ruiz-Irastorza G, Egurbide MV, et al. Transiently positive anticardiolipin antibodies and risk of thrombosis in patients with systemic lupus erythematosus. Lupus. 2007;16:810-816.
[15] de Laat HB, Derksen RH, Urbanus RT, Roest M, de Groot PG. beta2-glycoprotein I-dependent lupus anticoagulant highly correlates with thrombosis in the antiphospholipid syndrome. Blood. 2004;104:3598-3602.
[16] Arad A, Proulle V, Furie RA, Furie BC, Furie B. beta-Glycoprotein-1 autoantibodies from patients with antiphospholipid syndrome are sufficient to potentiate arterial thrombus formation in a mouse model. Blood;117:3453-3459.
[17] de Laat B, de Groot PG. Autoantibodies directed against domain I of beta2-glycoprotein I. Curr Rheumatol Rep;13:70-76.
[18] Pengo V, Biasiolo A, Pegoraro C, Cucchini U, Noventa F, Iliceto S. Antibody profiles for the diagnosis of antiphospholipid syndrome. Thromb Haemost. 2005;93:1147-1152.
[19] Ruffatti A, Calligaro A, Hoxha A, et al. Laboratory and clinical features of pregnant women with antiphospholipid syndrome and neonatal outcome. Arthritis Care Res (Hoboken);62:302-307.
[20] Rosenberg RD, Aird WC. Vascular-bed--specific hemostasis and hypercoagulable states. N Engl J Med. 1999;340:1555-1564.
[21] Cervera R, Piette JC, Font J, et al. Antiphospholipid syndrome: clinical and immunologic manifestations and patterns of disease expression in a cohort of 1,000 patients. Arthritis Rheum. 2002;46:1019-1027.
[22] Rosove MH, Brewer PM. Antiphospholipid thrombosis: clinical course after the first thrombotic event in 70 patients. Ann Intern Med. 1992;117:303-308.
[23] Cervera R, Khamashta MA, Shoenfeld Y, et al. Morbidity and mortality in the antiphospholipid syndrome during a 5-year period: a multicentre prospective study of 1000 patients. Ann Rheum Dis. 2009;68:1428-1432.
[24] Cervera R. Lessons from the "Euro-Phospholipid" project. Autoimmun Rev. 2008;7:174-178.
[25] Galli M, Luciani D, Bertolini G, Barbui T. Anti-beta 2-glycoprotein I, antiprothrombin antibodies, and the risk of thrombosis in the antiphospholipid syndrome. Blood. 2003;102:2717-2723.
[26] Zoghlami-Rintelen C, Vormittag R, Sailer T, et al. The presence of IgG antibodies against beta2-glycoprotein I predicts the risk of thrombosis in patients with the lupus anticoagulant. J Thromb Haemost. 2005;3:1160-1165.
[27] Ruiz-Irastorza G, Crowther M, Branch W, Khamashta MA. Antiphospholipid syndrome. Lancet;376:1498-1509.

[28] Urbanus RT, Siegerink B, Roest M, Rosendaal FR, de Groot PG, Algra A. Antiphospholipid antibodies and risk of myocardial infarction and ischaemic stroke in young women in the RATIO study: a case-control study. Lancet Neurol. 2009;8:998-1005.

[29] Rodrigues CE, Carvalho JF, Shoenfeld Y. Neurological manifestations of antiphospholipid syndrome. Eur J Clin Invest;40:350-359.

[30] Sanna G, D'Cruz D, Cuadrado MJ. Cerebral manifestations in the antiphospholipid (Hughes) syndrome. Rheum Dis Clin North Am. 2006;32:465-490.

[31] Hughes GR. Migraine, memory loss, and "multiple sclerosis ". Neurological features of the antiphospholipid (Hughes') syndrome. Postgrad Med J. 2003;79:81-83.

[32] Tektonidou MG, Varsou N, Kotoulas G, Antoniou A, Moutsopoulos HM. Cognitive deficits in patients with antiphospholipid syndrome: association with clinical, laboratory, and brain magnetic resonance imaging findings. Arch Intern Med. 2006;166:2278-2284.

[33] Fakhouri F, Noel LH, Zuber J, et al. The expanding spectrum of renal diseases associated with antiphospholipid syndrome. Am J Kidney Dis. 2003;41:1205-1211.

[34] Gigante A, Gasperini ML, Cianci R, et al. Antiphospholipid antibodies and renal involvement. Am J Nephrol. 2009;30:405-412.

[35] Sikara MP, Routsias JG, Samiotaki M, Panayotou G, Moutsopoulos HM, Vlachoyiannopoulos PG. {beta}2 Glycoprotein I ({beta}2GPI) binds platelet factor 4 (PF4): implications for the pathogenesis of antiphospholipid syndrome. Blood. 2010;115:713-723.

[36] Tektonidou MG, Sotsiou F, Nakopoulou L, Vlachoyiannopoulos PG, Moutsopoulos HM. Antiphospholipid syndrome nephropathy in patients with systemic lupus erythematosus and antiphospholipid antibodies: prevalence, clinical associations, and long-term outcome. Arthritis Rheum. 2004;50:2569-2579.

[37] Erkan D, Erel H, Yazici Y, Prince MR. The role of cardiac magnetic resonance imaging in antiphospholipid syndrome. J Rheumatol. 2002;29:2658-2659.

[38] Hojnik M, George J, Ziporen L, Shoenfeld Y. Heart valve involvement (Libman-Sacks endocarditis) in the antiphospholipid syndrome. Circulation. 1996;93:1579-1587.

[39] Tenedios F, Erkan D, Lockshin MD. Cardiac involvement in the antiphospholipid syndrome. Lupus. 2005;14:691-696.

[40] Roman MJ, Salmon JE, Sobel R, et al. Prevalence and relation to risk factors of carotid atherosclerosis and left ventricular hypertrophy in systemic lupus erythematosus and antiphospholipid antibody syndrome. Am J Cardiol. 2001;87:663-666, A611.

[41] Vaarala O, Manttari M, Manninen V, et al. Anti-cardiolipin antibodies and risk of myocardial infarction in a prospective cohort of middle-aged men. Circulation. 1995;91:23-27.

[42] Frances C. Dermatological manifestations of Hughes' antiphospholipid antibody syndrome. Lupus;19:1071-1077.

[43] Toubi E, Shoenfeld Y. Livedo reticularis as a criterion for antiphospholipid syndrome. Clin Rev Allergy Immunol. 2007;32:138-144.

[44] Toubi E, Krause I, Fraser A, et al. Livedo reticularis is a marker for predicting multi-system thrombosis in antiphospholipid syndrome. Clin Exp Rheumatol. 2005;23:499-504.

[45] Krause I, Leibovici L, Blank M, Shoenfeld Y. Clusters of disease manifestations in patients with antiphospholipid syndrome demonstrated by factor analysis. Lupus. 2007;16:176-180.
[46] Uthman I, Godeau B, Taher A, Khamashta M. The hematologic manifestations of the antiphospholipid syndrome. Blood Rev. 2008;22:187-194.
[47] Cuadrado MJ, Mujic F, Munoz E, Khamashta MA, Hughes GR. Thrombocytopenia in the antiphospholipid syndrome. Ann Rheum Dis. 1997;56:194-196.
[48] Pullarkat V, Ngo M, Iqbal S, Espina B, Liebman HA. Detection of lupus anticoagulant identifies patients with autoimmune haemolytic anaemia at increased risk for venous thromboembolism. Br J Haematol. 2002;118:1166-1169.
[49] Pierangeli SS, Liu XW, Barker JH, Anderson G, Harris EN. Induction of thrombosis in a mouse model by IgG, IgM and IgA immunoglobulins from patients with the antiphospholipid syndrome. Thromb Haemost. 1995;74:1361-1367.
[50] Pierangeli SS, Colden-Stanfield M, Liu X, Barker JH, Anderson GL, Harris EN. Antiphospholipid antibodies from antiphospholipid syndrome patients activate endothelial cells in vitro and in vivo. Circulation. 1999;99:1997-2002.
[51] Jankowski M, Vreys I, Wittevrongel C, et al. Thrombogenicity of beta 2-glycoprotein I-dependent antiphospholipid antibodies in a photochemically induced thrombosis model in the hamster. Blood. 2003;101:157-162.
[52] Mehdi AA, Uthman I, Khamashta M. Antiphospholipid syndrome: pathogenesis and a window of treatment opportunities in the future. Eur J Clin Invest;40:451-464.
[53] Meroni PL, Del Papa N, Raschi E, et al. Beta2-glycoprotein I as a 'cofactor' for anti-phospholipid reactivity with endothelial cells. Lupus. 1998;7 Suppl 2:S44-47.
[54] Martinez-Sales V, Vila V, Mico L, Contreras MT, Escandell A, Reganon E. [Circulating endothelial cells and microparticles in patients with antiphospholipid antibodies.]. Med Clin (Barc);136:431-433.
[55] Dignat-George F, Camoin-Jau L, Sabatier F, et al. Endothelial microparticles: a potential contribution to the thrombotic complications of the antiphospholipid syndrome. Thromb Haemost. 2004;91:667-673.
[56] Simantov R, LaSala JM, Lo SK, et al. Activation of cultured vascular endothelial cells by antiphospholipid antibodies. J Clin Invest. 1995;96:2211-2219.
[57] Del Papa N, Guidali L, Spatola L, et al. Relationship between anti-phospholipid and anti-endothelial cell antibodies III: beta 2 glycoprotein I mediates the antibody binding to endothelial membranes and induces the expression of adhesion molecules. Clin Exp Rheumatol. 1995;13:179-185.
[58] Meroni PL, Papa ND, Beltrami B, Tincani A, Balestrieri G, Krilis SA. Modulation of endothelial cell function by antiphospholipid antibodies. Lupus. 1996;5:448-450.
[59] Pierangeli SS, Liu X, Espinola R, et al. Functional analyses of patient-derived IgG monoclonal anticardiolipin antibodies using in vivo thrombosis and in vivo microcirculation models. Thromb Haemost. 2000;84:388-395.
[60] Pierangeli SS, Espinola RG, Liu X, Harris EN. Thrombogenic effects of antiphospholipid antibodies are mediated by intercellular cell adhesion molecule-1, vascular cell adhesion molecule-1, and P-selectin. Circ Res. 2001;88:245-250.
[61] Kaplanski G, Cacoub P, Farnarier C, et al. Increased soluble vascular cell adhesion molecule 1 concentrations in patients with primary or systemic lupus

erythematosus-related antiphospholipid syndrome: correlations with the severity of thrombosis. Arthritis Rheum. 2000;43:55-64.

[62] Espinola RG, Liu X, Colden-Stanfield M, Hall J, Harris EN, Pierangeli SS. E-Selectin mediates pathogenic effects of antiphospholipid antibodies. J Thromb Haemost. 2003;1:843-848.

[63] Forastiero RR, Martinuzzo ME, de Larranaga GF. Circulating levels of tissue factor and proinflammatory cytokines in patients with primary antiphospholipid syndrome or leprosy related antiphospholipid antibodies. Lupus. 2005;14:129-136.

[64] Zhou H, Wolberg AS, Roubey RA. Characterization of monocyte tissue factor activity induced by IgG antiphospholipid antibodies and inhibition by dilazep. Blood. 2004;104:2353-2358.

[65] Meroni PL, Raschi E, Testoni C, et al. Statins prevent endothelial cell activation induced by antiphospholipid (anti-beta2-glycoprotein I) antibodies: effect on the proadhesive and proinflammatory phenotype. Arthritis Rheum. 2001;44:2870-2878.

[66] Lopez-Pedrera C, Ruiz-Limon P, Aguirre MA, et al. Global effects of fluvastatin on the prothrombotic status of patients with antiphospholipid syndrome. Ann Rheum Dis;70:675-682.

[67] Agmon-Levin N, Blank M, Zandman-Goddard G, et al. Vitamin D: an instrumental factor in the anti-phospholipid syndrome by inhibition of tissue factor expression. Ann Rheum Dis;70:145-150.

[68] Dieude M, Senecal JL, Raymond Y. Induction of endothelial cell apoptosis by heat-shock protein 60-reactive antibodies from anti-endothelial cell autoantibody-positive systemic lupus erythematosus patients. Arthritis Rheum. 2004;50:3221-3231.

[69] Bouma B, de Groot PG, van den Elsen JM, et al. Adhesion mechanism of human beta(2)-glycoprotein I to phospholipids based on its crystal structure. Embo J. 1999;18:5166-5174.

[70] Zhang J, McCrae KR. Annexin A2 mediates endothelial cell activation by antiphospholipid/anti-beta2 glycoprotein I antibodies. Blood. 2005;105:1964-1969.

[71] Cesarman-Maus G, Rios-Luna NP, Deora AB, et al. Autoantibodies against the fibrinolytic receptor, annexin 2, in antiphospholipid syndrome. Blood. 2006;107:4375-4382.

[72] Raschi E, Testoni C, Bosisio D, et al. Role of the MyD88 transduction signaling pathway in endothelial activation by antiphospholipid antibodies. Blood. 2003;101:3495-3500.

[73] Vega-Ostertag M, Casper K, Swerlick R, Ferrara D, Harris EN, Pierangeli SS. Involvement of p38 MAPK in the up-regulation of tissue factor on endothelial cells by antiphospholipid antibodies. Arthritis Rheum. 2005;52:1545-1554.

[74] Fischetti F, Durigutto P, Pellis V, et al. Thrombus formation induced by antibodies to beta2-glycoprotein I is complement dependent and requires a priming factor. Blood. 2005;106:2340-2346.

[75] Pierangeli SS, Girardi G, Vega-Ostertag M, Liu X, Espinola RG, Salmon J. Requirement of activation of complement C3 and C5 for antiphospholipid antibody-mediated thrombophilia. Arthritis Rheum. 2005;52:2120-2124.

[76] Guerin J, Sheng Y, Reddel S, Iverson GM, Chapman MG, Krilis SA. Heparin inhibits the binding of beta 2-glycoprotein I to phospholipids and promotes the plasmin-mediated inactivation of this blood protein. Elucidation of the consequences of the

two biological events in patients with the anti-phospholipid syndrome. J Biol Chem. 2002;277:2644-2649.
[77] Martinuzzo ME, Maclouf J, Carreras LO, Levy-Toledano S. Antiphospholipid antibodies enhance thrombin-induced platelet activation and thromboxane formation. Thromb Haemost. 1993;70:667-671.
[78] Forastiero R, Martinuzzo M, Carreras LO, Maclouf J. Anti-beta2 glycoprotein I antibodies and platelet activation in patients with antiphospholipid antibodies: association with increased excretion of platelet-derived thromboxane urinary metabolites. Thromb Haemost. 1998;79:42-45.
[79] Urbanus RT, de Laat HB, de Groot PG, Derksen RH. Prolonged bleeding time and lupus anticoagulant: a second paradox in the antiphospholipid syndrome. Arthritis Rheum. 2004;50:3605-3609.
[80] Espinola RG, Pierangeli SS, Gharavi AE, Harris EN. Hydroxychloroquine reverses platelet activation induced by human IgG antiphospholipid antibodies. Thromb Haemost. 2002;87:518-522.
[81] Pierangeli SS, Vega-Ostertag ME, Gonzalez EB. New targeted therapies for treatment of thrombosis in antiphospholipid syndrome. Expert Rev Mol Med. 2007;9:1-15.
[82] Hulstein JJ, Lenting PJ, de Laat B, Derksen RH, Fijnheer R, de Groot PG. beta2-Glycoprotein I inhibits von Willebrand factor dependent platelet adhesion and aggregation. Blood. 2007;110:1483-1491.
[83] Joseph JE, Harrison P, Mackie IJ, Isenberg DA, Machin SJ. Increased circulating platelet-leucocyte complexes and platelet activation in patients with antiphospholipid syndrome, systemic lupus erythematosus and rheumatoid arthritis. Br J Haematol. 2001;115:451-459.
[84] Lutters BC, Derksen RH, Tekelenburg WL, Lenting PJ, Arnout J, de Groot PG. Dimers of beta 2-glycoprotein I increase platelet deposition to collagen via interaction with phospholipids and the apolipoprotein E receptor 2'. J Biol Chem. 2003;278:33831-33838.
[85] de Groot PG, Derksen RH, Urbanus RT. The role of LRP8 (ApoER2') in the pathophysiology of the antiphospholipid syndrome. Lupus;19:389-393.
[86] Romay-Penabad Z, Aguilar-Valenzuela R, Urbanus RT, et al. Apolipoprotein E receptor 2 is involved in the thrombotic complications in a murine model of the antiphospholipid syndrome. Blood;117:1408-1414.
[87] Shi T, Giannakopoulos B, Yan X, et al. Anti-beta2-glycoprotein I antibodies in complex with beta2-glycoprotein I can activate platelets in a dysregulated manner via glycoprotein Ib-IX-V. Arthritis Rheum. 2006;54:2558-2567.
[88] Vega-Ostertag M, Harris EN, Pierangeli SS. Intracellular events in platelet activation induced by antiphospholipid antibodies in the presence of low doses of thrombin. Arthritis Rheum. 2004;50:2911-2919.
[89] Reverter JC, Tassies D, Font J, et al. Effects of human monoclonal anticardiolipin antibodies on platelet function and on tissue factor expression on monocytes. Arthritis Rheum. 1998;41:1420-1427.
[90] Satta N, Kruithof EK, Fickentscher C, et al. Toll-like receptor 2 mediates the activation of human monocytes and endothelial cells by antiphospholipid antibodies. Blood.

[91] Zhou H, Yan Y, Xu G, et al. Toll-like receptor (TLR)-4 mediates anti-beta2GPI/beta2GPI-induced tissue factor expression in THP-1 cells. Clin Exp Immunol;163:189-198.
[92] Doring Y, Hurst J, Lorenz M, et al. Human antiphospholipid antibodies induce TNFalpha in monocytes via Toll-like receptor 8. Immunobiology;215:230-241.
[93] Miesbach W, Matthias T, Scharrer I. Identification of thrombin antibodies in patients with antiphospholipid syndrome. Ann N Y Acad Sci. 2005;1050:250-256.
[94] Rahgozar S, Yang Q, Giannakopoulos B, Yan X, Miyakis S, Krilis SA. Beta2-glycoprotein I binds thrombin via exosite I and exosite II: anti-beta2-glycoprotein I antibodies potentiate the inhibitory effect of beta2-glycoprotein I on thrombin-mediated factor XIa generation. Arthritis Rheum. 2007;56:605-613.
[95] Pengo V, Denas G, Bison E, et al. Prevalence and significance of anti-prothrombin (aPT) antibodies in patients with Lupus Anticoagulant (LA). Thromb Res;126:150-153.
[96] Schousboe I, Rasmussen MS. Synchronized inhibition of the phospholipid mediated autoactivation of factor XII in plasma by beta 2-glycoprotein I and anti-beta 2-glycoprotein I. Thromb Haemost. 1995;73:798-804.
[97] Takeuchi R, Atsumi T, Ieko M, Amasaki Y, Ichikawa K, Koike T. Suppressed intrinsic fibrinolytic activity by monoclonal anti-beta-2 glycoprotein I autoantibodies: possible mechanism for thrombosis in patients with antiphospholipid syndrome. Br J Haematol. 2002;119:781-788.
[98] Morrison C, Radmacher M, Mohammed N, et al. MYC amplification and polysomy 8 in chondrosarcoma: array comparative genomic hybridization, fluorescent in situ hybridization, and association with outcome. J Clin Oncol. 2005;23:9369-9376.
[99] Ames PR, Tommasino C, Iannaccone L, Brillante M, Cimino R, Brancaccio V. Coagulation activation and fibrinolytic imbalance in subjects with idiopathic antiphospholipid antibodies--a crucial role for acquired free protein S deficiency. Thromb Haemost. 1996;76:190-194.
[100] Ieko M, Ichikawa K, Atsumi T, et al. Effects of beta2-glycoprotein I and monoclonal anticardiolipin antibodies on extrinsic fibrinolysis. Semin Thromb Hemost. 2000;26:85-90.
[101] Shi T, Iverson GM, Qi JC, et al. Beta 2-Glycoprotein I binds factor XI and inhibits its activation by thrombin and factor XIIa: loss of inhibition by clipped beta 2-glycoprotein I. Proc Natl Acad Sci U S A. 2004;101:3939-3944.
[102] Shi T, Giannakopoulos B, Iverson GM, Cockerill KA, Linnik MD, Krilis SA. Domain V of beta2-glycoprotein I binds factor XI/XIa and is cleaved at Lys317-Thr318. J Biol Chem. 2005;280:907-912.
[103] Krone KA, Allen KL, McCrae KR. Impaired fibrinolysis in the antiphospholipid syndrome. Curr Rheumatol Rep;12:53-57.
[104] Atsumi T, Khamashta MA, Andujar C, et al. Elevated plasma lipoprotein(a) level and its association with impaired fibrinolysis in patients with antiphospholipid syndrome. J Rheumatol. 1998;25:69-73.
[105] Chen PP, Yang CD, Ede K, Wu CC, FitzGerald JD, Grossman JM. Some antiphospholipid antibodies bind to hemostasis and fibrinolysis proteases and promote thrombosis. Lupus. 2008;17:916-921.
[106] Cugno M, Cabibbe M, Galli M, et al. Antibodies to tissue-type plasminogen activator (tPA) in patients with antiphospholipid syndrome: evidence of interaction between

the antibodies and the catalytic domain of tPA in 2 patients. Blood. 2004;103:2121-2126.
[107] Yang CD, Hwang KK, Yan W, et al. Identification of anti-plasmin antibodies in the antiphospholipid syndrome that inhibit degradation of fibrin. J Immunol. 2004;172:5765-5773.
[108] Yasuda S, Atsumi T, Ieko M, et al. Nicked beta2-glycoprotein I: a marker of cerebral infarct and a novel role in the negative feedback pathway of extrinsic fibrinolysis. Blood. 2004;103:3766-3772.
[109] Horbach DA, van Oort E, Lisman T, Meijers JC, Derksen RH, de Groot PG. Beta2-glycoprotein I is proteolytically cleaved in vivo upon activation of fibrinolysis. Thromb Haemost. 1999;81:87-95.
[110] Bu C, Gao L, Xie W, et al. beta2-glycoprotein i is a cofactor for tissue plasminogen activator-mediated plasminogen activation. Arthritis Rheum. 2009;60:559-568.
[111] Brouwer JL, Bijl M, Veeger NJ, Kluin-Nelemans HC, van der Meer J. The contribution of inherited and acquired thrombophilic defects, alone or combined with antiphospholipid antibodies, to venous and arterial thromboembolism in patients with systemic lupus erythematosus. Blood. 2004;104:143-148.
[112] Liestol S, Sandset PM, Mowinckel MC, Wisloff F. Activated protein C resistance determined with a thrombin generation-based test is associated with thrombotic events in patients with lupus anticoagulants. J Thromb Haemost. 2007;5:2204-2210.
[113] Nojima J, Kuratsune H, Suehisa E, Iwatani Y, Kanakura Y. Acquired activated protein C resistance associated with IgG antibodies against beta2-glycoprotein I and prothrombin as a strong risk factor for venous thromboembolism. Clin Chem. 2005;51:545-552.
[114] Kassis J, Neville C, Rauch J, et al. Antiphospholipid antibodies and thrombosis: association with acquired activated protein C resistance in venous thrombosis and with hyperhomocysteinemia in arterial thrombosis. Thromb Haemost. 2004;92:1312-1319.
[115] Membre A, Wahl D, Latger-Cannard V, et al. The effect of platelet activation on the hypercoagulability induced by murine monoclonal antiphospholipid antibodies. Haematologica. 2008;93:566-573.
[116] de Laat B, Eckmann CM, van Schagen M, Meijer AB, Mertens K, van Mourik JA. Correlation between the potency of a beta2-glycoprotein I-dependent lupus anticoagulant and the level of resistance to activated protein C. Blood Coagul Fibrinolysis. 2008;19:757-764.
[117] Lin WS, Chen PC, Yang CD, et al. Some antiphospholipid antibodies recognize conformational epitopes shared by beta2-glycoprotein I and the homologous catalytic domains of several serine proteases. Arthritis Rheum. 2007;56:1638-1647.
[118] Dahlback HS, Brandal P, Meling TR, Gorunova L, Scheie D, Heim S. Genomic aberrations in 80 cases of primary glioblastoma multiforme: Pathogenetic heterogeneity and putative cytogenetic pathways. Genes Chromosomes Cancer. 2009;48:908-924.
[119] Brachvogel B, Dikschas J, Moch H, et al. Annexin A5 is not essential for skeletal development. Mol Cell Biol. 2003;23:2907-2913.
[120] Davis WD, Brey RL. Antiphospholipid antibodies and complement activation in patients with cerebral ischemia. Clin Exp Rheumatol. 1992;10:455-460.

[121] Holers VM, Girardi G, Mo L, et al. Complement C3 activation is required for antiphospholipid antibody-induced fetal loss. J Exp Med. 2002;195:211-220.

[122] Romay-Penabad Z, Liu XX, Montiel-Manzano G, Papalardo De Martinez E, Pierangeli SS. C5a receptor-deficient mice are protected from thrombophilia and endothelial cell activation induced by some antiphospholipid antibodies. Ann N Y Acad Sci. 2007;1108:554-566.

[123] Rauch J, Dieude M, Subang R, Levine JS. The dual role of innate immunity in the antiphospholipid syndrome. Lupus;19:347-353.

[124] Giannakopoulos B, Mirarabshahi P, Krilis SA. New insights into the biology and pathobiology of beta2-glycoprotein I. Curr Rheumatol Rep;13:90-95.

[125] Agar C, van Os GM, Morgelin M, et al. Beta2-glycoprotein I can exist in 2 conformations: implications for our understanding of the antiphospholipid syndrome. Blood;116:1336-1343.

[126] Ioannou Y, Zhang JY, Qi M, et al. Novel assays of thrombogenic pathogenicity for the antiphospholipid syndrome based on the detection of molecular oxidative modification of the major autoantigen ss2-glycoprotein I. Arthritis Rheum.

[127] Pierangeli SS, Chen PP, Raschi E, et al. Antiphospholipid antibodies and the antiphospholipid syndrome: pathogenic mechanisms. Semin Thromb Hemost. 2008;34:236-250.

[128] Meroni PL, Borghi MO, Raschi E, Tedesco F. Pathogenesis of antiphospholipid syndrome: understanding the antibodies. Nat Rev Rheumatol;7:330-339.

[129] Greinacher A. Heparin-induced thrombocytopenia. J Thromb Haemost. 2009;7 Suppl 1:9-12.

[130] Rauova L, Zhai L, Kowalska MA, Arepally GM, Cines DB, Poncz M. Role of platelet surface PF4 antigenic complexes in heparin-induced thrombocytopenia pathogenesis: diagnostic and therapeutic implications. Blood. 2006;107:2346-2353.

11

Adverse Pregnancy Outcome in Antiphospholipid Antibodies Syndrome: Pathogenic Mechanisms and Clinical Management

Nicoletta Di Simone and Chiara Tersigni
Department of Obstetrics and Gynaecology, Catholic University of Sacred Heart, Rome Italy

1. Introduction

The term antiphospholipid antibodies syndrome (APS) defines an autoantibody induced thrombophilia, associated to recurrent thrombosis and pregnancy complications (Hughes, 1993). Diagnosis of APS requires both serological positivity for antiphospholipid antibodies (aPL), a heterogeneous family of autoantibodies directed against protein phospholipid complexes, and the onset of the diagnostic clinical manifestations (see more below). Indeed, it has been widely shown that aPL are not sufficient *per se* to determine clinical manifestations of APS and that the likelihood that aPL may contribute to the pathogenesis of thrombosis or pregnancy complications, or both, varies between clinical settings (Meroni et al., 2004).

To better define this complex syndrome, it must clarify that APS is commonly distinguished between "primary APS", not associated to other autoimmune diseases, and "secondary APS", when aPL serological positivity and clinical features of APS occur in the context of a known autoimmune disease. The majority of patients with secondary APS are affected from Systemic Lupus Erythematosus (SLE) and develop aPL serological positivity. About 40% of patients with SLE have aPL positivity (Mok et al., 2005) but less than 40% of them will eventually have thrombotic events (Ruiz-Irastorza et al., 2004; Tektonidou et al., 2009). Actually, it is still unknown if APS and SLE are two manifestations of the same disease or if underlying SLE could favour the development of APS (Miyakis et al., 2006). Accordingly, distinction between primary or secondary APS it is not so easy and have to be made carefully (Miyakis et al., 2006).

2. Clinical manifestations of APS

2.1 Systemic features

Venous thrombosis, or embolism, are the most frequent manifestations of APS and might occur in any vascular vessel while, in congenital thrombophilias, mostly involve venous bed (Cervera, 2002). Among the arterial vessels, the central nervous system is the district most often affected, usually in the form of stroke or transient ischaemic attack (Cervera et al., 2002). aPL have also been associated with venous sinus thrombosis, myelopathy, chorea, migraine, and epilepsy (Sanna et al., 2003). Furthermore, in patients with SLE an association between serum anticardiolipin antibodies and cognitive impairment has been found (Hanly et al., 1999; Menon et al., 1999) as well as a mild cognitive dysfunction in more than 40% of patients with APS (Tektonidou et al., 2006).

Cardiovascular features of APS include valvular disease, coronary artery disease, intracardiac thrombus formation, pulmonary hypertension and dilated cardiomyopathy (Koniari et al., 2010). Cardiac valvular pathology commonly affects the mitral valve, followed by the aortic and tricuspid ones, determining irregular thickening of the valve leaflets due to deposition of immune complexes that may lead to vegetations and valve dysfunction. These lesions are almost frequent and may be a significant risk factor for stroke (Khamashta et al., 1990; Koniari et al., 2010).

Renal manifestations of APS generally took place as hypertension with proteinuria and renal insufficiency (Amigo et al., 1992; Tektonidou et al., 2004) with the most frequent renal histopathological features associated being thrombotic microangiopathy or, less often, fibrous intimal hyperplasia, focal cortical atrophy and arterial occlusions (Tektonidou et al., 2004).

Other clinical features associated to APS are haematological alterations, like thrombocytopenia and haemolytic anaemia, skin ulcers, avascular bone necrosis and also the endocrinologic manifestation of adrenal insufficiency (Cervera et al., 2002). Livedo reticularis, found in about a quarter of patients with APS, represents a physical sign that often suggests to the clinician the right diagnosis and, among patients with APS, it also identifies those at a higher risk for arterial thrombosis (Ruiz-Irastorza et al., 2010; Francès et al., 2005).

2.2 Adverse pregnancy outcomes associated to APS

Beyond thromboses, obstetric complications are the other main features of APS. Such association is confirmed by several epidemiological studies and experimental models showing that passive transfer of aPL IgG induces foetal loss and growth retardation in pregnant naive mice, giving the proof that aPL are involved in determining the clinical manifestations of the syndrome (Meroni et al., 2010).

The most common adverse pregnancy outcome associated to APS is recurrent miscarriage, defined as three or more unexplained consecutive miscarriages before the 10th week of gestation. Other obstetric features of APS are unexplained foetal deaths, occurring at or beyond the 10th week of gestation, and premature births of a morphologically healthy newborn baby before the 34th week of gestation because of eclampsia or severe pre-eclampsia (Miyakis et al., 2006).

Recurrent miscarriage occurs in about 1% of the general population attempting to have children (Stirrat, 1990) and about 10-15% of women with recurrent miscarriage are diagnosed with APS (Rai et al., 1995; Yetman & Kutteh, 1996). Foetal death in the second or third trimesters of pregnancy occurs in up to 5% of unselected pregnancies (Silver , 2007) but it is less likely as pregnancy advances (Smith et al., 2004). Although foetal death occurs significantly most often in APS (Oshiro et al., 1996), the overall contribution to the pathogenesis of this syndrome is unknown, because of the effect of other possible contributing factors such as underlying hypertension or pre-existing comorbidities, like SLE or renal diseases.

Pregnant women with diagnosis of APS are at increased risk for developing preeclampsia or placental insufficiency, but it is still unknown the precise relationship between aPL and the occurrence of such clinical manifestations (Clark et al., 2007). Furthermore, aPL seem to be detectable in 11 - 29% of women with preeclampsia, compared with 7% or less in controls and in 25% of women delivering growth restricted foetuses (Clark et al., 2007). Finally, results from prospective cohort studies indicate that of pregnant women with high concentrations of aPL, 10 - 50% develop preeclampsia, and more than 10% of these women deliver infants who are small for gestational age (Clark et al., 2007).

3. Diagnostic criteria

According to the last International consensus statement for APS diagnostic criteria, in order to make diagnosis of the syndrome the combination of at least one clinical and one laboratory criterion is required (Miyakis et al., 2006) (Table 1).

Clinical criteria	Laboratory criteria
Vascular thrombosis • One or more clinical episodes of arterial, venous, or small vessel thrombosis, in any tissue or organ. • Thrombosis should be supported by objective validated criteria—ie, unequivocal findings of appropriate imaging studies or histopathology. For histopathological support, thrombosis should be present without substantial evidence of inflammation in the vessel wall. **Pregnancy morbidity, defined by one of the following criteria:** • One or more unexplained deaths of a morphologically healthy foetus at or beyond the 10th week of gestation, with healthy foetal morphology documented by ultrasound or by direct examination of the fetus. • One or more premature births of a morphologically healthy newborn baby before the 34th week of gestation because of: eclampsia or severe preeclampsia defined according to standard definitions or recognized features of placental failure. • Three or more unexplained consecutive spontaneous abortions before the 10th week of gestation, with maternal anatomical or hormonal abnormalities and paternal and maternal chromosomal causes excluded. In studies of populations of patients who have more than one type of pregnancy morbidity, investigators are strongly encouraged to stratify groups of patients according to one of the three criteria.	• Lupus anticoagulant present in plasma, on two or more occasions at least 12 weeks apart, detected according to the guidelines of the International Society on Thrombosis and Hemostasis (Scientific Subcommittee on lupus anticoagulant/ phospholipid- dependent antibodies). • Anticardiolipin antibody of IgG or IgM isotype, or both, in serum or plasma, present in medium or high titres (ie, >40 GPL or MPL, or greater than the 99th percentile) on two or more occasions, at least 12 weeks apart, measured by a standardized ELISA. • Anti-β2-gycoprotein 1 antibody of IgG or IgM isotype, or both, in serum or plasma (in titres greater than the 99th percentile), present on two or more occasions, at least 12 weeks apart, measured by a standardized ELISA, according to recommended procedures.

Table 1. Revised diagnostic criteria of APS (Miyakis et al., 2006).

4. Pathogenetic mechanisms mediated by aPL

4.1 Vascular thrombosis

The molecular mechanisms underlying thrombosis and foetal death in APS have long been investigated. The main target antigens reported in patients with APS include beta-2-glycoprotein-1 (β2GPI), prothrombin and annexin V (Galli et al., 2003). Other putative antigens are thrombin, protein C, protein S, thrombomodulin, tissue plasminogen activator, kininogens (high or low molecular), prekallikrein, factor VII/VIIa, factor XI, factor XII, complement component C4, heparan sulfate proteoglycan, heparin, oxidised low-density lipoproteins (Galli et al., 2003; Rand et al., 2010). The main autoantigens are attracted to negatively charged phospholipids exposed on the outer side of cell membranes in great amounts only under special circumstances such as damage or apoptosis (e.g. endothelial cell) or after activation (e.g. platelets) (Galli et al., 2003).
Endothelial cells, activated by aPL with anti-β2GPI activity, express adhesion molecules such as intercellular cell adhesion molecule-1, vascular cell adhesion molecule-1, E-selectin, and both endothelial cells and monocytes upregulate the production of tissue factor (TF) (Pierangeli et al., 2008). All at once, activated platelets increase expression of glycoprotein IIb-IIIa and synthesis of thromboxane A2, determining a procoagulant state (Figure 1). (Pierangeli et al., 2006; Pierangeli et al., 2008; Lopez-Pedrera et al., 2008; Montiel-Manzano et al., 2007; Vega-Ostertag et al., 2005). Additional mechanisms promoting clot formation could be represented by interaction of aPL with proteins implicated in clotting regulation; such as annexin A5, prothrombin, factor X, protein C and plasmin (de Groot & Derksen, 2005; Pierangeli et al., 2008; Rand et al., 2010).

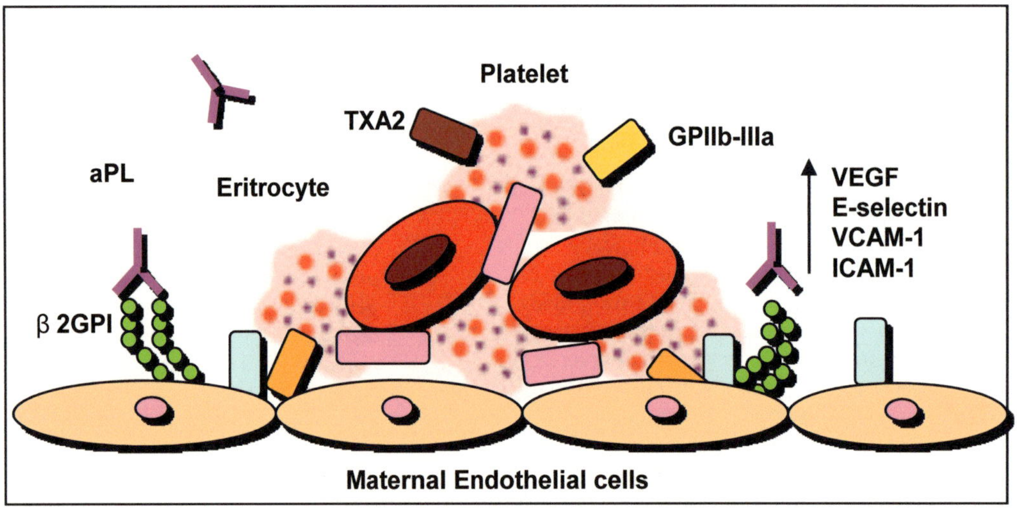

Fig. 1. aPL-mediated mechanism of trombosis.
aPL are able to activate endothelial cells and platelets leading to a procoagulant state (first hit). The occurrence of a second hit, like inflammation, can lead to clot formation.

Recent results from studies in mice highlight the role of inflammation in the pathogenesis of APS, showing a central role for complement activation in thrombosis and foetal loss induced by aPL (Pierangeli et al., 2005; Girardi et al., 2004). Because many individuals with high aPL antibody titers remain asymptomatic, a second hit hypothesis have been proposed. It is likely that in the aPL-induced vascular procoagulant state, activation of the complement cascade might close the loop and provoke thrombosis, often in the presence of a second hit, like tobacco, inflammation, or oestrogens (Meroni et al., 2004; de Groot & Derksen, 2005; Ruiz-Irastorza et al., 2010).

4.2 Placental thrombosis

Based on the knowledge of the process of intravascular aPL-mediate clot formation (Figure 1), initially intraplacental thrombosis was considered the main pathogenic mechanism mediating foetal loss in APS. This hypothesis of placental damage was supported by the finding of thrombosis and infarction in placentas from women with APS and by the demonstration of aPL capability to induce a procoagulant state *in vitro* through several mechanisms including the ability of the aPL antibodies (specifically, anti-β2GPI antibodies) to disrupt the anticoagulant annexin A5 shield on trophoblast and endothelial cell monolayers (Peaceman & Rehnberg, 1993; Nayar & Lage, 1996; Rand et al., 2010). Supporting the *in vitro* findings, a significantly lower distribution of annexin A5 covering the intervillous surfaces was found in the placentas of aPL-positive women in comparison with normal controls (Rand et al., 1994). Nevertheless, thrombotic events cannot account for all of the histopathologic findings in placentae from women with APS and other mechanisms of reproductive impairment are likely to be involved (Out et al., 1991; Park, 2006).

4.3 Defective placentation

4.3.1 Trophoblast invasiveness impairment

New aPL-mediated pathogenic mechanisms have been proposed during the last ten years: anti-β2GPI antibodies seem to bind directly the maternal decidua and the invading trophoblast, determining defective placentation.

On the foetal side, β2GPI has been shown to be expressed on trophoblast cell membranes, explaining the placental tropism of anti-β2GPI antibodies. Being a cationic plasma protein, β2GPI has been suggested to bind to exposed phosphatidylserine on the external cell membranes of trophoblasts undergoing syncitium formation (Meroni et al., 2010).

β2GPI-dependent antibodies can adhere to human trophoblast cells *in vitro* (Di Simone et al., 2000), consistently with the hypothesis that the visibility of anionic PLs on the external cell surface during intertrophoblastic fusion might offer a useful substrate for the cation PL-binding site (Katsuragawa et al., 1997; Rote et al., 1998). The binding to anionic structures induces the expression of new cryptic epitopes and/or increases the antigenic density, two events that are apparently pivotal for the antibody binding (Wang S.X. et al., 2000). *In vitro* studies with both murine and human monoclonal antibodies as well as with polyclonal IgG antibodies from APS patients have clearly demonstrated a binding to trophoblast monolayers (Lyden et al., 1992; Di Simone et al., 2000). Interestingly, once bound antibodies obtained from patients with APS can affect the trophoblast functions *in vitro*, inducing cell injury and apoptosis, inhibition of proliferation and syncitia formation, decreased production of human chorionic gonadotrophin, defective secretion of growth factors and impaired invasiveness (Figure 2) (Di Simone et al., 2000). β2GPI-dependent aPL seem, therefore, to represent the main pathogenic autoantibodies in obstetrical APS. Accordingly, it has been hypothesized that most of these potentially pathogenic autoantibodies should be absorbed at the placental level, where β2GPI is expressed, and should not be transferred to the fetus.

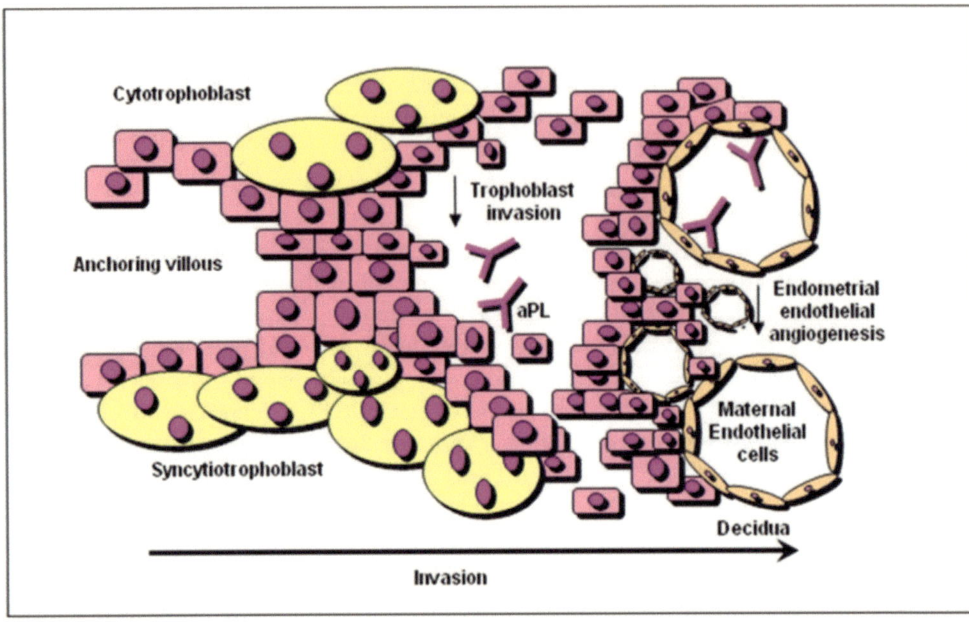

Fig. 2. aPL-mediated inhibition of trophoblast invasiveness and endometrial angiogenesis. Placental development has been proposed to be impaired by aPL direct binding to trophoblast cells, reducing its invasiveness and inhibiting cell proliferation, syncitia formation, secretion of human chorionic gonadotrophin and growth factors. Furthermore, aPL have also been suggested to inhibit maternal decidual angiogenesis, providing an additional mechanism able to explain placental failure associated to APS.

Recent findings have underlined a further mechanism by which aPL binding to human trophoblast could affect its functions: the aPL-mediated reduction of placental Heparin-Binding Epidermal Growth Factor–like growth factor (HB-EGF) expression. HB-EGF is a member of the EGF family (Raab & Klagsbrun, 1997; Iwamoto & Mekada, 2000). It has been shown to induce an invasive trophoblast phenotype in human and mouse blastocysts (Martin et al., 1998; Wang J., 2000) and to initiate molecular and cellular changes characteristic of decidualization in mice (Paria et al., 2001). HB-EGF is expressed in the human placenta during the first trimester, primarily within the villous trophoblast, but also in the extravillous cytotrophoblast, predominantly at the sites of cytotrophoblast extravillous invasion (Leach et al., 1999). Women with preeclampsia and infants small for gestational age display decreased placental expression of HB-EGF (Leach et al., 2002), strongly suggesting an association between HB-EGF down-regulation, poor trophoblast invasion, and failed physiologic transformation of the spiral arteries occurring in these disorders.

Interestingly, also in placental tissue obtained from women with APS, reduced expression of HB-EGF has been found (Di Simone et al., 2010a). Furthermore, polyclonal and monoclonal aPL have been shown to bind trophoblast monolayers *in vitro* significantly reducing the synthesis and the secretion of HB-EGF (Di Simone et al., 2010a). The ability of exogenous recombinant HB-EGF to reduce the aPL mediated effects on trophoblast cells supports the hypothesis of a key pathogenic role of this molecule in mediating APS-related adverse pregnancy outcomes. The experimental conditions did not involve complement activation, indicating that aPL may also affect placental tissue through direct, complement-independent effects, as previously suggested (Pierangeli et al., 2008).

4.3.2 Endometrial angiogenesis inhibition

On the maternal side, endometrial endothelial angiogenesis inhibition has been suggested to be an additional aPL-mediated mechanism of placental damage (Figure 2). aPL seem to selectively bind *in vitro* to endothelial cells isolated from human endometrium (HEEC) and to inhibit endothelial cell differentiation into capillary-like tubular structures, by reducing MMP-2 activity and VEGF secretion, via a suppression of NFKB DNA binding activity. Such an aPL-mediated inhibition of angiogenesis has also been confirmed *in vivo* in murine models showing a reduced angiogenesis in subcutaneous implanted angioreactors in aPL-inoculated mice (Di Simone et al., 2010b). Since it is well known that endometrial angiogenesis and decidualization, as well as trophoblast invasion, are fundamental prerequisites for successful implantation and the beginning of pregnancy, aPL-inhibition of such a central process in human placental development provides an important additional mechanism able to explain the association between APS and pregnancy complications associated to placental failure, like miscarriage, foetal growth restriction and preeclampsia.

4.4 Inflammation

It is widely accepted that a physiological pregnancy development requires a fine regulation of the maternal immune response during embryo implantation. Acute inflammatory events are recognized causes of a negative pregnancy outcome, and proinflammatory mediators, such as complement, tumor necrosis factor (TNF), and CC chemokines, have been shown to play a role in animal models of aPL-induced foetal loss (Chaouat, 2007). Intraperitoneal injections of large amounts of human IgG with aPL activity to pregnant naive mice after embryo implantation induce considerable placental inflammatory damage that results in foetal loss and growth retardation. An inflammation-mediated aPL damage has also been demonstrated by immunohistochemical and histological examination of murine deciduas, showing deposition of human IgG and mouse complement, neutrophil infiltration and local TNF secretion, in association with a transient but significant increase in blood TNF levels (Holers et al., 2002; Girardi et al., 2003; Berman et al., 2005). Furthermore, it has been demonstrated that in response to aPL-generated C5a, neutrophils express TF potentiating inflammation in the deciduas and leading to miscarriages in mice (Figure 3). Importantly, TF in myeloid cells, but not trophoblasts, seem to be associated with foetal injury, suggesting that the site for pathologic TF expression is neutrophils (Redecha et al., 2007). The pathogenic mechanism of complement-mediated foetal loss induced by aPL is also supported by the protection that deficiency in complement components confers on the animals, or that follows from *in vivo* inhibition of complement (Thurman et al., 2005; Girardi et al., 2006).

In another experimental model of foetal loss, mice deficient in chemokine-binding protein D6, a placental receptor that recognizes the majority of inflammatory CC chemokines and targets them for degradation, were more susceptible to foetal loss when passively infused with a small amount of human aPL IgG than wild-type mice or mice infused with normal IgG (Martinez de la Torre et al., 2007). Altogether, these findings suggest that a local acute inflammatory response might have a role in experimental aPL-mediated foetal loss.

Although C4d and C3b fragments have been shown to be deposited in the placentas of patients with APS, analysis of abortive material or full-term placentae from women with APS has not provided conclusive information about the pathogenic contributions of acute local inflammatory events and complement deposition (Park, 2006; Shamonki et al., 2007). In order to confirm this hypothesis more studies on human placentas are required.

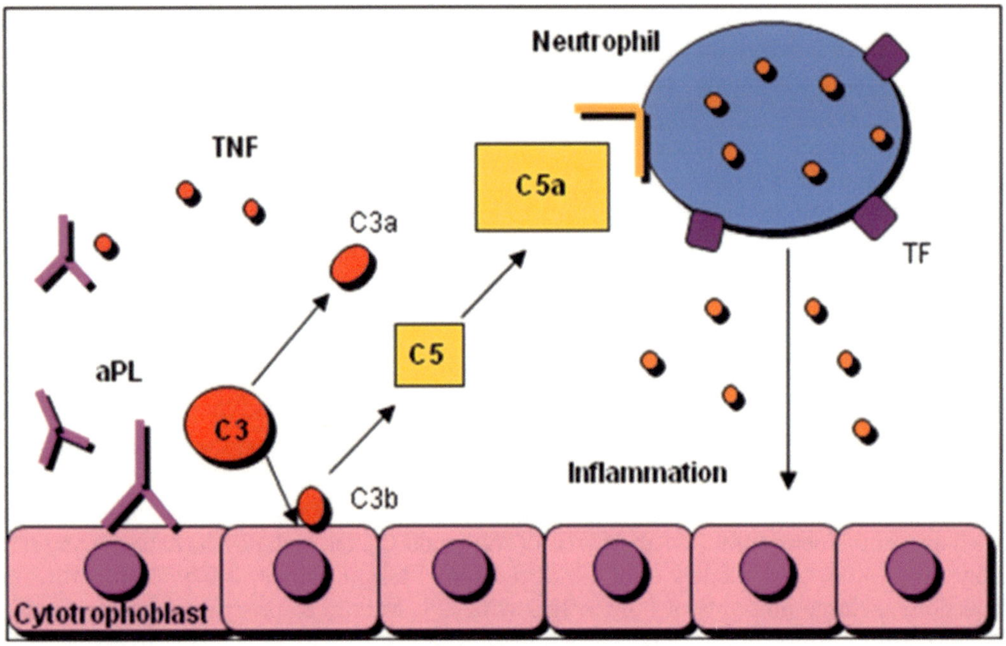

Fig. 3. aPL-mediated activation of complement system and foetal loss.
Endothelial cells, activated by aPL, express adhesion molecules and activated platelets increase expression of glycoprotein IIb-IIIa and synthesis of thromboxane A2, determining a procoagulant state (first hit). The occurrence of a second hit, like inflammation, can lead to clot formation.

5. Pregnancy management

Women with APS should be carefully managed by the physician during pregnancy. A clinical manifestations of APS associated to a high risk for maternal health in pregnancy is severe pulmonary hypertension, representing a contraindication to pregnancy. Furthermore, women with APS should be suggested to delay pregnancy when uncontrolled increase of blood pressure or recent thrombotic events have occurred (Ruiz-Irastorza et al., 2008, 2010).

More than 70% of pregnant women with APS properly managed will have a good pregnancy outcome (Bramhan et al., 2010). However, a complete profile of aPL should be performed before planning of pregnancy. These tests do not need to be repeated during pregnancy, since subsequent negative results after diagnosis do not eliminate the risk of complications (Ruiz-Irastorzaet al., 2008, 2010). Frequent prenatal visits and obstetric ultrasound, every 2-4 weeks, should be done in order to early detect pregnancy complications like maternal hypertension, proteinuria and other features of preeclampsia, placental insufficiency, foetal loss, foetal growth restriction and the need for iatrogenic preterm birth (Branch & Khamashta, 2003). Surveillance testing should begin at 32 weeks' gestation, or earlier if placental insufficiency is suspected, and should continue at least every week until delivery. Uterine and umbilical artery Doppler assessments are used for the high risk for preeclampsia, placental insufficiency, and foetal growth restriction after the 24th week of gestation in this category of patients and normal examinations have high negative predictive values (Le Thi Huong et al., 2006).

Nowadays, despite the controversies raised by clinical trials (Kutteh, 1996; Rai et al., 1997; Farquharson et al., 2002; Laskin et al., 2009; Noble et al., 2005; Stephenson et al., 2004), the gold standard treatment of patients with APS and history of recurrent early miscarriage is a combination of either low-dose heparin or low-molecular weight heparin and low-dose aspirin (Empson et al., 2005, Bates et al., 2008). Best pregnancy outcomes are achieved with heparin started in the early first trimester when a live embryo is detectable by ultrasound. For pregnant women with APS who have had a previous thrombotic event, low-dose aspirin and therapeutic dose heparin or low-molecular weight heparin anticoagulation are recommended (Bates et al., 2008).

Results from randomised trials do not define optimum treatment for women with foetal death (>10 weeks'gestation) or previous early delivery (<34 weeks'gestation) due to severe preeclampsia or placental insufficiency. Most experts recommend low-dose aspirin and either prophylactic or intermediate-dose heparin (Branch & Khamashta, 2003; Empson et al., 2005; Bates et al., 2008).

Use of glucocorticoids to treat pregnant women with APS have been shown to be less effective than heparin plus aspirin (Silver et al., 1993; Cowchock et al., 1992) as well as administration of intravenous immunoglobulins, either when added to heparin or used alone, do not ameliorate pregnancy outcome. However, intravenous immunoglobulins treatment should be considered whether classic treatment with aspirin plus heparin is not effective (Triolo et al., 2003; Branch et al., 2000; Vaquero et al., 2001), although it has been associated to an increased risk of pregnancy loss or premature birth, compared with heparin and low-dose aspirin (Empson et al., 2005).

Vitamin K antagonists (warfarin) are the gold standard treatment of APS clinically manifested with thromboses but, because of teratogenic risk, should be avoided between 6 and 12 weeks' of gestation. To avoid risk of foetal bleeding, warfarin after 12 weeks' gestation should be given only in exceptional circumstances (Bates et al., 2008; Østensen et al., 2004). Furthermore, women with APS should be treated with antithrombotic drug also during the post-partum period (Bates et al., 2008). Women with history of thrombosis need long-term anticoagulation, and it would be better to switch the treatment to warfarin, as soon as possible after delivery. In patients with no previous thrombosis, prophylactic dose heparin or low-molecular-weight heparin therapy for 6 weeks after delivery are recommended (Bates et al., 2008). Finally, both heparin and warfarin are safe for breastfeeding mothers (Østensen et al., 2004).

6. Conclusions

Although modern management and treatment of APS in pregnancy significantly ameliorate pregnancy outcome, more efforts are needed in order to unravel aPL-mediated pathogenic mechanisms still not understood and to open new perspective of therapies of this complex and multifactorial syndrome.

7. References

Amigo M.C., Garcia-Torres R., Robles M., Bochicchio T. & Reyes P.A. (1992). Renal involvement in primary antiphospholipid syndrome. *J Rheumatol,* Vol. 19, No. 8, (Aug 1992), pp. 1181-1185.

Bates S.M., Greer I.A., Pabinger I., Sofaer S. & Hirsh J; American College of Chest Physicians. (2008). Venous thromboembolism, thrombophilia, antithrombotic therapy, and pregnancy: American College of Chest Physicians Evidence-Based Clinical Practice Guidelines (8th edn). *Chest,* Vol. 133, No. 6 (Jun 2008), pp. 844 - 886.

Berman J., Girardi G. & Salmon J.E. (2005). TNF-α is a critical effector and a target for therapy in antiphospholipid antibody-induced pregnancy loss. *J Immunol,* Vol. 174, No. 1, (Jan 2005), pp. 485–490.

Bramham K., Hunt B.J., Germain S., Calatayud I., Khamashta M., Bewley S. & Nelson-Piercy C. (2010). Pregnancy outcome in different clinical phenotypes of antiphospholipid syndrome. *Lupus,* Vol. 19, No. 1, (Jan 2010), pp. 58 - 64.

Branch D.W., Peaceman A.M., Druzin M., Silver RK, El-Sayed Y., Silver R.M., Esplin M.S., Spinnato J. & Harger J. (2000). Peaceman AM, Druzin M, et al. A multicenter, placebo-controlled pilot study of intravenous immune globulin treatment of antiphospholipid syndrome during pregnancy. *Am J Obstet Gynecol,* Vol. 182, No. 1, (Jan 2000), pp. 122-127.

Branch D.W. & Khamashta M.A. (2003). Antiphospholipid syndrome: Obstetric diagnosis, management and controversies. Obstet Gynecol, Vol. 101, No. 6, (Jun 2003), pp. 1333-1344.

Cervera R., Piette J.C., Font J., Khamashta M.A., Shoenfeld Y., Camps M.T., Jacobsen S., Lakos G., Tincani A., Kontopoulou-Griva I., Galeazzi M., Meroni P.L., Derksen R.H., de Groot P.G., Gromnica-Ihle E., Baleva M., Mosca M., Bombardieri S., Houssiau F., Gris J.C, Quéré I., Hachulla E., Vasconcelos C., Roch B., Fernández-Nebro A., Boffa M.C., Hughes G.R. & Ingelmo M. Euro-Phospholipid Project Group. (2002). Antiphospholipid syndrome: clinical and immunologic manifestations and patterns of disease expression in a cohort of 1,000 patients. *Arthritis Rheum,* Vol. 46, No.4, (Apr 2002), pp. 1019-1027.

Chaouat G. (2007). The Th1/Th2 paradigm: still important in pregnancy? *Semin Immunopathol* Vol. 29, No. 2, (Jun 2007), pp. 95–113.

Clark E.A., Silver R.M. & Branch D.W. (2007). Do antiphospholipid antibodies cause preeclampsia and HELLP syndrome? *Curr Rheumatol Rep,* Vol. 9, No. 3, (Jun 2007), pp. 219-225.

Cowchock F.S., Reece E.A., Balaban D., Branch D.W. & Plouffe L. (1992). Repeated foetal losses associated with antiphospholipid antibodies: a collaborative randomized trial comparing prednisone with low-dose heparin. *Am J Obstet Gynecol,* Vol. 166, No. 5, (May 1992), pp. 1318-1323.

de Groot P.G. & Derksen R.H. Pathophysiology of the antiphospholipid syndrome. *J Thromb Haemost,* Vol. 3, No. 8, (Aug 2005), pp. 1854-1860.

Di Simone N., Meroni P.L., de Papa N., Raschi E., Caliandro D., De Carolis C.S., Khamashta M.A., Atsumi T., Hughes G.R., Balestrieri G., Tincani A., Casali P. & Caruso A. (2000). Antiphospholipid antibodies affect trophoblast gonadotropin secretion and invasiveness by binding directly and through adhered beta2-glycoprotein I. *Arthritis Rheum,* Vol. 43, No. 1, (Jan 2000), pp. 140-150.

Di Simone N., Marana R., Castellani R., Di Nicuolo F., D'Alessio M.C., Raschi E., Borghi M.O., Chen P.P., Sanguinetti M., Caruso A. & Meroni P.L. (2010a). Decreased expression of heparin-binding epidermal growth factor-like growth factor as a newly identified pathogenic mechanism of antiphospholipid-mediated defective placentation. *Arthritis Rheum,* Vol. 62, No. 5, (May 2010), pp. 1504-1512.

Di Simone N., Di Nicuolo F., D'Ippolito S., Castellani R., Tersigni C., Caruso A., Meroni P. & Marana R. (2010b). Antiphospholipid antibodies affect human endometrial angiogenesis. *Biol Reprod,* Vol. 83, No. 2, (Aug 2010), pp. 212-219.

Empson M., Lassere M., Craig J. & Scott J. (2005). Prevention of recurrent miscarriage for women with antiphospholipid antibody or lupus anticoagulant. *Cochrane Database Syst Rev,* Vol. 18, No. 2, (Apr 2005), CD002859.

Farquharson R.G., Quenby S. & Greaves M. (2002). Antiphospholipid syndrome in pregnancy: a randomized, controlled trial of treatment. *Obstet Gynecol,* Vol. 100, No. (2002), pp. 408 - 413.

Francès C., Niang S., Laffitte E., Pelletier F., Costedoat N. & Piette J.C. (2005). Dermatologic manifestations of the antiphospholipid syndrome: two hundred consecutive cases. *Arthritis Rheum,* Vol. 52, No. 6, (Jun 2005), pp. 1785-93.

Galli M., Luciani D., Bertolini G. & Barbui T. (2003). Anti-beta 2-glycoprotein I, antiprothrombin antibodies, and the risk of thrombosis in the antiphospholipid syndrome. *Blood,* 2003, Vol. 102, No. 8, (Oct 2003), pp. 2717-2723.

Girardi G., Berman J., Redecha P., Spruce L., Thurman J.M., Kraus D., Hollmann T.J., Casali P., Caroll M.C., Wetsel R.A., Lambris J.D., Holers V.M. & Salmon JE. (2003). Complement C5a receptors and neutrophils mediate foetal injury in the antiphospholipid syndrome. *J Clin Invest,* Vol. 112, No. 11, (Dec 2003), pp. 1644-1654.

Girardi G., Redecha P. & Salmon J.E. (2004). Heparin prevents antiphospholipid antibody-induced foetal loss by inhibiting complement activation. *Nat Med,* Vol. 10, No.11, (Nov 2004), pp. 1222-1226.

Girardi G., Yarilin D., Thurman J.M., Holers V.M. & Salmon J.E. (2006). Complement activation induces dysregulation of angiogenic factors and causes foetal rejection and growth restriction. *J Exp Med,* Vol. 203, No. 9, (Sep 2006), pp. 2165-2175.

Hanly J.G., Hong C., Smith S. & Fisk J.D. (1999). A prospective analysis of cognitive function and anticardiolipin antibodies in systemic lupus erythematosus. *Arthritis Rheum,* Vol. 42, No.4, (Apr 1999), pp. 728-734.

Holers V.M., Girardi G., Mo L., Guthridge J.M., Molina H., Pierangeli S.S., Espinola R., Xiaowei L.E., Mao D., Vialpando C.G. & Salmon J.E. (2002). Complement C3 activation is required for antiphospholipid antibody-induced foetal loss. *J Exp Med,* Vol. 195, No. 2, (Jan 2002), pp. 211-220.

Hughes, G.R.V. (1993) The antiphospholipid syndrome: ten years on. Lancet, Vol. 7, No. 342, (Aug 1993), pp. 341 - 344.

Iwamoto R. & Mekada E. (2000). Heparin-binding EGF-like growth factor: a juxtacrine growth factor. *Cytokine Growth Factor Rev,* Vol. 11, No. 4, (Dec 2000), pp. 335-344.

Katsuragawa H., Kanzaki H., Inoue T., Hirano T., Mori T. & Rote N.S. (1997). Monoclonal antibody against phosphatidylserine inhibits in vitro human trophoblastic hormone production and invasion. *Biol Reprod,* Vol. 56, No. 1, (Jan 1997), pp. 50–58.

Khamashta M.A., Cervera R., Asherson R.A., Font J., Gil A., Coltart D.J., Vázquez J.J., Paré C., Ingelmo M. & Oliver J. (1990). Association of antibodies against phospholipids with heart valve disease in systemic lupus erythematosus. *Lancet,* Vol. 335, No. , (1990), pp. 1541-1544.

Koniari I., Siminelakis S.N., Baikoussis N.G., Papadopoulos G., Goudevenos J. & Apostolakis E. (2010). Antiphospholipid syndrome; its implication in cardiovascular diseases: a review. *J Cardiothorac Surg,* Vol. 5, No. 101 (Nov 2010), pp. 1-10.

Kutteh W.H. (1996). Antiphospholipid antibody-associated recurrent pregnancy loss: treatment with heparin and low-dose aspirin is superior to low-dose aspirin alone. *Am J Obstet Gynecol,* Vol. 174, No. (1996), pp. 1584 - 1589.

Laskin C.A., Spitzer K.A., Clark C.A., Crowther M.R., Ginsberg J.S., Hawker G.A., Kingdom J.C., Barrett J. & Gent M. (2009). Low molecular weight heparin and aspirin for recurrent pregnancy loss: results from the randomized, controlled HepASA trial. *J Rheumatol,* Vol. 36, No. (May 2009), pp. 279 - 287.

Le Thi Huong D., Wechsler B., Vauthier-Brouzes D., Duhaut P., Costedoat N., Andreu M.R., Lefebvre G. & Piette J.C. (2006). The second trimester Doppler ultrasound examination is the best predictor of late pregnancy outcome in systemic lupus erythematosus and/or the antiphospholipid syndrome. *Rheumatology,* Vol. 45, No. 3, (Mar 2006), pp. 332-338.

Leach R.E., Khalifa R., Ramirez N.D., Das S.K., Wang J., Dey S.K., Romero R. & Armant D.R. (1999). Multiple roles for heparin-binding epidermal growth factor-like growth factor are suggested by its cell-specific expression during the human endometrial cycle and early placentation. *J Clin Endocrinol Metab,* Vol. 84, No. 9, (Sep 1999), pp. 3355–63.

Leach R.E., Romero R., Kim Y.M., Chaiworapongsa T., Kilburn B., Das S.K., Dey S.K., Johnson A., Qureshi F., Jacques S. & Armant D.R. (2002). Pre-eclampsia and expression of heparin-binding EGF-like growth factor. *Lancet* , Vol. 360, No. 9341, (Oct 2002), pp. 1215–1219.

Lyden T.W., Vogt E., Ng A.K., Johnson P.M. & Rote N.S. (1992). Monoclonal antiphospholipid antibody reactivity against human placental trophoblast. *J Reprod Immunol,* Vol. 22, No. 1, (Jun 1992), pp. 1-14.

Lopez-Pedrera C., Cuadrado M.J., Herández V., Buendïa P., Aguirre M.A., Barbarroja N., Torres L.A., Villalba J.M., Velasco F. & Khamashta M. (2008). Proteomic analysis in monocytes of antiphospholipid syndrome patients: Deregulation of proteins related to the development of thrombosis. Arthritis Rheum, Vol. 58, No. 9, (Sep 2008), pp. 2835 - 2844.

Martin K.L., Barlow D.H. & Sargent I.L. (1998). Heparin-binding epidermal growth factor significantly improves human blastocyst development and hatching in serum-free medium. *Hum Reprod,* Vol. 13, No. 6, (Jun 1998), pp. 1645-1652.

Martinez de la Torre Y., Buracchi C., Borroni E.M., Dupor J., Bonecchi R., Nebuloni M., Pasqualini F., Doni A., Lauri E., Agostinis C., Bulla R., Cook D.N., Haribabu B., Meroni P., Rukavina D., Vago L., Tedesco F., Vecchi A., Lira S.A., Locati M. &

Mantovani A. (2007). Protection against inflammation- and autoantibody-caused foetal loss by the chemokine decoy receptor D6. *Proc Natl Acad Sci*, Vol. 104, No. 7, (Feb 2007), pp. 2319–2324.

Menon S., Jameson-Shortall E., Newman S.P., Hall-Craggs M.R., Chinn R. & Isenberg D.A. (2005). A longitudinal study of anticardiolipin antibody levels and cognitive functioning in systemic lupus erythematosus. *Arthritis Rheum*, Vol. 42, No.4, (Apr 1999), pp. 735-741.

Meroni P.L., Borghi M.O., Raschi E., Ventura D., Sarzi Puttini P.C., Atzeni F., Lonati L., Parati G., Tincani A., Mari D. & Tedesco F. (2004). Inflammatory response and the endothelium. *Thromb Res*, Vol. 114, No.5-6, (2004), pp. 329-334.

Meroni P.L., Tedesco F., Locati M., Vecchi A., Di Simone N., Acaia B., Pierangeli S.S. & Borghi M.O. (2010). Anti-phospholipid antibody mediated foetal loss: still an open question from a pathogenic point of view. *Lupus*, Vol. 19, No.4, (Apr 2010), pp. 453-456.

Mok C.C., Tang S.S., To C.H. &, Petri M. (2005). Incidence and risk factors of thromboembolism in systemic lupus erythematosus: a comparison of three ethnic groups. *Arthritis Rheum*, Vol. 52, No.9, (Sep 2005), pp. 2774-2782.

Miyakis S., Lockshin M.D., Atsumi T., Branch D.W., Brey R.L., Cervera R., Derksen R.H., DE Groot P.G., Koike T., Meroni P.L., Reber G., Shoenfeld Y., Tincani A., Vlachoyiannopoulos P.G. & Krilis S.A. (2006). International consensus statement on an update of the classification criteria for definite antiphospholipid syndrome (APS). *J Thromb Haemost*, Vol. 4, No.2, (Feb 2006), pp. 295-306.

Montiel-Manzano G., Romay-Penabad Z., Papalardo de Martínez E., Meillon-García L.A., García-Latorre E., Reyes-Maldonado E. & Pierangeli S.S. (2007). In vivo effects of an inhibitor of nuclear factor-kappa B on thrombogenic properties of antiphospholipid antibodies. *Ann N Y Acad Sci*, No. 1108, (Jun 2007), pp. 540-553.

Nayar R. & Lage J.M. (1996). Placental changes in a first trimester missed abortion in maternal systemic lupus erythematosus with antiphospholipid syndrome; a case report and review of the literature. *Hum Pathol*, Vol. 27, No. 2, (Feb 1996), pp. 201–206.

Noble L.S., Kutteh W.H., Lashey N., Franklin R.D. & Herrada J. (2005). Antiphospholipid antibodies associated with recurrent pregnancy loss: prospective, multicenter, controlled pilot study comparing treatment with low-molecular weight heparin versus unfractionated heparin. *Fertil Steril*, Vol. 83, No. (2005), pp. 684 - 690.

Oshiro B.T., Silver R.M., Scott J.R., Yu H. & Branch D.W. (1996). Antiphospholipid antibodies and foetal death. *Obstet Gynecol*, Vol. 87, No. 4, Apr 1996), pp. 489 - 493.

Østensen M., Khamashta M., Lockshin M., Parke A., Brucato A., Carp H., Doria A., Rai R., Meroni P., Cetin I., Derksen R., Branch W., Motta M., Gordon C., Ruiz-Irastorza G., Spinillo A., Friedman D., Cimaz R., Czeizel A., Piette J.C., Cervera R., Levy R.A., Clementi M., De Carolis S., Petri M., Shoenfeld Y., Faden D., Valesini G. & Tincani A. (2006). Anti-inflamatory and immunosuppressive drugs and reproduction. *Arthritis Res Ther*, Vol. 8, No. 3 (May 2006), pp. 209 - 227.

Out H.J., Kooijman C.D., Bruinse H.W. & Derksen R.H. (1991). Histopathological finding from patient with intrauterine foetal death and antiphospholipid antibodies. *Eur J Obstet Gynecol*, Vol. 41, No. 3, (Oct 1991), pp. 179-186.

Park A.L. (2006). Placental pathology in antiphospholipid syndrome, In: *Hughes' Syndrome*, Khamashta M. A. pp. 362–374, Springer-Verlag, London.

Paria B.C., Ma W., Tan J., Raja S., Das S.K., Dey S.K. & Hogan B.L. (2001). Cellular and molecular responses of the uterus to embryo implantation can be elicited by locally applied growth factors. *Proc Natl Acad Sci U S A*, Vol. 98, No. 3, (Jan 2001), pp. 1047-1052.

Peaceman, A.M. & Rehnberg, K.A. (1993). The effect of immunoglobulin G fractions from patients with lupus anticoagulant on placental prostacyclin and thromboxane production. *Am J Obstet Gynecol*, Vol. 169, No. 6, (Dec 1993), pp. 1403–1406

Pierangeli S.S., Girardi G., Vega-Ostertag M., Liu X., Espinola R.G. & Salmon J. (2005). Requirement of activation of complement C3 and C5 for antiphospholipid antibody mediated thrombophilia. *Arthritis Rheum*, Vol. 52, No.7, (Jul 2005), pp. 2120-2124.

Pierangeli S.S., Chen P.P., González E.B. (2006). Antiphospholipid antibodies and the antiphospholipid syndrome: an update on treatment and pathogenic mechanisms. *Curr Opin Hematol*, Vol. 13, No. 5, (Sep 2006), pp. 366-375.

Pierangeli S.S., Chen P.P., Raschi E., Scurati S., Grossi C., Borghi M.O., Palomo I., Harris E.N. & Meroni P.L. (2008). Antiphospholipid antibodies and the antiphospholipid syndrome: pathogenic mechanisms. *Semin Thromb Hemost*, Vol. 34, No.3, (Apr 2008), pp. 236-250.

Raab G. & Klagsbrun M. (1997). Heparin binding EGF growth factor. Biochim Biophys Acta, Vol. 1333, No. 3, (Dec 1997), pp. 179–99.

Rai R.S., Regan L., Clifford K., Pickering W., Dave M., Mackie I., McNally T. & Cohen H. (1995). Antiphospholipid antibodies and ß2-glycoprotein-I in 500 women with recurrent miscarriage: results of a comprehensive screening approach. *Hum Reprod*, Vol. 10, No. 8, (Aug 1995), pp. 2001-2005.

Rai R., Cohen H., Dave M. & Regan L. (1997). Randomised controlled trial of aspirin and aspirin plus heparin in pregnant women with recurrent miscarriage associated with phospholipid antibodies (or antiphospholipid antibodies). *BMJ*, Vol. 314, No. (1997), pp. 253 - 257.

Rand, J.H., Wu X.X., Guller S., Gil J., Guha A., Scher J. & Lockwood C.J. (1994). Reduction of annexin-V (placental anticoagulant protein-I) on placental villi of women with antiphospholipid antibodies and recurrent spontaneous abortion. *Am J Obstet Gynecol*, Vol. 171, No. 6, (Dec 1994), pp. 1566–1572.

Rand, J.H., Wu X.X., Quinn A.S. & Taatjes D.J. (2010). The annexin A5-mediated pathogenic mechanism in the antiphospholipid syndrome: role in pregnancy losses and thrombosis. *Lupus*, Vol. 19, No. 4, (Apr 2010), pp. 460–469.

Redecha P., Tilley R., Tencati M., Salmon J.E., Kirchhofer D., Mackman N. & Girardi G. (2007). Tissue factor: a link between C5a and neutrophil activation in antiphospholipid antibody induced foetal injury. *Blood*, Vol. 110, No. 7, (Oct 2007), pp. 2423-2431.

Rote N.S., Vogt E., DeVere G., Obringer A.R. & Ng A.K. (1998) The role of placental trophoblast in the pathophysiology of the antiphospholipid antibody syndrome. *Am J Reprod Immunol*, Vol. 39, No. 2, (Feb 1998), pp. 125-136.

Ruiz-Irastorza G., Egurbide M.V., Ugalde J. & Aguirre C. (2004). High impact of antiphospholipid syndrome on irreversible organ damage and survival of patients with systemic lupus erythematosus. *Arch Intern Med,* Vol. 164, No. 1, (Jan 2004), pp. 77-82.

Ruiz-Irastorza G. & Khamashta M.A. Lupus and pregnancy: ten questions and some answers. *Lupus,* Vol. 17, No. 5, (May 2008), pp. 416-420.

Ruiz-Irastorza G., Crowther M., Branch W. & Khamashta M.A. (2010). Antiphospholipid syndrome. Lancet, Vol. 76, No. 9751, (Oct 2010), pp. 1498-1509.

Sanna G., Bertolaccini M.L., Cuadrado M.J., Khamashta M.A. & Hughes G.R. (2003). Central nervous system involvement in the antiphospholipid (Hughes) syndrome. *Rheumatology,* Vol. 42, No. 2, (Feb 2003), pp. 200 - 213.

Shamonki J.M., Salmon J.E., Hyjek E. & Baergen R.N. Excessive complement activation is associated with placental injury in patients with antiphospholipid antibodies. *Am J Obstet Gynecol,* Vol. 196, No. 2, (Feb 2007), p. 167. e1-5.

Silver R.K., MacGregor S.N., Sholl J.S., Hobart J.M., Neerhof M.G. & Ragin A. (1993). Comparative trial of prednisone plus aspirin versus aspirin alone in the treatment of anticardiolipin antibody-positive obstetric patients. *Am J Obstet Gynecol,* Vol. 169, No. 6, (Dec 1993), pp. 1411 - 1417.

Silver R.M. (2007). Foetal death. Obstet Gynecol, Vol. 109, No. 1, (Jan 2007), pp. 153-167.

Smith G.C.S., Crossley J.A., Aitken D.A., Pell J.P., Cameron A.D., Connor J.M. & Dobbie R. (2004). First-trimester placentation and the risk of antepartum stillbirth. *JAMA,* Vol. 292, No. 18, (Nov 2004), pp. 2249 - 2254.

Stephenson M.D., Ballem P.J., Tsang P., Purkiss S., Ensworth S., Houlihan E. & Ensom M.H. (2004). Treatment of antiphospholipid antibody syndrome (APS) in pregnancy: a randomized pilot trial comparing low molecular weight heparin to unfractionated heparin. *J Obstet Gynaecol Can,* Vol. 26, No. (2004), pp. 729 - 734.

Stirrat G.M. (1990). Recurrent miscarriage I: definition and epidemiology. *Lancet,* Vol. 336, No. 8716, (Sep 1990), pp. 673-675.

Tektonidou M.G., Sotsiou F., Nakopoulou L., Vlachoyiannopoulos P.G. & Moutsopoulos H.M. (2004). Antiphospholipid syndrome nephropathy in patients with systemic lupus erythematosus and antiphospholipid antibodies: prevalence, clinical associations, and long-term outcome. *Arthritis Rheum,* Vol. 50, No. 8, (Aug 2004), pp. 2596-2579.

Tektonidou M.G., Varsou N., Kotoulas G., Antoniou A. & Moutsopoulos H.M. (2006). Cognitive deficits in patients with antiphospholipid syndrome: association with clinical, laboratory, and brain magnetic resonance imaging findings. *Arch Intern Med,* Vol. 166, No. 20, (Nov 2006), pp. 2278-2284.

Tektonidou M.G., Laskari K., Panagiotakos D.B. &, Moutsopoulos H.M. (2009). Risk factors for thrombosis and primary thrombosis prevention in patients with systemic lupus erythematosus with or without antiphospholipid antibodies. *Arthritis Rheum,* Vol. 61, No. 1, (Jan 2009), pp. 29-36.

Thurman, J.M., Kraus D.M., Girardi G., Hourcade D., Kang H.J., Royer P.A., Mitchell L.M., Giclas P.C., Salmon J., Gilkeson G. & Holers V.M. (2005). A novel inhibitor of the alternative complement pathway prevents antiphospholipid antibody-induced pregnancy loss in mice. *Mol Immunol,* Vol. 42, No. 1, (Jan 2005), pp. 87–97.

Triolo G., Ferrante A., Ciccia F., Accardo-Palumbo A., Perino A., Castelli A., Giarratano A. & Licata G. (2003). Randomized study of subcutaneous low molecular weight heparin plus aspirin versus intravenous immunoglobulin in the treatment of recurrent foetal loss associated with antiphospholipid antibodies. *Arthritis Rheum,* Vol. 166, No. 5, (Mar 2003), pp. 728-731.

Vaquero E., Lazzarin N., Valensise H., Menghini S., Di Pierro G., Cesa F. & Romanini C. (2001). Pregnancy outcome in recurrent spontaneous abortion associated with antiphospholipid antibodies: a comparative study of intravenous immunoglobulin versus prednisone plus low-dose aspirin. *Am J Reprod Immunol,* Vol. 45, No. 3, (Mar 2001), pp. 174-179.

Vega-Ostertag M., Casper K., Swerlick R., Ferrara D., Harris E.N. & Pierangeli SS. (2005). Involvement of p38 MAPK in the up-regulation of tissue factor on endothelial cells by antiphospholipid antibodies. *Arthritis Rheum,* Vol. 52, No. 5, (May 2005), pp. 1545-1554.

Wang S.X., Sun Y.T. & Sui S.F. (2000). Membrane-induced conformational change in human apolipoprotein. *H Biochem J,* Vol. 348, (May 2000), pp. 103–106.

Wang J., Mayernik L., Schultz J.F. & Armant D.R. (2000). Acceleration of trophoblast differentiation by heparinbinding EGF-like growth factor is dependent on the stage-specific activation of calcium influx by ErbB receptors in developing mouse blastocysts. *Development,* Vol. 127, No. 1, (Jan 2000), pp. 33–44.

Yetman D.L. & Kutteh W.H. (1996). Antiphospholipid antibody panels and recurrent pregnancy loss: prevalence of anticardiolipin antibodies compared with other antiphospholipid antibodies. *Fertil Steril,* Vol. 66, No. 4, (Oct 1996), pp. 540-546.

12

Fetal Thrombophilia

Stefano Raffaele Giannubilo and Andrea Luigi Tranquilli
Department of Clinical Sciences – Università Politecnica delle Marche - Ancona Italy

1. Introduction

Pregnancy is physiologically characterized by an increased procoagulant activity; in fact, pregnant women have two- to fivefold higher risk for venous thromboembolism compared with nonpregnant women (Grandone et al., 1998). Coagulation factors VII, X, VIII, fibrinogen, von Willebrand factor, prothrombin fragment 1 and 2, and thrombin-antithrombin complexes increase (Bremme, 2003). In parallel, there is a decrease of physiologic anticoagulants such as protein S and the acquisition of activated protein C resistance. These physiologic changes appear to relate to the development of an adequate placental perfusion and provide a protective mechanism for hemostasis during delivery. A hypercoagulable state may expose, however, the pregnant women to thrombotic risk during pregnancy and the immediate postpartum period. This risk is higher in women with multiple thrombophilic defects (Tranquilli et al., 2004). Congenital thrombophilia includes deficiency or defects of some factors such as antithrombin, protein C and S, and in the case of genetic specific mutations of one or more genes among these indicated: methylenetetrahydrofolate reductase (MTHFR C677 T), Prothrombin (FII G20210A), Factor V (FV G1691A), and Plasminogen activator inhibitor-1 (PAI-1 4G/5G). In the literature, thrombophilia has been reported as related to obstetric pathology; in particular, the association with intrauterine fetal death (IUFD), a complication that ranged from 4.9 to 10.4 babies in each 1,000, and where in the 12% to 50% of cases the cause remains unknown, has been confirmed (Martinelli et al., 2003; Kupferminc et al., 1999; Preston et al. 1996) or not confirmed (Gonen et al., 2005). Although thrombophilia is extensively studied for its implications in pregnancy complications, the role of different factors, the gestational age at which those factors may intervene, has not been completely elucidated, nor has it been given enough relevance to the weight of fetal thrombophilia in the origin of some specific form of those obstetric complications (Tranquilli et al., 2006). Most of the actual studies in the literature have focused their attention on maternal biologic samples and considering exclusively the genetic contribution of the mother.

2. Placental genetics and biology

The placenta is the highly specialised organ of pregnancy that supports the normal growth and development of the fetus. Changes in placental development and function have dramatic effects on the fetus and its ability to cope with the intrauterine environment. Implantation and the formation of the placenta is a highly coordinated process involving interaction between maternal and embryonic cells. Trophoblast cell invasion of uterine tissues and remodelling of uterine spiral arterial walls ensures that the developing feto-placental unit receives the necessary supply of blood and that efficient transfer of nutrients and gases and the removal of wastes can take place. Different types of placentation are categorised according to the number and types of layers between the maternal and fetal circulations, the human placenta is defined as a "haemochorial" villous organ, In the hemochorial placentation the wall of maternal blood vessels going towards the implantation site is breached and maternal blood bathes placental cells. In this process, maternal blood passes through channels that are lined by placental trophoblast cells (Georgiades et al., 2002). This situation contrasts with all other vascular beds where the blood vessel endothelium lies at the blood tissue interface. The human trophoblast cells express a range of gene products that are expressed normally by the endothelium and that regulate the hemostatic function. These include molecules that regulate thrombin activity (thrombomodulin, endothelial protein C receptor, tissue factor pathway inhibitor), regulators of vasodilation and platelet function (nitric oxide synthase 2, cyclooxygenase 2 and prostacyclin synthase) and some regulators of fibrinolysis (plasminogen activator inhibitor, tissue plasminogen activator). These findings suggest that, although derived from a distinct developmental lineage, trophoblast cells mimic endothelial cells in their ability to partake in anticoagulant and fibrinolytic activities. Trophoblast cells are derived from the zygote and are genetically identical to the fetus (Sood, 2009). The development of gene "knock-out" and transgenic animal models indicate that complete absence of tissue factor, tissue factor pathway inhibitor or prothrombin is lethal in the developing mouse embryo. Placental thrombi resulting in placental infarction may also occur on either side of the maternal-fetal interface and may have serious implications for the mother or her fetus, including an increased risk for perinatal morbidity and mortality (Fuke et al., 1994; Redline et al., 1995). A placental infarct is an area of placental parenchyma that has undergone ischemic necrosis; it may occur on either side of the maternal-fetal interface. Development of the fetal arterial blood supply to the placenta begins as early as 18 to 20 days after conception. The fetal placental vessels vary little from vessels of other organs and are lined by endothelial cells. Endothelium-lined vessels are dependent on the normal balance of procoagulant and anticoagulant mechanisms for damage repair and maintaining blood fluidity. Failure to maintain this delicate balance in the presence of a fetal hypercoagulable state may result in placental infarction in the distribution of fetal vessels and may even result in early spontaneous miscarriage. Furthermore placental infarction is more common in women with severe preeclampsia (Salafia et al., 1995) but it is not known whether it precedes the onset of disease or develops as a consequence. Because vascular features of the placenta seem to be involved, and because the placenta is of fetal origin, fetal genes related to vascular conditions could be relevant. In cases of maternal thrombophilia associated with fetal growth restriction (FGR), maternal floor infarction of the placenta, which is characterized by deposition of fibrinoid material, could be found not only in the maternal surface but also in intervillous spaces of the placenta (Adams-Chapman et al., 2002). Thus, both maternal thrombophilia and infarction of intervillous spaces of the placenta could be causes of fetal growth restriction. Antiphospholipid antibodies syndrome (APS) represents a singular case of maternal and fetal thrombophilia since the antiphospholipid antibodies cross the placental wall. The hypothesis that hypercoagulability of APS was in some way impacting the utero-placental circulation is supported by the finding of intervillous thrombosis, extensive villous fibrosis, or rather marked infarction in some placentas of APS pregnancies. Numerous possible mechanisms of thrombosis in the intervillous space have been considered such as increased tissue factor (Branch et al., 1993; Dobado-Berrios et al., 1999) or prostacyclin-thromboxane pathway (Peaceman et al., 1993). If the thrombotic tendency may explain the later placental insufficiency, a particularly attractive candidate mechanism for early pregnancy loss as well as placental insufficiency in later pregnancy is aPL-mediated inhibition of trophoblast invasion (Di Simone et al., 2000).

3. Fetal and neonatal genetics

Despite the number of studies that have confirmed or not confirmed an association between inherited thrombophilias and pregnancy complications, it remains difficult to establish the exact risk figures for particular adverse events in the presence of genetic thrombophilic mutations. The complexity of the placental disorders of pregnancy has led more Authors to speculate that a feto-maternal genome interaction is plausible (Lie et al., 1998). When the fetus itself has an inherited risk of thrombosis, pregnancy is also more prone to placental infarction at the maternal–fetal interface resulting in an increased risk for intrauterine death as compared with fetuses from uncomplicated pregnancies. This is consistent with the observation that women who are homozygous of factor V Leiden mutation, an inherited risk for thrombosis, are even more prone to fetal loss (Meinardi et al., 1999). A higher prevalence of fetal genetic risk factors for thrombosis (factor V Leiden or prothrombin 20210A allele) was found in fetuses born from a pregnancy complicated with intrauterine fetal death as compared with the prevalence of a historic control group (Dekker et al., 2004). It has been speculated that the Factor V Leiden mutation could contribute to the development of obstetric complications by promoting the formation of microthrombi in the placenta, thus compromising fetomaternal circulation (Younis et al., 1997). By the results of Tranquilli et al. (Tranquilli et al. 2010) no higher risk was observed when a singular gene mutation occurs. On the contrary, the mutation of Factor V is significantly more frequent when an intrauterine fetal demise occurs. The results obtained by the PAI-1 and MTHFR gene analysis are particularly interesting because was observed a cumulative higher risk for intrauterine fetal demise when a double condition of homozigosity occurs relative to the two genes, according to other investigators (Alonso et al., 2002; Pickering et al., 2001). The association between homozygosity for polymorphism of MTHFR and PAI-1 with the thrombotic phenomenons is controversial, but seem to be in accord with Nelen et al. (Nelen et al., 1997), who described the double condition of homozygosity MTHFRT/Tand PAI-1 4 G/4 G as a cause contributing to the pregnancy loss. The common mutation analyzed in the MTHFR gene has been reported to reduce the enzymatic activity. This variant is responsible of elevated plasmatic levels of homocysteine mainly after an oral load of methionine: the condition of homozygosity for MTHFR T/T predisposes to the onset of blood hyperomocisteine (Jacques et al., 1996). PAI-1 is the main factor of the regulation of the Plasminogen activators, and homozigosity for PAI 4 G/4 G is associated with increased PAI-1 levels and decrease fibrinolitic activity, which lead to a reduction of the trophoblast's ability to invade into the endometrium and compromise the successful placentation. The underling hypothesis is that thrombophilia mediated by the physiologic hyperestrogenemia of pregnancy may be synergistic, with a genetic thrombophilic pattern promoting thrombus formation in the spiral arteries of the placenta, placental insufficiency, and pregnancy loss (Paidas et al., 2004). Jivraj et al. (16) reported that only multiple thrombophilic mutations in either partner of recurrent miscarriage couples increased the risk of miscarriages in subsequent pregnancies 1.9-fold. Evidence suggests that preeclampsia has a maternal genetic component. Preeclampsia is more common in mothers, daughters, and sisters of women who experience preeclampsia, suggesting a role of inherited susceptibility of preeclampsia through maternal genes (Lie et al., 1998). Men who have fathered one preeclamptic pregnancy are nearly twice as likely to father a preeclamptic pregnancy in a different woman (Lie et al., 1998). Fathers who themselves came from a preeclamptic pregnancy are also at increased risk of fathering a preeclamptic pregnancy (Esplin et al., 2001). Numerous casecontrol studies of affected and unaffected mothers indicate an association between genes expressing thrombophilia and genes expressing preeclampsia (Powers et al., 1999; van Pampus et al., 1999; Kupferminc et al., 2000; Kim et al., 2001), but none of the 27 such studies covered in a recent review (Alfirevic et al., 2002) assessed or adjusted for possible effects of fetal alleles. In fact compared with controls, preeclamptic women from 16 studies were more heterozygous for the FVL (RR=1.6; CI=1.2 to 2.1) or homozygous for the MTHFR variant (RR=1.7; CI=1.2 to 2.3) Because mothers with variant alleles also more often have children with variant alleles, adjustment for fetal alleles could be essential for correct estimation of the effects of maternal alleles (Vefring et al., 2004). Small case series suggest concordance for preeclampsia in identical twins (Lachmeijer et al., 1998; O'Shaughnessey et al., 2000), but a large cohort study found no evidence of concordance (Thornton & Macdonald, 1999). Thus, it is clear that maternal genes alone do not determine the risk. Changing paternity, and thus changing maternal–paternal genomic expression in the fetus, is associated with an increased risk of preeclampsia (Lie et al., 1998). Kajantie et al. reported that people born after pregnancies complicated by preeclampsia are at increased risk of stroke in adult life (Kajantie et al., 2009). Fetal thrombophilia may result from low birth weight. In a retrospective analysis, von-Kries and colleagues (Von-Kries et al., 2001) stated that a higher odds ratio for birth weight in the lowest quartile was observed among children carrying prothrombotic risk factors. This conclusion was not supported by Rivard and colleagues (Infante-Rivard et al., 2002) in a large case-controlled study. The placenta, which has its own hemostatic mechanisms, is probably an important locus of pathology in perinatal arterial ischemic stroke (PAS). Association between thrombosis and infarction in the placenta and peri- and neonatal infarction, the most commonly presumed mechanism being embolization to the fetus, has been reported in literature (Adams-Chapman et al., 2002). Pregnancy itself is a prothrombotic state as shift toward prothrombotic reactions is seen in women as gestation progresses through the second and third trimesters and just after gestation (Clark et al., 2003). In cases reviewed for litigation because of cerebral palsy in the child, thrombotic lesions were the most common pathology found in the placenta (Kraus et al., 1999). In a study in a national inpatient sample (James et al., 2005) reported risk factors for pregnancy-related stroke to include postnatally identified infection (OR 25); migraine (OR 16.9); thrombophilia, including history of thrombosis and the antiphospholipid syndrome (OR 16.0); systemic lupus (OR 15.2); heart disease (OR 13.2); preeclampsia (OR 4.4); diabetes (OR 2.5); and smoking (OR 1.9). A number of reports describe acquired thrombophilias in women whose pregnancies resulted in the birth of a child with perinatal stroke (Nelson, 2007). Antiphospholipid antibodies can pass from mother to child via the placenta and can alter the placenta itself, changing its function. In one of the few studies limited to perinatal arterial ischemic stroke, Gunther and colleagues (Gunther et al., 2000) found at least 1 of the 6 examined prothrombotic risk factors in 68% of affected children and in 24% of controls. Factor V Leiden mutation, the prothrombin mutation, hyperhomocystinemia, and elevated lipoprotein (a) levels have been described with increased frequency in infants who have PAS when compared with healthy control subjects (Hogeveen et al., 2003; Golomb, 2003) . In a cohort study from the UK of Mercuri and coll. (Mercuri et al., 2001). among 24 infants with perinatal cerebral infarction confirmed by neonatal magnetic resonance imaging, 10 (42%) had at least one prothrombotic risk factor. There are some reports on an increased incidence of thrombophilic risk factors in selective cohorts of neonates who have vascular complications, such as intraventricular hemorrhage (Pet et al., 2001), retinopathy of prematurity, and necrotizing enterocolitis. Hypercoagulability may also be associated with late neurologic sequelae (Smith et al., 1976). Necrotizing enterocolitis (NEC) is associated to hematologic abnormalities, including evidence for intravascular coagulation (Hutter et al., 1976). Nonetheless, whether thrombophilic risk factors promote the occurrence of NEC or its severity remains to be proven (Kenet et al., 2006). Furthermore, neonatal posthemorrhagic ventriculomegaly, following fetal germinal matrix-intraventricular hemorrhage (GMH-IVH) diagnosed in utero by means of NMR, was recently described in a neonate found to be heterozygous for two thrombophilic patterns, factor V Leiden and methylenetetrahydrofolate reductase mutation (Ramenghi et al., 2005). The possible pathogenesis of intraventricular hemorrhage (IVH)may be vessel occlusion triggering high-pressure bleeding. The incidence of Factor V of Leiden was increased among infants reported in two case-series with IVH and as hydrocephalus (Aronis et al., 1998); however, the occurrence of periventricular leukomalacia (PVL) in patients who had IVH was not increased among FVL-heterozygous patients (Aronis et al., 1998). In a series of 29 cases Redline and Pappin demonstrated that neonatal death, intrauterine growth restriction, birth asphyxia, major thrombotic events and thrombocytopenia were the major neonatal complications associated with avascular villi (Redline et al., 1995). Retinopathy of prematurity (ROP) is considered as a multifactorial disease and was reported to be associated with hypoxia-induced angiogenesis. Since vasculogenesis may be influenced by the presence of thrombophilic risk factors Kenet et al. (Kenet et al., 2003) studied the incidence and severity of ROP was similar among premature infants who had thrombophilia as compared with nonthrombophilic infants of the study group. The prevalence of genetic prothrombotic markers (FVL, MTHFR, FII20210A) and plasma omocysteine levels were assayed in 166 premature and low-birth-weight infants but the prevalence of perinatal complications and the severity of diseases were similar among infants with or without thrombophilia, although the numbers of patients within any subgroup of complications was small.

4. Therapy

A successful pregnancy requires the development of adequate placental circulation, thrombophilia may be hypothesised to be a risk factor for the placenta mediated pregnancy complications and anticoagulants (heparin and aspirin) may be of interest to prevent these complications. In clinical trials the effects of some of these drugs on the development of preeclampsia have already been investigated in pregnant women. Low-molecular-weight heparins, fractions of crude heparin with high bioavailability and a relatively long half-life, are produced by the enzymatic or chemical breakdown of unfractionated heparin and have been widely used during the last decade. It has been shown that they do not cross the human placenta in vivo. Two general hypotheses have been proposed to explain how heparin and aspirin attenuate miscarriage rates: The first involves prevention of aberrant coagulation, reducing placental ischemia and the second involves direct modulation of cell biology, preventing apoptosis and maintaining trophoblast proliferation (Yacobi et al., 2002). Since the aspirin cross the placental wall its effect may act also on the fetal side. In randomized placebo-controlled studies, administration of aspirin throughout the first trimester, but not later than 16 weeks, or of LMWH starting at 10-11 weeks of gestation or even before conception, lowered the risk of developing hypertensive disorders and intrauterine growth restriction in pregnancy (Rey et al., 2009; Duley et al., 2007). The potential effect of aspirin in improving pregnancy outcomes is due to the selective inhibition of thromboxane synthesis without impairing prostacyclin synthesis. However the placenta effect of aspirin can vary between individuals because liver metabolism, adding a reason to the why aspirin may not be good for all patients. The interplay between the coagulation system and the placenta mediated pregnancy complications may not be isolated to thrombotic effects at a vascular level leading to placental insufficiency. Recent evidence demonstrates that coagulation activation may directly impact on trophoblast cell growth and differentiation at a cellular level without thrombosis at a vascular level as an intermediary. That is, coagulation activation may play a role in the development of placental insufficiency through abnormal placental development rather than placental vascular thrombosis. The anticoagulant activity of heparin is mediated by both antithrombin dependent and independent pathways, but the role of heparin as an anti-inflammatory agent has been the subject of much investigation. Inflammation is known to play a key role in pathogenesis of preeclampsia and other obstetric complications. The immunological mechanism involves the regulation of Th1/ Th2 balance, production of inflammatory cytokines and leuckocyte activation. Animal models have shown that heparin disacchrides inhibit TNF α production by macrophages, and hence decrease immune mediated inflammation (Tyrell et al., 1995). The anti inflammatory effect is mediated by antithrombin and a TFPI independent pathway, by inhibition of matrix degrading enzymes, proteases and also by Selectin modulation. Mello et al. reported that the absolute risk of pre-eclampsia was reduced from 28.2% (11/39) in the no drug intervention group to 7.3% (3/41) in the dalteparin group. The absolute risk of early onset preeclampsia (≤34 weeks gestation) was similarly reduced from 20.5% (8/39) in the no drug intervention group to 2.4% (1/41) as was fetal growth restriction from 43.6% (17/39) in the no drug intervention group to 9.8% (4/41) in the dalteparin group (Mello et al., 2005). Further prospective studies are needed to assess whether inherited or acquired thrombophilia increases the risk of development and recurrence Placental mediated disorders of pregnancy. The administration of prophilactic doses of low-molecular weight heparin from the beginning of pregnancy may reduce the recurrence rate of these disorders. If the use of antithrombotic therapy will be proven to be effective in reducing maternal and perinatal morbidity and mortality, acceptable, and cost effective, then a screening program should be planned to identify women and fetus with thrombophilia and a past history of severe complications of pregnancy.

5. Conclusions

Inherited and acquired factors may determine thrombophilia. Given that some complications of pregnancy are not always associated with maternal thrombophilia, controversy still exists on the exact impact of the disorders with the adverse pregnancy outcomes. While we are convinced that thrombophilias are extensively implicated in pregnancy complications, we feel that there has not been completely elucidated the role of the different factors, the gestational age at which those factors may intervene, nor has been given enough relevance to the weight of fetal thrombophilias in the origin of some specific form of those obstetric complications. The homozygosity of polymorphism in placental tissue necessarily includes a role of the father's genetic pattern in pregnancy destiny, and may identify a "fetal thrombophilic status" inherited from both parents. Maternal thrombophilias may be responsible for venous thromboembolism, preeclampsia HELLP syndrome and eclampsia, whereas fetal thrombophilia, may account for fetal growth restriction or stillbirth. This last would also explain some stillbirth or repeated late miscarriage observed in non-thrombophilic mothers. The two sides of thrombophilia may, of course, concur, resulting in the more severe clinical presentations. The clinical implications of these hypothesis need to be addressed in future research to answer the question of whether or not maternal/paternal/fetal thrombophilia should be treated with low molecular-weight heparin and/or low dose aspirin.

6. References

Adams-Chapman, I., Vaucher, Y.E., Bejar, R.F., Benirschke, K., Baergen, R.N., & Moore, T.R. (2002). Maternal floor infarction of the placenta: association with central nervous system injury and adverse neurodevelopmental outcome. *J Perinatol*, Vol.22, No. 3, pp. 236-241, ISSN 0743-8346

Alfirevic, Z., Roberts, D., & Martlew, V. (2002). How strong is the association between maternal thrombophilia and adverse pregnancy outcome? A systemic review. Eur J *Obstet Gynecol Reprod Biol*, Vol.101, No.1, pp.6-14, ISSN 0301-2115

Alonso, A., Soto, I., Urgelles, M.F., Corte, J.R., Rodriguez, M.J., & Pinto, C.R. (2002). Acquired and inherited thrombophilia in women with unexplained fetal losses. *Am J Obstet Gynecol*, Vol.187, No.5. pp. 1337–1342, ISSN 0002-9378

Aronis, S., Platokouki, H., Photopoulos, S., Adamtziki, E., & Xanthou, M. (1998). Indications of coagulation and/or fibrinolytic system activation in healthy and sick very low birth weight neonates. *Biol Neonate*, Vol.74, No.5, pp. 337-344, ISSN 0006-3126

Branch, D.W., & Rodgers, G.M. (1993). Induction of endothelial cell tissue factor activity by sera from patients with antiphospholipid syndrome: a possible mechanism of thrombosis. *Am J Obstet Gynecol*, Vol.168, No.1, pp. 206-210, ISSN 0002-9378

Bremme, K.A. (2003) Hemostatic changes in pregnancy. *Best Pract Res Clin Haematol*, Vol.16, No.2, pp.153-158, ISSN 1521-6926

Clark P. (2003). Changes of hemostasis variables during pregnancy. *Semin Vasc Med*, Vol.3, No.1, pp.13-24, ISSN 1528-9648

Dekker, J.W.T., Lind, J., Bloemenkamp, K.W.M., Quint, V.G.W., Kuijpers, J.C., van Doorn, L.J., & de Groot, C.J.M. (2004). Inherited risk of thrombosis of the fetus and intrauterine fetal death. *Eur J Obstet Gynecol Reprod Biol*, Vol.117, No.1, pp.45-48, ISSN 0301-2115

Di Simone, N., Meroni, P.L., de Papa, N., Raschi, E., Caliandro, D., De Carolis, C.S., Khamashta, M.A., Atsumi, T., Hughes, G.R., Balestrieri, G., Tincani, A., Casali, P., & Caruso, A. (2000). Antiphospholipid antibodies affect trophoblast gonadotropin secretion and invasiveness by binding directly and through adhered beta2-glycoprotein I. *Arthritis Rheum*, Vol.43, No.1, pp.140-150, ISSN 0004-3591

Dobado-Berrios, P.M., Lopez-Pedrera, C., Velasco, F., Aguirre, M.A., Torres, A., & Cuadrado, M.J. (1999). Increased levels of tissue factor mRNA in mononuclear blood cells of patients with primary antiphospholipid syndrome. *Thromb Haemost*, Vol.82, No.6, pp.1578-1582, ISSN 0340-6245

Duley, L., Henderson-Smart, D.J., Meher, S., & King, J.F. (2007). Antiplatelets agents for preventing pre-eclampsia and its complications. *Cochrane Database Syst Rev*; CD004659

Esplin, M.S., Fausett, M.B., Fraser, A., Kerber, R., Mineau, G., Carrillo, J., & Varner, M.W. (2001). Pat.ernal and maternal components of the predisposition to preeclampsia. *N Engl J Med*, Vol.344, No.12, pp.867-872, ISSN 0028-4793

Fuke, Y., Aono, T., Imai, S., Suehara, N., Fujita, T., & Nakayama, M. (1994). Clinical significance and treatment of massive intervillous fibrin deposition associated with recurrent fetal growth retardation. *Gynecol Obstet Invest*, Vol.38, No.1, pp.5-9, ISSN 0378-7346

Georgiades, P., Ferguson-Smith, A.C., & Burton, G.J. (2002). Comparative developmental anatomy of the murine and human definitive placentae. *Placenta*, Vol.23, No.1, pp. 3-19 ISSN 0143-4004

Golomb, M.R. (2003). The contribution of prothrombotic disorders to peri and neonatal ischemic stroke. *Semin Thromb Hemost*, Vol.29, No.4, pp. 415-424, ISSN 0094-6176

Gonen, R., Lavi, N., Attias, D., Schliamser, L., Borochowitz, Z., Toubi, E., & Ohel, G. (2005). Absence of association of inherited thrombophilia with unexplained third-trimester intrauterine fetal death. *Am J Obstet Gynecol*, Vol.192, No. 3, pp. 742–746, ISSN 0002-9378

Grandone, E., Margaglione, M., Colaizzo, D,, D'Andrea, G., Cappucci, G., Brancaccio, V., Di & Minno, G. (1998). Genetic susceptibility to pregnancy-related venous thromboembolism: roles of factor V Leiden, prothrombin G20210A, and methylenetetrahydrofolate reductase C677 T mutations. *Am J Obstet Gynecol*, Vol.179, No.5, pp. 1324–1328, ISSN 0002-9378

Gunther, G., Junker, R., Strater, R., Schobess, R., Kurnik, K., Heller, C., Kosch, A., & Nowak-Gottl, U., for the Childhood Stroke Study Group. (2000). Symptomatic ischemic stroke in full-term neonates: role of acquired and genetic prothrombotic risk factors. *Stroke*, Vol. 31, No, 10, pp.2437–2441, ISSN 0039-2499

Hogeveen, M., Blom, H.J., Van Amerongen, M., Boogmans, B., Van Beynum, I.M., & Van De Bor, M. (2002). Hyperhomocysteinemia as risk factor for ischemic and hemorrhagic stroke in newborn infants. *J Pediatr*, Vol.141, No. 3, pp. 429-431, ISSN 0022-3476

Hutter, J.J., Hathaway, W.E., & Wayne, ER. (1976). Hematologic abnormalitiesin severe neonatal necrotizing enterocolitis. *J Pediatr*, Vol.88, No.6, pp. 1026-1031, ISSN 0022-3476

Infante-Rivard, C., Rivard, G.E., Yotov, W.V., Génin, E., Guiguet, M., Weinberg, C., Gauthier, R., & Feoli-Fonseca, J.C. (2002). Absence of association of thrombophilia polymorphisms with intrauterine growth restriction. *N Engl J Med*, Vol.347. No.1, pp. 19-25, ISSN 0028-4793

Jacques, P.F., Bostom, A.G., Williams, R.R., Ellison, R.C., Eckfeldt, J.H., Rosenberg, I.H., Selhub, J., & Rozen, R. (1996). Relation between folate status, a common mutation in methylenetetrahydrofolate reductase, and plasma homocysteine concentrations. *Circulation*, Vol.93, No.1, pp. 7-9, ISSN 0009-7322

James, A.H., Bushnell, C.D., Jamison, M.G., & Myers, ER. (2005). Incidence and risk factors for stroke in pregnancy and the puerperium. *Obstet Gynecol*, Vol.106, No.3, pp.509-516, ISSN 0029-7844

Kajantie, E., Eriksson, J.G., Osmond, C., Thornburg, K., & Barker, D.J.P. (2009). Pre-eclampsia is associated with increased risk of stroke in the adult offspring: the Helsinki birth cohort study. *Stroke*, Vol.40, No.4, pp.1176-1180, ISSN 0039-2499

Kenet, G., Maayan-Metzger, A., Rosenberg, N., Sela, B.A., Mazkereth, R., Ifrah, A., & Kuint, J. (2003). Thrombophilia does not increase risk for neonatal complications in preterm infants. *Thromb Haemost*, Vol.90, No.5, pp.823-828, ISSN 0340-6245

Kenet, G., & Nowak-Gottl, U. (2006). Fetal and Neonatal Thrombophilia. *Obstet Gynecol Clin N Am*, Vol.33, No.3, pp.457-466, ISSN 0889-8545

Kim, Y.J., Williamson, R.A., Murray, J.C., Andrews, J., Pietscher, J.J., Peraud, P.J., & Merrill, D.C. (2001). Genetic susceptibility to pre-eclampsia: Roles of cytosine-to-thymine substitution at nucleotide 677 of the gene for methylenetetrahydrofolate reductase, 68-base pair insertion at nucleotide 844 of the gene for cystathionine -synthase, and factor V Leiden mutation. *Am J Obstet Gynecol*, Vol.184, No.6, pp.1211–1217, ISSN 0002-9378

Kraus, F.T., & Acheen, V.I. (1999). Fetal thrombotic vasculopathy in the placenta: cerebral thrombi and infarcts, coagulopathies, and cerebral palsy. *Hum Pathol*, Vol.30, No.7, pp.759-769, ISSN 0046-8177

Kupferminc, M.J., Eldor, A., Steinman, N., Many, A., Bar-Am, A., Jaffa, A., Fait, G., & Lessing, J.B. (1999). Increased frequency of genetic thrombophilia in women with complications of pregnancy. *N Engl J Med*, Vol.340, No.1, pp. 9-13, ISSN 0028-4793

Kupferminc, M.J., Fait, G., Many, A., Gordon, D., Eldor, A., & Lessing, J.B. (2000). Severe preeclampsia and high frequency of genetic thrombophilic mutations. *Obstet Gynecol*, Vol.96, No.1, pp.45-49, ISSN 0029-7844

Lachmeijer, A.M., Aarnoudse, J.G., ten Kate, L.P., Pals, G., & Dekker, G.A. (1998). Concordance for pre-eclampsia in monozygous twins. *Br J Obstet Gynaecol*, Vol.105, No.12, pp.1315–1317, ISSN 0306-5456

Lie, R.T., Rasmussen, S., Brunborg, H., Gjessing, H.K., Lie-Nielsen, E., & Irgens, L.M. (1998). Fetal and maternal contributions to the risk of pre-eclampsia: population based study. *BMJ*, Vol.316, No.7141, pp.1343-1347, ISSN 0959-8138

Martinelli, I., Taioli, E., Cetin, I., Marinoni, A., Gerosa, S., Villa, M.V., Bozzo, M., & Mannucci, P.M. (2000). Mutations in coagulation factors in women with unexplained late fetal loss. *N Engl J Med*, Vol.343, No.14, pp.1015–1018, ISSN 0028-4793

Meinardi, J.R., Middeldorp, S., de Kam, P.J., Koopman, M.M., van Pampus, E.C., Hamulyák, K., Prins, M.H., Büller, H.R., & van der Meer, J. (1999). Increased risk for fetal loss in carriers of the factor V Leiden mutation. *Ann Int Med*, Vol.130, No.9, pp.736-739, ISSN 0003-4819

Mello, G., Parretti, E., Fatini, C., Riviello, C., Gensini, F., Marchionni, M., Scarselli, G.F., Gensini, G.F., & Abbate, R. (2005). Low molecular-weight heparin lowers the recurrence rate of preeclampsia and restores the physiological vascular changes in angiotensin-converting enzyme DD women. *Hypertension*, Vol.45, No.1, pp.86-91, ISSN 0194-911X

Mercuri, E., Cowan, F., Gupte, G., Manning, R., Laffan, M., Rutherford, M., Edwards, A.D., Dubowitz, L., & Roberts, I. (2001). Prothrombotic disorders and abnormal neurodevelopmental outcome in infants with neonatal cerebral infarction. *Pediatrics*, Vol.107, No.6, pp.:1400-1404, ISSN 0031-4005

Nelen, W.L., Steegers, E.A., Eskes, T.K., & Blom, H.J. (1997). Genetic risk factor unexplained recurrent early pregnancy loss. *Lancet*, Vol.350, No.9081, p.861, ISSN 0140-6736

Nelson, K.B. (2007). Perinatal Ischemic Stroke. *Stroke*,Vol.38, No. 2 suppl., pp.742-745, ISSN 0039-2499

O'Shaughnessey, K.M., Ferraro, F., Fu, B., Downing, S., & Morris, N.H. (2000). Identification of monozygotic twins that are concordant for pre-eclampsia. *Am J Obstet Gynecol*, Vol.182, No.5, pp.1156-1157, ISSN 0002-9378

Paidas, M.J., Ku, D.H., & Arkel, Y.S. (2004). Screening and management of inherited thrombophilias in the setting of adverse pregnancy outcome. *Clin Perinatol*, Vol.31, No.4, pp. 783-805, ISSN 0095-5108

Peaceman, A.M., & Rehnberg, KA. (1993). The effect of immunoglobulin G fractions from patients with lupus anticoagulant on placental prostacyclin and thromboxane production. *Am J Obstet Gynecol*, Vol169, No.6, pp.1403-1406, ISSN 0002-9378

Petäjä, J., Hiltunen, L., & Fellman, V. (2001). Increased risk of intraventricular hemorrhage in preterm infants with thrombophilia. *Ped Res*, Vol.49, No.5, pp.643-646, ISSN 0031-3998

Pickering, W., Marriott, K., & Regan, L. (2001). G20210A prothrombin gene mutation: prevalence in recurrent miscarriage population. *Clin Appl Thromb Hemost*, Vol.7, No.1, pp. 25-28, ISSN 1076-0296

Powers, R.W., Minich, L.A., Lykins, D.L., Ness, R.B., Crombleholme, W.R., & Roberts, J.M. (1999). Methylenetetrahydrofolate reductase polymorphism, folate, and susceptibility to preeclampsia. *J Soc Gynecol Investig*, Vol.6, No.2, pp.74-79, ISSN 1071-5576

Preston, F.E., Rosendaal, F.R., Walker, I.D., Briët, E., Berntorp, E., Conard, J., Fontcuberta, J., Makris, M., Mariani, G., Noteboom, W., Pabinger, I., Legnani, C., Scharrer, I., Schulman, S., & van der Meer, F.J. (1996). Increased fetal loss in women with heritable thrombophilia. *Lancet*, Vol.348, No.9032, pp.913–916, ISSN 0140-6736

Ramenghi, L.A., Fumagalli, M., Righini, A., Triulzi, F., Kustermann, A., & Mosca, F. (2005). Thrombophilia and fetal germinal matrixintraventricular hemorrhage: does it matter? *Ultrasound Obstet Gynecol*, Vol.26, No.5, pp.574-576, ISSN 0960-7692

Redline, R.W., & Pappin, A. (1995). Fetal thrombotic vasculopathy: the clinical significance of extensive avscular villi. *Hum Pathol*, Vol.26, No.1, pp.80-85, ISSN 0046-8177

Rey, E., Garneau, P., David, M., Gauthier, R., Leduc, L., Michon, N., Morin, F., Demers, C., Kahn, S.R., Magee, L.A., & Rodger, M. (2009). Dalteparin for the prevention of recurrence of placental-mediated complications of pregnancy in women without thrombophilia: a pilot randomized controlled trial. *J Thromb Haemost*, Vol.7, No.1, pp. 58-64, ISSN 1538-7933

Riikonen, R., & Kekomki, R. Resistance to activated protein C in childhood hydrocephalus. *Thromb Hemost*, Vol.79, No.5, pp. 1059-60, ISSN 0340-6245

Salafia, C.M., Pezzullo, J.C., Lopez-Zeno, J.A., Simmens, S., Minior, V.K., & Vintzileos, A.M. (1995). Placental pathologic features of preterm preeclampsia. *Am J Obstet Gynecol*, Vol.173, No.4, pp.1097-1105, ISSN 0002-9378

Smith, R.A., Skelton, M., Howard, M., & Levene, M. (2001). Is thrombophilia a factor in the development of hemiplegic cerebral palsy? *Dev Med Child Neurol*, Vol.43, No.11, pp.724-730, ISSN 0012-1622

Sood, R. (2009). Thrombophilia and fetal loss: Lessons from gene targeting in mice. *Thromb Res*, Vol.123, No. suppl 2, pp. 79-84, ISSN 0049-3848

Thornton, J.G., & Macdonald, A.M. (1999). Twin mothers, pregnancy hypertension and pre-eclampsia. *Br J Obstet Gynaecol*, Vol.106, No.6, pp.570-575, ISSN 0306-5456

Tranquilli, A.L., & Emanuelli, M. (2006). The thrombophilic fetus. *Med Hypotheses*, Vol.67, No.5, pp. 1226–1229, ISSN 0306-9877

Tranquilli, A.L., Giannubilo, S.R., Dell'Uomo, B., & Grandone, E. (2004). Adverse pregnancy outcomes are associated with multiple maternal thrombophilic factors. *Eur J Obstet Gynecol Reprod Biol*, Vol.117, No.2, pp. 144-147, ISSN 0301-2115

Tranquilli, A.L., Saccucci, F., Giannubilo, S.R., Cecati, M., Nocchi, L., Lorenzi, S., & Emanuelli, M. (2010). Unexplained fetal loss: the fetal side of thrombophilia. *Fertil Steril*, Vol.94, No.1, pp.378-380, ISSN 0015-0282

Tyrell, D.J., Kilfeather, S., & Page, CP. (1995). Therapeutic uses of heparin beyond its traditional role as an anticoagulant. *Trends Pharmacol Sci*, Vol.16, No.6, pp. 198-204, ISSN 0165-6147

van Pampus, M.G., Dekker, G.A., Wolf, H., Huijgens, P.C., Koopman, M.M., von Blomberg, B.M., & Büller H.R. (1999). High prevalence of hemostatic abnormalities in women with a history of severe preeclampsia. *Am J Obstet Gynecol*, Vol.180, No.5, pp.1146–1150, ISSN 0002-9378

Vefring H, Lie RT, Ødegård R, Mansoor MA, Nilsen ST. (2004). Maternal and Fetal Variants of Genetic Thrombophilias and the Risk of Preeclampsia. *Epidemiology*, Vol.15, No.3, pp. 317-322, ISSN 1044-3983

von Kries, R., Junker, R., Oberle, D., Kosch, A., & Nowak-Göttl, U. (2001). Foetal growth retardation in children with prothrombotic risk factors. *Thromb Haemost*, Vol.86, No.4, pp. 1012-1016, ISSN 0340-6245

Yacobi, S., Ornoy, A., Blumenfeld, Z., & Miller, R.K. (2002). Effect of sera from women with systemic lupus erythematosus or antiphospholipid syndrome and recurrent abortions on human placental explants in culture. Teratology, Vol.66, No. 6, pp. 300-308, ISSN 0040-3709

Younis, J.S., Ohel, G., Brenner, B., & Ben-Ami, M. (1997). Familial thrombophilia the scientific rationale for thrombophylaxis in recurrent pregnancy loss? *Hum Reprod*, Vol.12, No.7, pp. 1389-1390, ISSN 0268-1161